MECHANISMS OF
CANCER METASTASIS

DEVELOPMENTS IN ONCOLOGY

F.J. Cleton and J.W.I.M. Simons, eds.: Genetic Origins of Tumour Cells. 90-247-2272-1.
J. Aisner and P. Chang, eds.: Cancer Treatment and Research. 90-247-2358-2.
B.W. Ongerboer de Visser, D.A. Bosch and W.M.H. van Woerkom-Eykenboom, eds.: Neuro-oncology: Clinical and Experimental Aspects. 90-247-2421-X.
K. Hellmann, P. Hilgard and S. Eccles, eds.: Metastasis: Clinical and Experimental Aspects. 90-247-2424-4.
H.F. Seigler, ed.: Clinical Management of Melanoma. 90-247-2584-4.
P. Correa and W. Haenszel, eds.: Epidemiology of Cancer of the Digestive Tract. 90-247-2601-8.
L.A. Liotta and I.R. Hart, eds.: Tumour Invasion and Metastasis. 90-247-2611-5.
J. Banoczy, ed.: Oral Leukoplakia. 90-247-2655-7.
C. Tijssen, M. Halprin and L. Endtz, eds.: Familial Brain Tumours. 90-247-2691-3.
F.M. Muggia, C.W. Young and S.K. Carter, eds.: Anthracycline Antibiotics in Cancer. 90-247-2711-1.
B.W. Hancock, ed.: Assessment of Tumour Response. 90-247-2712-X.
D.E. Peterson, ed.: Oral Complications of Cancer Chemotherapy. 0-89838-563-6.
R. Mastrangelo, D.G. Poplack and R. Riccardi, eds.: Central Nervous System Leukemia. Prevention and Treatment. 0-89838-570-9.
A. Polliack, ed.: Human Leukemias. Cytochemical and Ultrastructural Techniques in Diagnosis and Research. 0-89838-585-7.
W. Davis, C. Maltoni and S. Tanneberger, eds.: The Control of Tumor Growth and its Biological Bases. 0-89838-603-9.
A.P.M. Heintz, C. Th. Griffiths and J.B. Trimbos, eds.: Surgery in Gynecological Oncology. 0-89838-604-7.
M.P. Hacker, E.B. Double and I. Krakoff, eds.: Platinum Coordination Complexes in Cancer Chemotherapy. 0-89838-619-5.
M.J. van Zwieten. The Rat as Animal Model in Breast Cancer Research: A Histopathological Study of Radiation- and Hormone-Induced Rat Mammary Tumors. 0-89838-624-1.
B. Lowenberg and A. Hogenbeck, eds.: Minimal Residual Disease in Acute Leukemia. 0-89838-630-6.
I. van der Waal and G.B. Snow, eds.: Oral Oncology. 0-89838-631-4.
B.W. Hancock and A.M. Ward, eds.: Immunological Aspects of Cancer. 0-89838-664-0.
K.V. Honn and B.F. Sloane, eds.: Hemostatic Mechanisms and Metastasis. 0-89838-667-5.
K.R. Harrap, W. Davis and A.N. Calvert, eds.: Cancer Chemotherapy and Selective Drug Development. 0-89838-673-X.
V.D. Velde, J.H. Cornelis and P.H. Sugarbaker, eds.: Liver Metastasis. 0-89838-648-5.
D.J. Ruiter, K. Welvaart and S. Ferrone, eds.: Cutaneous Melanoma and Precursor Lesions. 0-89838-689-6.
S.B. Howell, ed.: Intra-Arterial and Intracavitary Cancer Chemotherapy. 0-89838-691-8.
D.L. Kisner and J.F. Smyth, eds.: Interferon Alpha-2: Pre-Clinical and Clinical Evaluation. 0-89838-701-9.
P. Furmanski, J.C. Hager and M.A. Rich, eds.: RNA Tumor Viruses, Oncogenes, Human Cancer and Aids: On the Frontiers of Understanding. 0-89838-703-5.
J.E. Talmadge, I.J. Fidler and R.K. Oldham: Screening for Biological Response Modifiers: Methods and Rationale. 0-89838-712-4.
J.C. Bottino, R.W. Opfell and F.M. Muggia, eds.: Liver Cancer. 0-89838-713-2.
P.K. Pattengale, R.J. Lukes and C.R. Taylor, eds.: Lymphoproliferative Diseases: Pathogenesis, Diagnosis, Therapy. 0-89838-725-6.
F. Cavalli, G. Bonadonna and M. Rozencweig, eds.: Malignant Lymphomas and Hodgkin's Disease. 0-89838-727-2.
L. Baker, F. Valeriote and V. Ratanatharathorn, eds.: Biology and Therapy of Acute Leukemia. 0-89838-728-0.
J. Russo, ed.: Immunocytochemistry in Tumor Diagnosis. 0-89838-737-X.
R.L. Ceriani, ed.: Monoclonal Antibodies and Breast Cancer. 0-89838-739-6.
D.E. Peterson, G.E. Elias and S.T. Sonis, eds.: Head and Neck Management of the Cancer Patient. 0-89838-747-7.
D.M. Green: Diagnosis and Management of Malignant Solid Tumors in Infants and Children. 0-89838-750-7.
K.A. Foon and A.C. Morgan, Jr., eds.: Monoclonal Antibody Therapy of Human Cancer. 0-89838-754-X.
J.G. McVie, et al, eds., Clinical and Experimental Pathology of Lung Cancer. 0-89838-764-7.

MECHANISMS OF CANCER METASTASIS

Potential Therapeutic Implications

edited by

Kenneth V. Honn
William E. Powers
Bonnie F. Sloane

Martinus Nijhoff Publishing
a member of the Kluwer Academic Publishers Group
Boston/Dordrecht/Lancaster

Distributors for North America:
Kluwer Academic Publishers
190 Old Derby Street
Hingham, Massachusetts 02043, USA

Distributors for the UK and Ireland:
Kluwer Academic Publishers
MTP Press Limited
Falcon House, Queen Square
Lancaster LA1 1RN, UNITED KINGDOM

Distributors for all other countries:
Kluwer Academic Publishers Group
Distribution Centre
Post Office Box 322
3300 AH Dordrecht, THE NETHERLANDS

Library of Congress Cataloging-in-Publication Data
Main entry under title:

Mechanisms of cancer metastasis.

(Developments in oncology)
Includes bibliographies and index.
1. Metastasis.   I. Honn, Kenneth V.   II. Powers,
William E.   III. Sloane, Bonnie F.   IV. Series.
[DNLM: 1. Neoplasm Metastasis.   2. Neoplasms—drug
therapy.   W1DE998N / QZ 202 M4854]
RC269.M44   1985   616.99'4071   85-21656
ISBN 0-89838-765-5

CONTENTS

CONTRIBUTORS

PETER P. ALEXANDER
Departments of Medical
  Oncology and Surgery
Centre Block CR99
University of Southampton and
  Southampton General Hospital
Southampton SO9 4XY
UNITED KINGDOM

SANFORD H. BARSKY
Laboratory of Pathology
Section of Tumor Invasion
  and Metastasis
National Cancer Institute
National Institutes of Health
Bethesda, Maryland 20205

EDWARD W. BLANK
Bruce Lyon Memorial Research
  Laboratory
Children's Hospital Medical
  Center
51st and Grove Streets
Oakland, California 94609

PHILIP G. CAVANAUGH
Department of Biological Sciences
210 Science Hall
Wayne State University
Detroit, Michigan 48202

ROBERTO L. CERIANI
Bruce Lyon Memorial Research
  Laboratory
Children's Hospital Medical
  Center
51st and Grove Streets
Oakland, California 94609

BRUCE CHABNER
Division of Cancer Treatment
National Cancer Institute
National Institutes of Health
Bethesda, Maryland 20205

RICHARD CLARKE
Departments of Medical
  Oncology and Surgery
Centre Block CF99
University of Southampton and
  Southampton General Hospital
Southampton SO9 4XY
UNITED KINGDOM

EVA CRAMER
Department of Microbiology
  and Immunology
SUNY Downstate Medical Center
Brooklyn, New York 11203

JOHN D. CRISSMAN
Department of Pathology
Wayne State University and
Harper-Grace Hospitals
Detroit, Michigan 48201

FRANCES DAVIS
Department of Pathology
University of Texas System
  Cancer Center
M.D. Anderson Hospital and
  Tumor Institute
6723 Bertner Avenue
Houston, Texas 77030

NANCY A. DAY
Department of Pharmacology
Wayne State University
Detroit, Michigan 48201

SANDRA FAIRBAIRN
Department of Microbiology
  and Immunology
Suny Downstate Medical Center
Brooklyn, New York 11203

x

ISAIAH J. FIDLER
Department of Cell Biology
University of Texas System
  Cancer Center
M.D. Anderson Hospital and
  Tumor Institute
6723 Bertner Avenue
Houston, Texas 77030

RICHARD J. FORD
Department of Pathology
University of Texas System
  Cancer Center
M.D. Anderson Hospital and
Tumor Institute
6723 Bertner Avenue
Houston, Texas 77030

RHONDA GILBERT
Department of Microbiology
  and Immunology
SUNY Downstate Medical Center
Brooklyn, New York 11203

RONALD H. GOLDFARB
Cancer Metastasis Research
  Group
Department of Immunology and
  Infectious Disease
Central Research Division
Pfizer Inc.
Groton, Connecticut 06340

STUART G. GORDON
Department of Medicine
University of Colorado
  Health Sciences Center
4200 East Ninth Avenue
Denver, Colorado 80262

RUSSELL GREIG
Smith Kline & French Laboratories
1500 Spring Garden Street
Philadelphia, Pennsylvania 19101

GLORIA H. HEPPNER
Department of Immunology
Michigan Cancer Foundation
Detroit, Michigan 48201

RONALD B. HERBERMAN
Frederick Cancer research Center
Biological Development Branch
National Cancer Institute
National Institutes of Health
Frederick, Maryland 21701

KENNETH V. HONN
Department of Radiation Oncology
210 Science Hall
Wayne State University
Harper-Grace Hospital
Detroit, Michigan 48202

TATSURO IRIMURA
Department of Tumor Biology
University of Texas System
  Cancer Center
M.D. Anderson Hospital and
  tumor Institute
6723 Bertner Avenue
Houston, Texas 77030

NICOLA KOUTTAB
Department of Pathology
University of Texas System
  Cancer Center
M.D. Anderson Hospital and
  Tumor Institute
6723 Bertner Avenue
Houston, Texas 77030

JANIS LACOVARA
Department of Microbiology
  and Immunology
SUNY Downstate Medical Center
Brooklyn, New York 11203

TAMARA T. LAH
Department of Pharmacology
Wayne State University
Detroit, Michigan 48201

VICTOR LING
Division of Biological Research
Ontario Cancer Institute
Toronto, Ontario M4X 1K9
CANADA

LANCE LIOTTA
Laboratory of Pathology
Section of Tumor Invasion
  and Metastasis
National Cancer Institute
National Institutes of Health
Bethesda, Maryland 20205

LAWRENCE J. MARNETT
Department of Chemistry
Wayne State University
Detroit, Michigan 48202

J. PHILIP MCCOY, JR.
Department of Pathology
The University of Michigan
Ann Arbor, Michigan 48109

SHASHI MEHTA
Department of Pathology
University of Texas System
  Cancer Center
M.D. Anderson Hospital and
  Tumor Institute
6723 Bertner Avenue
Houston, Texas 77030

DAVID G. MENTER
Department of Biological
  Sciences
210 Science Hall
Wayne State University
Detroit, Michigan 48202

PAUL MURPHY
Departments of Medical Oncology
  and Surgery
Centre Block CF99
University of Southampton and
  Southampton General Hospital
Southampton SO9 4XY
UNITED KINGDOM

MOTOWO NAKAJIMA
Department of Tumor Biology
University of Texas System
  Cancer Center
M.D. Anderson Hospital and
  Tumor Institute
6723 Bertner Avenue
Houston, Texas 77030

GARTH L. NICOLSON
Department of Tumor Biology
University of Texas System
  Cancer Center
M.D. Anderson Hospital and
  Tumor Institute
6723 Bertner Avenue
Houston, Texas 77030

GEORGE OJAKIAN
Department of Microbiology
  and Immunology
SUNY Downstate Medical Center
Brooklyn, New York 11023

JAMES M. ONODA
Department   of   Radiation
  Oncology
210 Science Hall
Wayne State University
Detroit, Michigan 48202

JERRY A. PETERSON
Bruce Lyon Memorial Research
  Laboratory
Children's Hospital Medical Center
51st Center and Grove Streets
Oakland, California 94609

GEORGE POSTE
Smith Kline & French Laboratories
1500 Spring Garden Street
Philadelphia, Pennsylvania 19101

WILLIAM E. POWERS
Department of Radiation Oncology
Wayne State University
Detroit, Michigan 48201

NELLIKUNJA J. PRAKASH
Merrell Dow Pharmaceuticals
  Inc.
Department of Chemotherapeutics
Cincinnati, Ohio 45215

JAMES QUIGLEY
Department of Microbiology
  and Immunology
SUNY Downstate Medical Center
Brooklyn, New York 11203

NAGESWARA C. RAO
Laboratory of Pathology
Section of Tumor Invasion and
  Metastasis
National Cancer Institute
National Institutes of Health
Bethesda, Maryland 20205

JURIJ ROZHIN
Department of Pathology
Wayne State University
Harper-Grace Hospitals
Detroit, Michigan 48201

RANDALL E. RYAN
Department of Pharmacology
Wayne State University
Detroit, Michigan 48201

ALAN J. SCHROIT
Department of Cell Biology
University of Texas System
  Cancer Center
M.D. Anderson Hospital and
  Tumor Institute
6723 Bertner Avenue
Houston, Texas 77030

RANDI SCHWIMMER
Department of Microbiology
  and Immunology
SUNY Downstate Medical Center
Brooklyn, New York 11203

PAUL V. SENIOR
Departments of Medical Oncology
  and Surgery
Centre Block CF99
University of Southampton and
  Southampton General Hospital
Southampton SO9 4XY
UNITED KINGDOM

BONNIE F. SLOANE
Department of Pharmacology
Wayne State University
Detroit, Michigan 48201

PRASAD S. SUNKARA
Merrell Dow Pharmaceuticals Inc.
Department of Chemotherapeutics
Cincinnati, Ohio 45212

JOHN D. TAYLOR
Department of Biological
  Sciences
210 Science Hall
Wayne State University
Detroit, Michigan 48202

TAINA M. TURPEENNIEMI-HUJANEN
Laboratory of Pathology
Section of Tumor Invasion and
  Metastasis
National Cancer Institute
national Institutes of Health
Bethesda, Maryland 20205

JAMES VARANI
Department of Pathology
The University of Michigan
  Medical School
Ann Arbor, Michigan 48109

LEONARD WEISS
Department of Experimental
  Pathology
Roswell Park Memorial Institute
Buffalo, New York 14263

LEO R. ZACHARSKI
Veterans Administration Medical
  Center and Dartmouth Medical
  School
White River Junction, Vermont 05001

PREFACE

The past twenty years have witnessed significant advances in the treatment of cancer by surgery and radiation therapy. Gains with cytotoxic chemotherapy have been much more modest. Of the approximately 900,000 newly diagnosed cases of cancer each year, 50% result in death of the patient. The primary cause of these deaths is metastasis.

Although the term metastasis was first coined by Recamier in 1829, only in the past ten years have there been intensive scientific investigations into the mechanisms by which tumor cells metastasize. What has emerged is a complex process of host-tumor cell interactions which has been termed the metastatic cascade. Due to the complexity of the metastatic process, the study of metastasis is multifaceted and involves elements of such areas as differentiation, enzymology, genetics, hematology, immunology, membrane biochemistry and molecular biology.

The major objectives of this book were to present the most recent advances in our understanding of how tumor cells metastasize to secondary sites by the leading experts in the biology of tumor invasion and metastasis. We hope that this book will lead to new concepts for the treatment of subclinical metastatic cancer. The chapters in this book address both the basic science of metastasis and potential clinical therapies directed toward interruption of the metastatic cascade or toward eradication of subclinical metastases. Many relevant topics have been omitted due to space considerations and thus the topics included reflect the prejudices of the editors. We thank the contributors for the excellence of their chapters and hope the readers will find this book of interest.

K.V. Honn
W.E. Powers
B.F. Sloane

CHAPTER 1. THE CANCER PROBLEM TODAY

WILLIAM E. POWERS

     A Gallup Poll survey in 1976 revealed that cancer is the most feared of all diseases in our society (Table 1). The fear seems justified when we recognize that in 1984 870,000 new patients were found to have invasive cancer and another 445,000 patients to have non-invasive skin cancer or carcinoma in situ of the cervix (Figure 1). The American Cancer Society estimated that 450,000 deaths would occur due to cancer in 1984; only 326,000 of the 870,000 newly diagnosed patients will survive for five years (Figure 2). The death rate due to cancer in the U.S. has increased over the past forty years despite many advances in early detection and treatment. The increasing incidence of cancer and of death due to cancer in our population presents a dismal picture.

Table 1. "Most Feared Diseases".

		Cancer	58%
Blindness	21%	Heart Disease	10%
Arthritis	2%	Polio	2%
Loss of Limb	2%	Tuberculosis	1%
Deafness	1%	Undecided	3%

Gallup Poll 1976 (N = 1548)

2

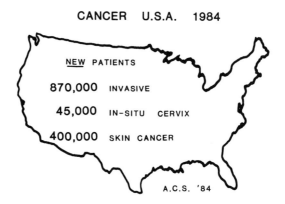

FIGURE 1. Predicted Cases of Cancer in 1984.

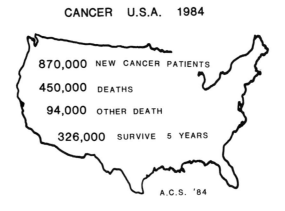

FIGURE 2. Mortality Predictions for New Cancer Patients in 1984.

The National Cancer Institute program entitled "Surveillance Epidemiology and End Results Reporting" has reported a significant improvement in relative survival rates for most types of cancer in the recent past. For example, relative survival rates increased from 40% in 1967-1973 to 45% in the period 1973-1979. The five year survival for almost all adult cancer patients has shown improvement (Table 2). Survival rates for specific diseases in children have also undergone a remarkable improvement (Table 3). These improvements have resulted in the survival (with a good chance of cure) of approximately 320,000 additional patients diagnosed as having invasive cancer in the decade of the 1970's. The appropriate question is can we save more lives? The American Cancer Society estimates that in 1984 an additional 148,000 of the newly diagnosed patients and in 1985 an additional 160,000 of the newly diagnosed patients who are fated to die of cancer could have been saved by earlier diagnosis and prompt appropriate treatment.

Table 2. Comparison of the Five Year Survival Rates for Adult Cancers.

Site of Cancer	1960-1963	1970-1973
Breast	63%	68%
Cervix	58%	64%
Bladder	53%	61%
Prostate	50%	63%
Colon	43%	49%
Rectum	38%	45%
Stomach	11%	13%
Lung	8%	10%
Pancreas	1%	1%

"SEER" NCI 1982.

Table 3. Comparison of the Five Year Survival Rates for Childhood
Cancers.

Type of Cancer	1960-1963	1970-1973
Acute Leukemia	4%	34%
Hodgkin's Disease	52%	90%
Bone Tumors	20%	30%

"SEER" NCI 1982.

Certain segments of our population, notably blacks, have not
shared in the rapid increase in survival, particularly in cases of
bladder, uterine, breast and prostate cancer. For uterine cancer the
1984 survival expectation for black patients is poorer than that
observed for white patients in 1960. The general level of cancer
awareness and cancer care of our black population needs improvement.

There has been a dramatic decrease in the age adjusted death rate
for stomach and uterine cancer. The death rate changed from over 30
per 100,000 population in 1930 to about 8 per 100,000 population in
1980 (Figure 3). This decrease in deaths is even more significant when
one considers the increasing age of the American population. The basis
for these decreases is not clearly understood; these decreases occurred
before improved treatment, screening programs or targeted behavior
modification, i.e., smoking, diet, had made any significant
contribution. There is a less dramatic reduction in the age adjusted
death rate for liver cancer (from 12 per 100,000 in 1930 to less than 6
per 100,000 in 1980). This reduction may reflect a decreased
prevalence of hepatitis. Since there is a high prevalence of liver
cancer worldwide, determining why liver cancer deaths in the United
States have decreased would be important. These decreases in cancer
death rates in the United States have been more than offset by the
great increase in the death rate due to lung cancer, a disease for
which the cause in at least 80% of cases is known, i.e., self-inflicted
exposure to cigarette smoke over a period of many years.

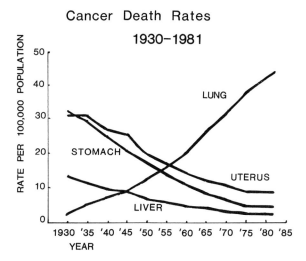

FIGURE 3. Major Reductions in Cancer Death Rate (Age Adjusted) have Occurred in Stomach and Uterine Cancer with a Lesser Reduction in Liver Cancer. These have been offset by an increase in death rate due to lung cancer. ACS 1985 - Cancer Facts & Figures.

Cancer at various sites is related to cultural, dietary and self-imposed exposures. For example, practicing Mormons are known to abstain from smoking, drinking stimulants including alcohol and coffee, etc. and their "Standardized mortality rate (among active Mormons) is 50% for all cancers, being 23% for smoking related sites and 68% for all other sites" (1). Such an example indicates that we have many reasons to believe that modification of our behavior will result in a decreased incidence of cancer.

Cancer has an impact not only in terms of early death and suffering but also in terms of the health care dollar. More than 10% of our gross national product is expended for health care; this amounted to 393 billion dollars in 1984. Since 20% of deaths in the United States are due to cancer, least 10% - 15% of health care costs must be related to the total direct costs of cancer care including prevention, detection, treatment and continuing followup. In the Detroit Metropolitan area in 1969-1970 the Third National Cancer Survey found that 15 days of hospitalization were required for cured patients and 55 days of hospitalization for patients who were not cured. As lives are prolonged the cost of cancer care is increasing more rapidly than most health care costs. The cost of palliative care of the patient with incurable cancer is probably more than the cost of curative treatment and the medical costs associated with subsequent death from other causes. Unfortunately, we do not have accurate studies of these costs. This topic deserves further study to allow rational allocation of health care resources.

6

The cost of cancer research is an investment which should reduce the cost of future cancer care. However, since there is no good way to estimate the costs of future cancer care, it is difficult to predict the return on our current investments in cancer research. It is estimated that the cost of cancer care is 30 to 40 billion dollars per year. This suggests that an investment of about 2 billion dollars per year in research and development (half from the NCI and half from other sources) is inadequate when one considers the major economic, scientific and social benefits that will be achieved by solving this problem. Since the initiation of the National Cancer Program in 1971 the actual number of dollars expended has increased continually. However, when corrected for inflation the number of dollars (constant) has actually decreased significantly since the peak in 1977 (Figure 4). Only by imaginative and courageous administration and reprogramming of less profitable endeavors has the creative impetus of the National Cancer Program been continued successfully in this era of diminished real dollars available for the research and development programs.

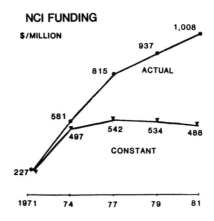

FIGURE 4. National Cancer Institute Funding 1971 to 1981 (3).

Future recommendations for the National Cancer Programs should include realistic projections to the public of the results which can be achieved. To a large extent this has been accomplished with a prediction of future incidence and mortality for the year 2000 in the absence of new initiatives. We need similar realistic estimates of cancer care costs such that the dollar costs as well as the "fear" and "social" costs are known to the public. With more realistic estimates and public expectations, requests for increased research funding are more easily justified since the predicted accomplishments can be evaluated in terms of the original estimates of lives and dollars saved.

The National Cancer Institute has recently instituted a program entitled "National Cancer Program: Goal For the Year 2000" with the aim of reducing cancer mortality in the year 2000 by a factor of 50%. In 1980 414,000 people died of cancer; in the year 2000 the National Cancer Institute projects 575,000 cancer deaths. The National Cancer Program seeks a 50% reduction from the expected cancer deaths to 288,000 deaths in the year 2000. Forty percent of the proposed reduction in mortality depends on the success in achieving cancer prevention and the other 60% on improved results of current and new treatment plans (Table 4). Improvement in the diagnosis, prevention and treatment of micro-metastases will contribute approximately 1/3 of the reduction in mortality.

Table 4. Factors in Mortality Reduction.

Strategy	Objective	Impact % Reduction
Prevention	Reduce smoking by 50%	15%
Prevention	Diet-reduce fat and increase fiber	5%
Treatment	State of art treatment	15%
Treatment	Continued improved treatment of micro-metastases	15%
TOTAL REDUCTION		50%

I propose that the prudent use of limited research dollars should include the sharing of expensive and unique facilities between the National Cancer Institute and the entire scientific community. The physics community has long recognized that the cost of facilities and resources for many investigations is out of reach of the individual laboratory or in fact of a large university. Therefore they developed the concept of national laboratories (generally operated by a consortium of universities) where individual investigators can use expensive facilities and resources for individual and/or collaborative programs that would not be otherwise possible. Two outstanding (and very expensive) resources are now operated by the National Cancer Institute. These are the "Surveillance Epidemiology and End Results" program and the "Frederick Research Program." Each of these represent a national resource available to NCI staff and investigators yet largely unavailable to researchers in the general scientific community. Utilization of these very expensive facilities and programs by qualified investigators from the general scientific community could provide support facilities for investigations that might otherwise not be possible. This usage could be an important contribution to the National Cancer Program.

Reports from the Department of Health and Human Services indicate a marked decrease in the age adjusted death rates for cardiovascular disease (Figure 5) and cerebrovascular disease (Figure 6). No such marked decrease has been observed for cancer (Figure 7). There is still some room for optimism; for cancer other than lung cancer, there has been a decrease. However, this is more than offset by the increase in the death rate due to lung cancer which has occurred in spite of an increased survival rate (see Table 2). The decrease in deaths due to

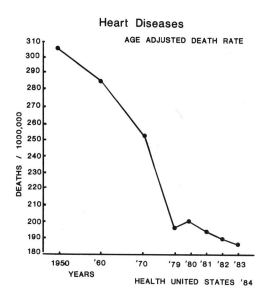

FIGURE 5. The Age Adjusted Death Rate for Heart Disease Has Demonstrated a Significant Decrease in the Period 1950 to 1979 and a Less Rapid Decrease in the Period 1980 to 1983.

9

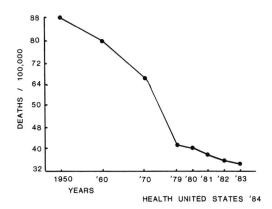

FIGURE 6. The Age Adjusted Death Rate for Cerebrovascular Disease Has Demonstrated a Significant Decrease in the Period 1950 to 1979 with a Less Rapid Decrease in the Period 1979 to 1983.

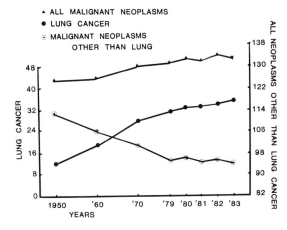

FIGURE 7. Age Adjusted Death Rates per 100,000 for Lung Cancer Have Increased from 12.8 in 1950 to 38.1 in 1983. The age adjusted death rates for cancers other than lung cancer have shown a decrease in the same interval from 112.6 in 1950 to 93.2 in 1983. Thus the steady increase in the age adjusted death rates for all cancers is due to the increase in the age adjusted death rate for lung cancer, which offsets any improvements in the reduction in death rates from other malignancies (4).

heart disease and stroke has resulted in improved health and increased
length of life. Life expectancy in the United States has increased
from 70.9 years in 1970 to 74.5 years in 1983. Because of the
increasing life expectancy we have a modest increase in the crude death
rate for all cancers excluding lung cancer (Figure 8). When the
increased death rate due to lung cancer is added, we observe an almost
35% increase in the crude death rate from cancer in the interval from
1950 to 1985 (Figure 8). In addition to the aging of our population
and a decreasing death rate from cardiovascular and cerebrovascular
disease, we have a constantly increasing population. It is probably
these several events occurring together that have resulted in the
observation by the American Cancer Society that in the past two decades
the number of new cancer patients each year has increased as has the
number of cancer patient deaths per year (Figure 9). Fortunately
deaths are not increasing as rapidly as the number of new cases.

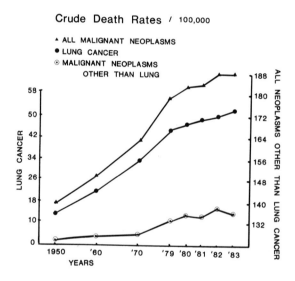

FIGURE 8. Crude Death Rates from Cancer have Shown an Increase from
1950 (139.8) to 1983 (188.3). This increase has to a significant
extent been due to an increase in lung cancer death rates which
increased from 14.1 to 51.6 in the same interval. The death rate from
cancer other than lung cancer has shown a modest increase from 125.7 to
136.7. Thus lung cancer represents the single largest contributor to
the increase in our death rate (4).

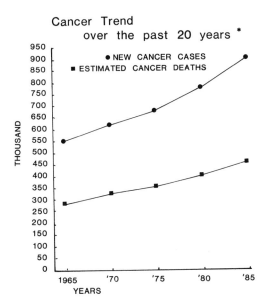

Cancer Trend
over the past 20 years *

● NEW CANCER CASES
■ ESTIMATED CANCER DEATHS

THOUSAND

YEARS

FIGURE 9. Data Provided by the American Cancer Society Indicate a 65% Increase in the Number of Patients with Invasive Cancer from 550,000 in 1965 to 910,000 in 1985. There was an associated increase in cancer deaths from 296,000 in 1965 to 462,000 in 1985 – a 56% increase. The incidence of cancer and the number of cancer deaths are both increasing, but fortunately the number of deaths is increasing at a more modest rate. (ACS Collected Data).

Unfortunately, in contrast to cardiovascular and cerebrovascular disease, there is no evidence of a decrease in the cancer death rate in the past two decades. Of even greater concern is the prediction by the American Cancer Society that one of three persons born in the United States will develop cancer at some time in their life – an increase from the previous prediction of one in four. We have reason for concern that we may not reach the goal of the National Cancer Program for the Year 2000 since we observe that in the 20 years since the Surgeon General's report on the possible ill effects of smoking cigarettes we have had only a modest decrease (from 42% of our adult population to 33%) in smoking (Table 5). The most significant concern is that there is no decrease in smoking in women and probably an increased overall use of tobacco in teenagers. Considerable evidence exists that the increased incidence of lung cancer is associated with

Table 5. Changes in Smoking.

	1964	1984
Adults	42%	33%
Men	52%	38%
Women	34%	33%

HHS, 1983.

tobacco smoking.   Figure 10 illustrates the relationship between consumption of cigarettes and the mortality from lung cancer. The increased smoking in women occurring in the decades of the 1940's through the 1960's and its persistence today leads to the prediction of a future increased mortality for women in the United States due to lung cancer. Lung cancer has clearly become the "Equal Opportunity Disease."   The American Cancer Society and The American Lung Association point out that in either 1985 or 1986 more women will die of lung cancer than breast cancer and even predict a future increase in the number of deaths each year (Figure 11).

Much of the data I have presented is foreboding, however, I call your attention to a new NCI booklet - "Good News-Better News and Best News". The "Good News" - not everyone gets cancer. The "Better News" - more people are being cured of cancer. The "Best News" - many cancers can be prevented by a prudent lifestyle, i.e., no smoking, prudent diet, avoidance of toxic substances. The "Very Best News" will be when research leads to nontoxic methods of predicting, treating or preventing cancer and metastases.

CANCER MORTALITY

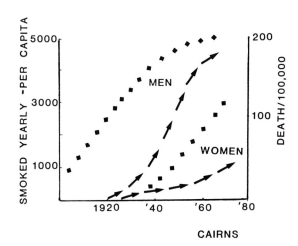

CAIRNS

FIGURE 10. The Relationship of Cancer Mortality in Men to Smoking
Demonstrates a Lag Period of Approximately 20 Years with an Apparent
Plateau Associated with a Reduction in or a Plateau in Smoking.
Unfortunately in women the increase in deaths appears to follow the
same lag period; therefore, with continued smoking we may reasonably
predict an increased mortality in women due to lung cancer (2).

14

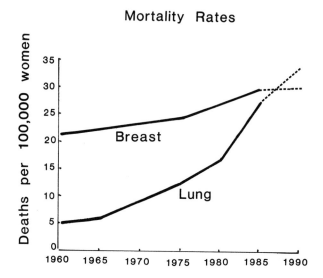

FIGURE 11. Mortality Rates in Women Due to Breast and Lung Cancers.

REFERENCES

1. Enstrom J: Cancer and total mortality among active Mormons.
    Cancer 42:1943-1951, 1978.
2. Cairns J: Cancer: Science and Society. W.H. Freeman:San
    Francisco, 1978.
3. NCI Fact Book, 1980. U.S. Department of Health and Human
    Services.
4. Health United States, 1984. U.S. Department of Health and Human
    Services.

CHAPTER 2. PRESENT STATUS AND FUTURE PROSPECTS FOR TREATMENT OF METASTATIC CANCER

BRUCE A. CHABNER

The problem of curing cancer is steadily coming into sharper focus and the picture emerging is the challenge of dealing with metastatic cancer in new ways. Of the 870,000 new cases of cancer each year, approximately half will be localized at presentation. The majority of these, about 400,000 patients per year, will be cured with either surgery or radiotherapy. The remainder will require some form of systemic therapy, either to prevent recurrence (adjuvant therapy) or to treat actual recurrent disease. Of this number about 50,000 will be cured. The remainder, constituting 50% of patient with cancer, will die. The primary cause of their deaths will be metastases.

I. CHEMOTHERAPY

To date our limited successes in treating metastatic disease have been with drugs. The alkylating agents, antimetabolites and natural products developed during the past 35 years have primarily been successful in treating the rapidly growing malignancies that afflict the younger population, such as childhood acute leukemia, Hodgkin's disease, testicular cancer and choriocarcinoma (Table 1). The majority of these patients can now be cured with drugs (1). The slower-growing solid tumors occur in patients of advanced age. These patients have decreased tolerance to the side effects of chemotherapy and have in the main proved at best responsive, yet rarely curable, with even the most intensive chemotherapy (Table 2). In treating metastatic adenocarcinomas with chemotherapy the most favorable results have been a high initial response rate in patients with ovarian cancer and breast cancer and an impact on overall survival in premenopausal breast cancer and in soft tissue sarcomas of the extremities in the adjuvant setting when tumor burden is low (Table 3). Few patients with metastatic ovarian cancer, breast cancer, lung cancer or gastrointestinal adenocarcinomas have been cured with drugs. Thus, although chemotherapy has had a truly remarkably beneficial effect on the survival of patients with hematologic malignancies and childhood cancers, its impact on the majority of tumors affecting the older age groups has primarily been palliative.

16

Table 1. Curability of Patients with Advanced Malignancy.
1973 - 1983.

Type of Cancer	Five-Year Disease-Free Survival		Number of Patients Potentially Curable per Year*
	1973	1983	
Acute lymphocytic leukemia	30%	50%	1000
Hodgkin's disease (Stage III-IV)	50%	60%	2400
Diffuse histiocytic lymphoma	5%	65%	4000
Testicular cancer (Stage II-III)	10%	70%	2200
Burkitt's lymphoma	20%	35%	100
Choriocarcinoma	80%	90%	1000
Ovarian cancer	< 5%	20%	2400
Acute nonlymphocytic leukemia	< 5%	15%	1000
Nodular mixed lymphoma	< 5%	--	500

*Based on estimates of the number of new cases each year in the United States as provided by the Biometric Research and Analytical Studies Section, Biometry Branch, Division of Cancer Prevention and Control, National Cancer Institute.

Table 2. Response of Patients to Chemotherapy[*].

	Response Rate	
	1973	1983
Small cell carcinoma of the lung	30%	90%
Nodular lymphocytic lymphoma	50%	90%
Breast cancer	75%	75%
Gastric cancer	20%	50%
Multiple myeloma	30%	60%
Chronic leukemia	90%	90%

[*]Tumors responsive to chemotherapy, but not cured.

Table 3. Change in Prognosis for Cancer Patients.

1973 - 1983

Adjuvant therapy prolongs survival

Breast cancer, Stage II

Soft tissue sarcoma, extremity

Childhood sarcomas

Adjuvant therapy possibly delays recurrence

Gastric cancer, stage II

Rectal cancer

Osteosarcoma

Head and neck cancer

How can we account for the difficulties in producing responses in these major categories of malignancy? More specifically, what biological properties of these tumors are responsible for the lack of sensitivity to chemotherapy? Goldie and Coldman (2) have developed an attractive model for explaining the emergence of drug resistance in genetic terms. Their work is based upon the hypothesis that drug-resistant mutants arise at a rate independent of drug exposure; the probability of such mutations lies, for most mammalian genes, in the range of 10^{-6} to 10^{-7}. Thus the chances of a drug-resistant mutant arising in a given tumor depend on this intrinsic mutation rate and the number of cells in the tumor (see also Chapters 5 and 6). For clinically apparent tumors, which contain at least 10^9 cells, the probability is high that such a mutant, drug-resistant clone exists. This theory, which has important ramifications for treatment strategy and combination drug usage (Table 4), is supported by studies of the genetics of drug resistance in cell culture experiments. Such

Table 4. Clinical Strategies Based upon Spontaneous Mutation Theory of Drug Resistance.

1. Treat early, especially in adjuvant situation.

2. Treat intensively to discourage outgrowth of lower degree resistance.

3. Use non-cross-resistant combinations in alternating cycles.

4. Reduce tumor bulk with surgery and/or radiotherapy.

experiments have demonstrated the ease with which drug-resistant mutants can be selected out from a drug-sensitive population by low-dose drug exposure. Unfortunately, the Goldie-Coldman hypothesis may have its greatest applicability and usefulness in improving the therapy of already responsive tumors, such as acute leukemia and Hodgkin's disease, in which the majority of cells are initially responsive to drugs, and for which a broad variety of agents are available for combination therapy. The theory appears to be less applicable to the problem of treating the major solid malignancies, for the following reasons:

    The assumption that the initial tumor cell clone is drug-sensitive may not be correct. At the time of clinical presentation the bulk of cells in these patients is clearly drug resistant. There are three possible explanations for this high-grade initial resistance: 1) the original clone was drug resistant, 2) the drug-resistant mutation occurred at a very early time point in the history of the tumor or 3) the growth rate of the resistant mutant was vastly greater than that of the drug-sensitive initial clone. The latter possibilities (2 and 3) are unlikely, since there is no reason to believe that drug-resistant mutations occur at rates approaching 10^{-1} or higher; secondly, most drug-resistant clones have slower growth rates, and lower metastatic potential, than the parent drug-sensitive clone (3). Thus, we are left with the likely possibility that most solid tumors that are initially insensitive to drugs arise from intrinsically insensitive malignant clones. Perhaps the drug resistance of these tumors is a reflection of an innate biological property, such as membrane transport characteristics, of the cell of origin of the tumor.

While basic differences may thus exist in the timing of development of drug resistance (compare potentially curable hematologic malignancies that acquire resistance to de novo drug-resistant solid tumors) there is no reason to believe that the biochemical mechanisms involved are intrinsically different. That is, the same changes in drug transport, target protein concentration, affinity for drug, or cellular kinetics may underlie "acquired" (late-occurring resistance in initially sensitive tumors and "intrinsic" (initial) resistance. The understanding of these processes holds the key to rational drug development and improved therapy of metastatic cancer. Our knowledge of drug resistance has progressed rapidly in recent years, due primarily to the use of tissue culture models for characterizing the genetic and biochemical changes responsible for resistance to specific drugs. Some of these changes are listed in Table 5. One of the most interesting and important findings has been the emergence of a general type of resistance which affects a broad group of natural products, termed pleotropic drug resistance (PDR). Included in this group are the vinca alkaloids, anthracyclines, epipodophyllotoxins and various other natural products. These drugs do not share a common mechanism of action, but all appear susceptible to a common mechanism of resistance that results from amplification of membrane glycoprotein(s) and decreased intracellular drug accumulation. Ling and co-workers have identified one such amplified protein, P-170, which is markedly amplified in PDR-type Chinese hamster ovary cells and human T-cell leukemia cells (CEM cells) (4; see also Chapter 6). This form of resistance appears to be genetically stable, although reversion to drug sensitivity does occur spontaneously. In some PDR cells, drug resistance may be reversed by calcium channel blockers, such as verapamil, a finding of great interest to clinical oncology (5). Whether this form of drug resistance occurs in clinical practice is not known at present, although its presence is suspected on the basis of clinical experience with drug-resistant tumors. The implications of its occurrence in the clinic would be far-reaching, and include:

1. The need to rethink accepted patterns of cross-resistance in the design of combination chemotherapy. Drugs such as adriamycin, vincristine, VP-16, and actinomycin-D cannot be considered to be unrelated in terms of potential cross-resistance.

2. The need to incorporate drug-resistant tumor models into drug
    screening systems in order to identify agents active against this
    type of cell.

Table 5. Biochemical Mechanisms of Drug Resistance.

Mechanism	Example
1. Transport deficiency	Methotrexate Melphalan Cytosine arabinoside
2. Increased target enzyme	Methotrexate N-phosphono-acetyl-L- aspartic acid
3. Decreased drug activation	6-Mercaptopurine 6-Thioguanine Cytosine arabinoside 5-Fluorouracil
4. Increased drug degradation	Cytosine arbinoside 6-Mercaptopurine
5. Increased competitive substrate	Cytosine arabinoside (dCTP)
6. "Pleotropic" drug resistance (decreased drug accumulation)	Adriamycin Actinomycin-D Vinca alkaloids VP-16 m-AMSA

3. The possibility of detecting PDR-type cells by pretreatment
    screening for P-170 or by pretreatment studies of drug accumulation
    or effect.

4. The possible use of calcium channel antagonists or calmodulin
    antagonists to reverse clinical drug resistance.

II. INNOVATIONS IN DRUG DISCOVERY

While research progresses toward an understanding of resistance to established drugs, we must also be alert to potential improvements in the process of discovering new drugs, which is ongoing in industry, academia and in research institutions such as the National Cancer Institute. New insights into the biochemical basis for processes such as cell differentiation and metastasis are providing alternatives to cytotoxic chemotherapy. Is it possible to treat cancer effectively by inducing terminal differentiation? Experience with low-dose cytosine arabinoside in treatment of preleukemia suggests, but does not prove, that induction of differentiation may be possible (6). Other cytidine analogs and unrelated differentiating agents, such as N-methyl formamide and hexamethylenebisacetamide (HMBA), will undergo clinical evaluation in our initial efforts to test this type of therapy, although neither of these is outstandingly potent as compared to retinoic acid derivatives. What is needed now is a preclinical in vivo model system for testing such drugs, because a crucial question - whether the high concentrations of drug required to induce differentiation in vitro can be tolerated by the whole animal - cannot be answered by any existing in vitro model.

The exciting possibility of basing cancer treatment approaches upon the unique biochemical features of metastatic tumors is discussed elsewhere in this volume. The challenge will be in demonstrating that such unique features do exist and can be exploited.

In a more empirical approach, the National Cancer Institute is supporting studies which ask the question of whether human tumor colony-forming cells can select agents missed by the more conventional murine leukemia screens (P388 and L1210) that will be active against human malignancy. The preliminary results of this study indicate that this type of screen, although fraught with technical problems and uncertainties, can identify agents otherwise missed by the traditional screen (7). The clinical efficacy of these drugs remains to be proved.

III. BIOLOGICALS AND IMMUNOTHERAPY

As an alternative to chemotherapy, the biological response modifiers offer the very attractive potential of greater selectivity and specificity. It is beyond the scope of this chapter to discuss the broad range of biological approaches now under development for cancer treatment. Suffice it to say that these approaches are certain to complement, if not displace conventional chemotherapy. This field, which once suffered from lack of biochemical characterization of immune factors, has rapidly progressed from the level of phenomenology to the isolation, purification and production (by genetic engineering) of lymphokines such as IL-2, lymphotoxins, tumor necrosis factor, interferons and others (see Chapters 13-16). Tumor growth factors are being identified, and they or their receptors may become useful targets for monoclonal antibodies. Oncogene products are now the object of efforts to inhibit tumor proliferation. Of perhaps ultimate importance, monoclonal antibodies offer exceptional promise, either as diagnostic tools or as therapeutic carriers for radionuclides or toxins (see Chapter 16). A revolution in cancer treatment is likely to emerge from this general area of research.

In summary, the past and present achievements in the treatment of metastatic cancer can be credited to chemotherapy. The future will be very different, and will largely be determined by the relative pace of scientific understanding of drug resistance and tumor biology. The rapid progress in understanding metastasis, differentiation, growth factors, and immunobiology may well lead to effective treatments which displace the less specific and more toxic conventional therapies. For the first time in the past three decades, chemotherapy has competition.

REFERENCES

1. Chabner BA, Fine RL, Allegra CJ, Yeh GC, Curt GA: Cancer chemotherapy: Progress and expectations. Cancer (In press).
2. Goldie JH, Coldman AJ: A mathematic model for relating the drug sensitivity of tumors to their spontaneous mutation rate. Cancer Treat. Rep. 63:1727-1733, 1979.
3. Biedler JF, Peterson PHF: Altered plasma membrane glycoconjugates of Chinese hamster cells with acquired resistance to actinomycin D, daunorubicin and vincristine. IN: Sartorelli AC, Lazlo JS and Bertino JR (eds.) Molecular Actions and Targets for Cancer Chemotherapeutic Agents. Academic Press, New York, pp. 453-482, 1981.
4. Kartner N, Riordan JR, Ling V: Cell surface P-glycoprotein associated with multi-drug resistance in mammalian cell lines. Science 221:1285-1288, 1983.
5. Tsuruo T, Iida H, Nojiri M, Tsukagoshi S, Sakurai Y: Circumvention of vincristine and adriamycin resistance in vitro and in vivo by calciun influx blockers. Cancer Res. 43:2905-2910, 1983.
6. Wisch JS, Griffin JD, Kufe DW: Response of preleukemic syndromes to continuous infusion of low-dose cytarabine. N. Engl. J. Med. 309:1599-1602, 1983.
7. Shoemaker RH, Wolpert-DeFilippes MK, Kern DH, Lieber MM, Makuch RW, Melnick NR, Miller WP, Salmon SE, Simon RM, Vendetti JM, Von Hoff DD: Application of human tumor colony-forming assay to new drug screening. Cancer Res. (In press).
8. Curt GA, Clendeninn NJ, Chabner BA: Drug resistance in cancer. Cancer Treat. Rep. 68:87-99, 1984.

CHAPTER 3. A CRITICAL OVERVIEW OF THE METASTATIC PROCESS

LEONARD WEISS

I. INTRODUCTION

In many patients with cancer, their primary lesion can be removed, but the patients eventually die as a consequence of metastasis. Thus, metastases are an important consideration in diagnosis, staging and treatment of cancer. A metastasis is a cancer which is not in contiguity with the original primary tumor. Thus, detachment of cancer cells is a fundamental part of the metastatic process. Detachment may occur before or after a cancer has gained access to blood or lymph vessels or to body cavities, often by invasion.

In order to progress into the next phase of metastasis, cancer cells must usually be arrested, and in the case of circulating cells, this occurs at the endothelium of the microvasculature. The interactions of cancer cells with vessel walls are exceptionally complex with respect to events occurring before, during and after arrest. It appears that these events are pivotal to the metastatic process, and culminate in the death and subsequent release of most of the temporarily arrested cancer cells. A few of the arrested cells survive, and sooner or later extravasate.

The extravasated cancer cells may proliferate to form micro-metastases which acquire a neovasculature from their host, and grow to form overt metastases which may in turn then metastasize (see Chapter 23). Other cancer cells do not develop a neovasculature and tend to remain in a micrometastatic, operationally dormant state, activation from which poses a constant threat to the patient. Yet other extravasated cells are killed as a consequence of a whole repertoire of interactions with host cells and humoral agents. It is important to recognize that at least some of these interactions associated with an inflammatory response may be injurious to the patient and may actually enhance parts of the metastatic process. For example, leukocyte sequestration following cancer cell arrest at a vessel wall may, on the one hand, be associated with cancer cell death due to oxygen radicals, but on the other hand, release of leukocyte lysosomal enzymes may result in histiolysis which serves to promote invasion by the surviving cancer cells.

Conceptually, it is helpful to compartmentalize the metastatic process in order to dissect out the various mechanisms involved. However, this is in a sense misleading because metastasis is an ongoing process, characterized by a series of repetitive, overlapping steps which are extremely inefficient and therefore, costly in terms of cancer cells.

For obvious reasons, many of the mechanisms of metastasis cannot be studied in people but require the use of in vivo and in vitro models, which may in themselves create additional interpretive problems. Individual parts of the metastatic process can be studied in model systems. Indeed we have no other options. However, it is doubtful whether there are rodent models which are adequate for all aspects of the metastatic process in people, and some of the so-called "models" are inadequate to account for metastasis in rodents. In many naturally occurring or induced cancers in rodents, when the host dies the tumor may commonly account for half of the animal's body weight in the absence of overt metastases. Analogous behavior is rare in humans! In many metastasis-related experiments, large numbers of cancer cells are injected into animals. This short-circuits any host-interactions, including adaptive or selective processes, that may occur during the natural uni- or paucicellular development of tumors. In the current wave of enthusiasm to make global statements about the mechanisms of metastasis in people, some of these disparities tend to be overlooked.

In this brief overview, I will focus on a few of the interpretive, practical problems of metastasis which I think are of importance.

II. PRIMARY CANCERS

The cancer cells in a tumor are heterogeneous; cellular pleomorphism has long been recognized by pathologists, and other types of heterogeneity in both benign and cancer cell populations are well known (see Chapter 5). The elegant studies of Fidler and his colleagues and others have shown that by use of repetitive and alternating in vivo and in vitro passages, lines of cancer cells can be developed which, when injected into the tail veins of animals, give rise to different numbers of pulmonary colonies (1). Quite apart from changes in cell characteristics occurring on repeated passage in animals and/or in culture (2) or the disparities between pulmonary colonization after intravenous injections of cancer cells and spontaneous pulmonary metastasis (3), the major problem is not in accepting the concepts of heterogeneity (4) and tumor progression (5), but in assessing their importance in, and relevance to, metastasis formation in the natural history of cancer. The term heterogeneity is almost meaningless unless it is qualified with respect to a specific parameter, and the different parameters need not coincide. The comments in this section are confined to heterogeneity with respect to metastatic capacity.

It would be generally agreed that most cancer cells entering the metastatic process fail to form metastases. Basically, two explanations are used to account for the "successful" fraction of metastasis-forming cells: Fidler and Kripke (6) advanced the hypothesis that metastases arise exclusively or predominantly from relatively stable subpopulations of cancer cells with a "pre-existing metastatic phenotype"; according to this hypothesis, metastasis is a non-random event. In contrast, it has been argued that many, if not all, cancer cells in a tumor have metastatic potential, and that these are recruited into "transient metastatic compartments" from which metastases are generated on an operationally random basis (7).

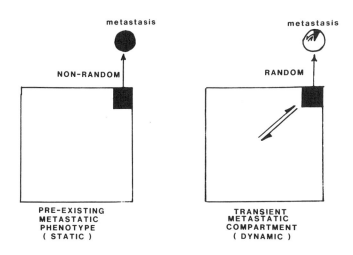

FIGURE 1. Basic Differences Between the Two Concepts That: (a) Metastases arise exclusively from subpopulations of cancer cells within a tumor which express a stable, pre-existing metastatic phenotype. A consequence of this non-random process would be that metastases are more metastatic than the whole cancer cell population of the primary lesion. (b) Metastases arise from a dynamic, transient metastatic compartment in a random manner, with the consequence that cancer cells in metastases have similar metastatic capacities to the cells in the primary lesion as a whole. The experimental evidence favors the latter concept.

Considerations affecting entry of cancer cells into transient compartments include topography. For example, it is expected that a cancer cell in a poorly vascularized, central part of a tumor has less chance of entering the metastatic process than a similar cell located in a well-vascularized, peripheral region. Many studies have shown that such metastatic-relevant cancer cell properties as adhesion, detachment and deformability are not static but are extremely dynamic properties which are coupled to metabolism and position in the cell cycle (8). Interactions between cancer cells and their environments, particularly their microenvironments which include other cells, can also produce changes in cancer host cell properties which are expected to be relevant to metastasis (9). The extent to which metastasis is dependent on transient, dynamic cancer cell properties as exemplified above, and on "pre-existing" metastatic subpopulations must be determined by experimentation. Recent studies have tended to support the concept of "transient metastatic compartments" based on genetic (10) and epigenetic events (7,11) and indicate that metastatic capacity is an unstable property. The evidence reviewed elsewhere has been interpreted by different authors to claim that at the cell level metastasis is either random (12), non-random (13), or both (14).

If metastases arise selectively from stable subpopulations of cancer cells, then on a per cell basis, metastases should be more metastatic on immediate reimplantation into new animal hosts after single passage than their parent primary tumors. This is not the general case (12,13)! One obvious interpretation of negative observations of this type is that metastases are not simply recruited exclusively from stable metastatic subpopulations. Other more complicated explanations invoke varying degrees of instability among these subpopulations after seeding (10,15), heterogeneity in phenotypic stability (16) and interactions between subpopulations in which the presence of a metastatic subpopulation can cause a relatively non-metastatic subpopulation to metastasize (17). Therefore, as predicted some time ago (8), the complex dynamism of this aspect of metastasis precludes dogmatic statements on possible underlying selective mechanisms. In spite of the many interpretive problems, the current literature abounds with uncritical and dogmatic statements to the effect that metastases arise exclusively from pre-existing, metastatic subpopulations.

Individual metastases ultimately develop from surviving cancer cells in either the single form or, more likely, in small clusters. Therefore, if, as suggested, the cancer cells in the transient metastatic compartments of primary tumors are heterogeneous, it is expected that individual metastases will have functionally different progenitors. The extent of the initial differences between the metastases themselves, and the differences in variation between the metastases and their parent tumors, would be influenced by the degree to which heterogeneity in expression of metastatic potential coincides with expression of heterogeneity in response to the therapeutic agents in question. Heppner et al. (19; also see Chapter 5) make special note of the lack of correlation between metastatic potential and drug sensitivity. In the paucicellular, micrometastatic stage of disease, any differences would tend to be maximal. However, as the secondary lesions increase in size, then on the one hand, genetic and epigenetic events will tend to increase the degree of cellular heterogeneity within individual tumors (15,20), and on the other hand, drug therapy may exert selective pressures, reducing subsequent heterogeneity in response. These potential differences between small ("young") and large ("old") lesions may be important. The net result of these considerations is that at different stages of their life histories, but particularly in the early (micrometastatic) stages, metastases may possibly be different from each other with respect to any parameter including drug-sensitivity, and the average properties of metastases may be different from the average properties of their parent primary lesions.

In a review of the literature (21), the evidence for general differential therapeutic responses by primary tumors and their metastases in vivo was not found to be compelling, and even in those cases where differences were documented in vivo, it was usually impossible to discriminate between those due to differences between cancer cells in the two situations and other causes including topographic factors, growth rate, drug delivery, etc. Although experiments with selected cell populations (22,23) have indicated the feasibility of such differences, they appear to be of little demonstrable clinical importance, and in treating patients cellular heterogeneity with respect to therapeutic response presents important but similar problems in both primary and metastatic lesions.

III. INVASION

Invasion is generally regarded as an essential part of the metastatic process, and is associated with the displacement or destruction of "normal" tissues by the advancing tumor. Invasion is involved in the "break-out" of cancers through confining basement membranes, intravasation and extravasation. Other things being equal, a proliferating tumor will expand in the direction of least resistance, as provided by natural anatomic (fascial) planes and cavities; the growth of renal carcinomas in the lumina of renal veins, for example.

It has been known since the late nineteenth century that cancer cells are capable of active locomotion, and the presence of single cancer cells in the tissues indicates that active cell movement also occurs in vivo. Morphometric analyses of sections of human malignant melanomas invading subcutaneous tissues suggest that the cancer cells actively migrate into these tissues for a distance of several hundred micrometers in advance of the main tumor body. Active translatory movements cease; the cancer cells then proliferate and come to occupy the previously tumor-free regions, and the migration/proliferation cycle is then repeated (24).

It is important to note that from a mechanical viewpoint, directionality can be imposed on invasion by local weaknesses in the tissue matrix. These weaknesses may be macroscopic, microscopic or at molecular levels. Thus, the strength of the intercellular matrix between parenchymal cells in the rat liver surrounding Walker 256 tumors shows an inverse relationship to distance from the tumor edge; however, in this situation there is no evidence for this change at macroscopic or microscopic levels (25).

28

Enzymes can cause host matrix degradation, and emphasis has justifiably been focused on the cancer cells themselves as a source of these invasion-related enzymes which produce a pericellular, sub-lethal autolysis (26). However, interactions involving cancer cells also involve the release of enzymes from other cell interactants, including polymorphonuclear leukocytes, macrophages and fibroblasts (27). Discrimination must be made between the enzymes themselves and agents inducing enzyme release (28). The relationship of enzymes to invasion is discussed elsewhere in this volume (see Chapters 18-22). However, there is not always a simple relationship between enzyme production by cancer cells and their invasive capacities either in vivo (29) or in vitro (30), and the critical issue may be the degree of inhibition of enzyme activity. Thus, Hakala et al. (29) showed that invasiveness in a series of intracranial tumors does not correlate with enzyme production, but rather that the invasive tumors tend to produce less tissue inhibitor of metalloproteinases (TIMP) than non-invasive tumors. This question of inhibitors is particularly relevant to the resistance to invasion by cartilage (31).

Enzymatic degradation of basement membrane is probably not an absolute requirement for intravasation and extravasation of all types of cancer cells in in vivo situations. Thus, in some sarcomas, intratumoral blood supply is provided by vascular clefts or channels which are lined by cancer cells, liberated into the bloodstream by direct shedding as distinct from an invasive process. In other cancers, entry into the bloodstream is via the tumor neovasculature which often consists of leaky, fenestrated vessels in which relatively little degradation is required for intravasation. Entry of carcinoma cells into the lymphatic system is a very common event, and the saccules and initial lymphatic channels do not possess a developed basement membrane. Extravasation in at least some tumors is accomplished by the intravascular proliferation of arrested or impacted cancer emboli, which burst out of the blood vessels confining them (32). While this latter process could be facilitated by enzymatic weakening of the vessel wall, it would not appear to be an absolute requirement for extravasation.

IV. INTERACTIONS OF CANCER CELLS WITH VESSEL WALLS

Arrest of circulating cancer cells, which is essential for metastasis formation, takes place mainly in the microcirculation of the first organ encountered. Studies on experimental animals show that in most host/cancer cell systems studied the vast majority of single cancer cells arriving in either the lungs (33) or the liver (34) are temporarily arrested and then released mostly in a non-viable state. In most cases, thousands of cancer cells must be delivered into the circulation of experimental animals in order to generate one tumor.

From a biophysical viewpoint, the events leading to arrest are exceptionally complex, and both the net negative electrical charge on cancer and vascular endothelial cells, and the boundary layers of plasma between them tend to prevent or retard arrest (35); however, arrest ultimately occurs.

Following contact with cancer cells, the vascular endothelium retracts exposing the subendothelium at which many of the biologically significant interactions involving cancer and other cells occur. Laminin is an important adhesion-protein in the exposed subendothelium, and in some cancer cells at least, attachment to type IV collagen of the basement membrane is enhanced by laminin and blocked by antibodies to laminin (36 and Chapter 19).

Due to their viscoelastic properties, cancer cells squeezed into small capillaries tend to expand against the vessel walls forcing out the very thin plasma (boundary) layer separating them. On the one hand, this promotes cancer cell arrest; on the other hand, the tight fit between moving cancer cells and the vessel walls may result in an increase in friction which may so raise the tension at the cancer cell surfaces that rupture could occur with consequent cancer cell death (37).

V. POST-EMBOLIC EVENTS

The arrest of emboli of any type at the luminal surfaces of blood vessels triggers a whole series of events coupling inflammatory response, complement activation, blood coagulation, fibrinolysis and tissue damage (38,39). Some of these post-embolic events are expected to kill arrested cancer cells but others, by causing vessel damage, enhance the extravasation of the survivors with increased risk of metastasis formation.

Within seconds of endothelial cell retraction following cancer cell arrest, circulating platelets interact with the exposed sub-endothelium and initiate fibrin deposition. Clot formation is also due to extravascular tissue products which initiate the extrinsic coagulation pathway. Over the years, it has been suggested that this fibrin "cocoon" protects arrested cancer cells. The cocoon is removed by a process of fibrinolysis, which is demonstrable soon after coagulation is completed. Attempts to reduce metastasis by the use of anticoagulants or fibrinolytic agents have not been successful, and the reported antimetastatic effects of coumarin derivatives are independent of their anticoagulant activity. Although platelets can interact directly with cancer cells, at least some of the major interactions involving platelets occur after interaction of cancer cells with the vascular endothelium. Platelet aggregation at these sites is inhibited by prostacyclin (PGI_2), which is produced by the vascular endothelium, and promoted by thromboxane (TXA_2), which is released from aggregated or damaged platelets. The regulation of PGI_2/TXA_2 balance by the vascular endothelium appears to be of wide biologic significance, and its therapeutic manipulation in favor of PGI_2 has been shown to reduce metastasis in mice and is discussed elsewhere by Honn et al. (see Chapter 9).

Possible specific factors contributing to post-embolic vascular damage include fibrin-induced fibrinolysis, leukocyte-mediated injury, platelet aggregation, serotonins, histamine, bradykinin and impaired organ function. These and other agents bear an often complex inter-relationship. For example, plasminogen activator released by cancer and endothelial cells ultimately induces fibrinolysis yet in addition may enhance invasion directly through stromal lysis, and indirectly by activation of collagenase through collagenolysis (see Chapter 20). Different polypeptide fragments of fibrinogen can increase microvascular permeability and can also cause endothelial cell retraction, thereby exposing the subendothelium and initiating more platelet induced changes. By virtue of their leukotactic activity, the fibrin degradation products may promote local collections of leukocytes.

The sequestration of leukocytes at sites of microembolism is partly due to the actions of TXA_2, the leukotrienes and 12-HETE. Although sequestration is part of a host defense-reaction, it must be remembered that such reactions can be injurious to the organism. Embolism triggers coagulation and fibrinolytic reaction cascades; in turn, plasmin activates complement, generating its C5a component which produces leukostasis, either directly through its chemotactic action, or indirectly by inducing macrophages to produce a chemotactic factor. The granulocytes injure both cancer cells and normal tissues with superoxide and related ions. On the one hand, leukocyte-mediated cancer cell damage could constitute an important component of host-defense and make major contributions to the inefficiency of the metastatic process. On the other hand, the vascular damage associated with leukocyte adhesion to the vessel walls and manifested as permeability increases could also facilitate extravasation of cancer cells.

Many of the enzymes implicated in invasion and often attributed solely to cancer cells are also released from sequestered leukocytes, including neutral proteinases, collagenase(s), elastase and cathepsin C.

VI. POST-EXTRAVASATION PHASE

A. Host-"Defense"

Arrested cancer cells which survive the trauma of short-term interactions at the walls of the microvasculature may or may not develop into metastases. Some of the subsequent interactions determining the fate of these survivors may be classified as defense reactions.

It is important to discriminate between defense reactions and immune reactions and between tumor antigenicity and immunogenicity. In human tumors, there is little direct evidence (of which I am aware) that the immune response affects the course of the disease. In human tumors, while antigenicity may be demonstrable, it often lacks specificity; there is great heterogeneity in antigenic expression among the cancer cell population of the various human tumors so far examined. I will not discuss in detail either humoral or cellular aspects of host-defense. However, in the case of human solid tumors a direct, effective T-lymphocyte-mediated attack seems unlikely, and the role of NK cells is controversial (see Chapters 13-15). Other cellular components of host-defense include macrophages and polymorphonuclear leukocytes. The macrophages can be activated by a variety of stimuli including lymphokines, and together with the polymorphs are frequently associated with host-cancer-specific inflammatory responses. The roles of the many surface receptors on macrophages and their interactions and control, particularly in antibody-dependent cellular cytotoxicity (ADCC) in specific anticancer cell responses, are not well understood (40).

Although a number of cytolytic agents are produced by activated macrophages (41) and polymorphs, much attention has been recently given to the reactive metabolites produced consequent to bursts of increased oxygen consumption associated with stimulation (42,43). Initially, superoxide anions (O_2^-) are formed, which give rise to H_2O_2 in a dismutation reaction:

$$O_2^- + O_2^- + 2H^+ \rightarrow O_2 + H_2O_2$$

In the presence of myeloperoxidase associated with the lysosomal granules of neutrophil polymorphs and monocytes, and of Fe^{2+}, the cytotoxicity of H_2O_2 is increased by the formation of hydroxyl radicals (OH·) as follows:

$$H_2O_2 + Fe^{2+} \rightarrow Fe^{3+} + O\bar{H} + OH\cdot$$

The toxicity of these reactions is reduced by breakdown of H_2O_2 by catalase and dissipation of O_2^- by superoxide dismutase. It must be emphasized, however, that toxicity mediated by oxygen-dependent pathways is not the only mechanism involved.

The localization of activity of the oxygen metabolites and other leukocyte products to regions close to their targets serves to both potentiate their target cytotoxicity and to limit their generalized toxicity. In addition, as a variety of cancer cells examined usually have lower levels of superoxide dismutase than their normal counterparts (43), these metabolites may well play an important role in killing cancer cells in the post-arrest phase of metastasis. Their preferential localized delivery has therapeutic potential. Poste and Fidler (44) have used the approach of delivering the macrophage activator muramyl dipeptide to the lungs in liposome-encapsulated form as effective therapy against certain lung tumors in mice (see Chapter 14). The types of cancers responding to this form of therapy

32

have yet to be determined, and the question of whether adequate local numbers of effector cells can be obtained in man remains unanswered. One problem appears to be that in mice part of the macrophage population around lesions is due to migration, whereas the other major part is derived from macrophage proliferation in these sites; the extent of on-site proliferation in man has yet to be determined.

B. DORMANCY

After extravasation subsequent growth of surviving cancer cells proceeds through micrometastases to metastases; this progression may be blocked by dormancy. Micrometastases may be very broadly defined as lesions which meet their nutritional requirements by diffusion, which serves to limit their diameters to approximately 1 to 2 mm. A cellular steady-state is maintained in these micrometastases when cell proliferation matches cell loss (pseudodormancy) or, alternatively, when the cancer cells are "locked" into the so called G_0 or G_2 phase of the cycle. Using this definition, a metastasis can be operationally defined as a tumor which satisfies its nutritional requirements via its own blood supply. Thus, according to this scheme, progression from micrometastasis to metastasis is neovasculature-dependent or associated, and dormancy could be associated with failure of neovascularization. Thus, when tumor fragments are implanted into the vitreous humor of animals' eyes, avascular tumor growth is very slow for some weeks. However, after the tumor fragments make contact with the retinal surface, vascularization occurs and is associated with rapid growth (45). Although vascularization is a major factor in metastasis growth, it is not the only factor.

Neovascularization of tumors occurs from capillary sprouts of mitotically active endothelial cells in nearby host vessels which respond to stimuli from the tumors. Although the factor producing this stimulation was first termed "tumor angiogenic factor," later work has shown that non-cancerous tissues exhibit similar angiogenic activities. Cells associated with postembolic events and inflammation in general, including activated macrophages, PMN and in some way, platelets also have angiogenic activity. Angiogenesis is stimulated by prostaglandin E_1 and mobilization of copper (46) and heparin (47), and is inhibited by inhibitors of prostaglandin synthesis, including aspirin and indomethacin (48), and protamine (47).

VII. METASTATIC INEFFICIENCY

Regardless of mechanism, interference at any step in the metastatic cascade can lead to "metastatic inefficiency" (49). This in essence refers to the disparity between the very large numbers of cancer cells available to participate in the metastatic process, compared with the relatively small numbers of overt metastases actually formed.

Basal cell carcinomas provide an excellent example of local invasive efficiency as indicated by sometimes massive tissue destruction in combination with metastatic inefficiency as indicated by the extreme rarity of metastases. This is associated with the failure of the basal cell carcinoma cells to intravasate.

In humans, it is well-recognized that the presence of circulating cancer cells is not synonymous with metastasis (50). Even on morphologic evidence, it appears that most of the cancer cells are killed in the microcirculation (51). Although quantitative data are lacking for humans, published data on the presence of cancer cells in the venous effluent from cancers (52) lead to the reasonable expectation that millions of cancer cells per day are released from primary cancers into the circulation. Even so at autopsy relatively few overt metastases can usually be identified.

A dramatic example of metastatic inefficiency is provided by the detailed autopsy data of Tarin et al. (53). In a patient dying as a result of ovarian carcinoma with peritoneal ascites, peritoneo-venus shunts were used to relieve the malignant ascites. After more than two years with functioning shunts, during which time millions of viable cancer cells must have been delivered directly into the bloodstream, the patient died without "established metastases in any organ."

Experiments with rats and mice show that most cancer cells injected into the bloodstream are temporarily arrested in the micro-vasculature of the first major organs encountered. The cancer cells are then killed following their interactions with vessel walls as a consequence of the pre- or post-embolic trauma. Most of the cancer cells subsequently released from these first major organs are therefore dead or moribund and the comparatively few viable cells arriving and surviving in the vascular bed of the next organ downstream may therefore be below the tumorigenic level (34,49). This type of metastatic inefficiency probably accounts for some of the complexities of metastatic patterns.

In attributing metastatic inefficiency to any particular mechanism, it is important to bear in mind that inefficiency at any step of the metastatic cascade may result in metastasis being a functionally slow process, which can therefore be interrupted by death of the patient due to a primary lesion or its treatment. An illustrative example is provided by cancers of the head and neck. At the beginning of this century less than 1% of patients died with visceral metastases, giving rise to the erroneous concept that head and neck cancers have an inherent tendency not to spread below the clavicle. However, with improvements in local therapy and the ability to treat infection, patients now survive longer, and the incidence of distant metastases at death now ranges from 10 to 52%. Metastases in the lungs, bones and viscera are now considered to be common sequelae of head and neck cancer.

VIII. METASTATIC PATTERNS

Organ patterns of metastasis of different primary cancers are important considerations in the diagnosis, treatment and prognosis of malignant diseases. One of the oldest problems in oncology lies in accounting for the different metastatic patterns exhibited by different types of cancers. Two deceptively simple hypotheses have been used to account for metastatic patterns of varying degrees of complexity. The first, the so-called "mechanical" hypothesis popularized by Ewing, focuses on the anatomic, hemodynamic and lymphodynamic factors determining the dose of cells delivered to target organs. The second, the "seed and soil" hypothesis popularized by Paget, focuses on the preferential growth of arrested emboli in different target organs subsequent to their delivery. The two hypotheses are not mutually exclusive.

Proponents of the "mechanical" hypothesis have argued that following dissemination in the arterial blood cancer cells must reach every organ. The fact that overt metastases are not detected in every organ indicates that tumorigenic doses are not delivered to them; metastatic patterns reflect vagaries in the delivery system. In view of recent studies on metastatic inefficiency, it seems likely that only small numbers of viable cancer cells enter the arterial blood, except in patients with advanced pulmonary lesions. In contrast, proponents of the "soil and seed" hypothesis argue that as the numbers of delivery systems - vascular, lymph drainage, body cavities, etc. - are limited and common to many different types of cancer, then the basic underlying mechanisms of their different metastatic patterns must lie in differential interactions between cancer emboli and target organs.

Before the role of the "seed and soil" hypothesis can be assessed, it is absolutely mandatory that the dose of viable cancer cells delivered to various organs be determined. Only when the incidence of metastases in a group of organs does <u>not</u> correlate with live cancer cell delivery is it permissible to invoke the "seed and soil" hypothesis. In many studies purporting to support the latter hypothesis, little attention has been given to cancer cell delivery.

It is now generally accepted that the mechanical hypothesis accounts for the high incidence of metastases in the first organs encountered by cancer cells after leaving their parent tumors, including liver, lungs, bone and lymph nodes. The clinical significance of the "mechanical hypothesis" therefore relates to the subsequent dissemination of cancer cells by the arterial route. The key question in this respect is whether the incidence of metastases in organs receiving cancer cells exclusively via the arterial route correlates with organ blood supply. In animals it is difficult to test the hypothesis directly because animals will die as a consequence of their primary tumors, or lung or liver metastases, before metastases can develop in other organs. Indirect tests have been performed in mice in which B16 cancer cells are injected directly into the arterial blood via the left ventricle; the proportions of the cardiac output going to the various target organs had previously been determined. In these experiments, target organs fall into two broad groups within which the incidence of tumor involvement correlates significantly with experimentally determined blood flow. Thus, both a "seed and soil" and a "mechanical" effect are demonstrated with this mouse tumor system (54). However, the latter is dominant.

In the case of humans, we find no recorded attempts to seek correlation between organ blood flow determined by modern "non-invasive" techniques and the incidence of metastasis. Our own preliminary studies of autopsy data on 15 types of primary cancers in 8 types of target organs for which blood flow data are available reveal suggestive correlations between published organ blood flow data and metastatic incidence. This is true for primary cancers in 4 of 5 primary sites in which initial main venous drainage is into the portal system, but in only one of 10 groups of primary cancers in sites in which initial main venous drainage is into the venae cavae (55). Analyses of the organ incidence of metastases in patients dying as a consequence of carcinomas of the upper rectum and lower esophagus indicates a predominant metastatic sequence. This sequence is along the lines of the type of metastatic cascade described by Viadana et al. (56), which represents metastasis of metastases (57; see also Chapter 23). The data indicated that distant metastases usually occur first in the liver; these secondary hepatic metastases then metastasize to the lungs, and these tertiary pulmonary metastases are then disseminated by the arterial route via the left ventricle. The incidence of organ involvement by the consequent quaternary metastases correlates closely with the blood flow per gram of target organ in accord with the "mechanical" hypothesis (58). The fact that the actual cancer cells involved in seeding the tertiary and quaternary metastases arise from secondary and tertiary metastases, respectively, as distinct from the primary cancers themselves, may well be a reflection of massive cancer cell death following direct transit through the microvasculature of the liver and lungs, as described above. In contrast, in primary adeno-carcinomas and squamous cell carcinomas in the lower rectum and upper esophagus, respectively, where initial main venous drainage is into the venae cavae, the organ incidence of metastasis does not correlate with blood flow. Therefore they are not in accord with the mechanical hypothesis (58).

The major differences between the two groups of primary cancers is that the former spread via metastatic sites in the liver and then the lungs, while the latter spread directly from lung metastases. This raises the question of whether residence of cancer cells in the liver modifies their subsequent arrest, retention, and growth patterns following arterial dissemination. In animals, organ-induced, irreversible selection (59) and reversible adaptation (60) in cancer cell peripheral structure have been observed, although the relationship of these changes to metastasis remains to be determined.

Studies in favor of the "seed and soil" hypothesis have followed the lines of Kinsey's (61) classical experiments, in which tumors selectively arise in specific embryonic transplants in the thigh muscles of mice, following intravenous or intra-arterial injections of cancer cells.   In addition, by stepwise procedures <u>in vivo</u> and <u>in vitro</u>, or <u>in vivo</u> only, organ-specific colonizing lines of cells have been selected (62).   The results indicate that factors over and above those related exclusively to delivery <u>can</u> play a part in tumor dissemination patterns, although their significance in natural metastasis requires clarification.

A note of caution is appropriate on the description of at least some of these organ-selective cell lines. For example, the M5076 reticulum cell sarcoma is often stated to metastasize selectively and virtually exclusively to the liver and ovaries of mice from subcutaneous and intravenous injections, and it has often been stated that the lungs are rarely involved. While this statement is true with respect to metastatic nodules visible to the naked eye, my colleague Dorothy Glaves has observed many small lung metastases in these animals in random histologic sections, indicating that organ preference is manifest as <u>variable</u> growth-rate, rather than as an all-or-none phenomenon. The degree of expression of this type of selectivity therefore depends on the length of time the animal survives.

In common with many other experimentalists, I think that short-term experiments with mice can be a misleading model for the development of metastatic patterns in people. In humans, metastasis is an ongoing and often lengthy process during the clinical course of which the cancer itself may "progress," the patient may change as evidenced, for example, by the emergence of paraneoplastic syndromes, and interactions between target organs and tumor emboli may change. The metastatic patterns may be complicated by tumor-bearing itself or by metastasis of metastases, and be perturbed by treatment. It therefore seems extremely unlikely that metastatic patterns can be explained in terms of the simplistic and static concept used in originally formulating the "mechanical" and "seed and soil" hypotheses.

IX. CONCLUSION

Although it would be convenient to present an overview of metastasis in a manner implying that there is consensus on the basic mechanisms involved, this could only be accomplished by ignoring large bodies of experimental evidence. The only conclusions which I can draw at present are: first, that metastasis is much more complex than initially supposed, and second, that at present many of the problems now appear to be defined, even if the answers are lacking.

REFERENCES

1.   Fidler IJ: Selection of successive tumor lines for metastasis. Nature (London) New Biol. 242:148-151, 1973.
2.   Rubin H: Adaptive changes in spontaneously transformed Balb/3T3 cells during tumor formation and subsequent cultivation. J. Natl. Cancer Inst. 72:375-382, 1984.
3.   Weiss L, Mayhew E, Rapp DG, Holmes JC: Metastatic inefficiency in mice bearing B16 melanomas. Br. J. Cancer 45:44-53, 1982.

4. Heppner GH, Miller BE: Tumor heterogeneity: Biological implications and therapeutic consequences. Cancer Metastasis Rev. 2:5-24, 1983.
5. Foulds L: Neoplastic Development. Academic Press, London, 1969.
6. Fidler IJ, Kripke ML: Metastasis results from preexisting variant cells within a malignant tumor. Science 197:893-895, 1977.
7. Weiss L: Dynamic aspects of cancer cell populations in metastasis. Am. J. Pathol. 97:601-608, 1979.
8. Weiss L: Membrane dynamics and the metastasis of cancer. Cell Biophys. 1:331-343, 1979.
9. Weiss L, Maslow DE: In vitro studies on the interactions of tumor and non-tumor cells. IN: Richards RJ and Rajan KT (eds.) Tissue Culture in Medical Research (II). Pergamon Press, Oxford, pp. 117-124, 1980.
10. Harris JF, Chambers AF, Hill RP, Ling V: Metastatic variants are generated spontaneously at a high rate in mouse KHT tumor. Proc. Natl. Acad. Sci. USA 79:5547-5551, 1982.
11. Frost P, Kerbel RS: On possible epigenetic mechanism(s) of tumor cell heterogeneity. Cancer Metastasis Rev. 2:375-378, 1983.
12. Weiss L: Random and nonrandom processes in metastasis and metastatic inefficiency. Invasion Metastasis 3:193-207, 1983.
13. Talmadge JE: The selective nature of metastasis. Cancer Metastasis Rev. 2:25-40, 1983.
14. Talmadge JE, Fidler IJ: Cancer metastasis is selective or random depending on the parent tumor population. Nature (London) 297:593-594, 1982.
15. Poste G, Greig R: On the genesis and regulation of cellular heterogeneity in malignant tumors. Invasion Metastasis 2:137-176, 1982.
16. Miller FR, Miller BE, Heppner GH: Characterization of metastatic heterogeneity among subpopulations of a single mouse mammary tumor: Heterogeneity in phenotypic stability. Invasion Metastasis 3:22-31, 1983.
17. Miller FR: Tumor subpopulation interactions in metastasis. Invasion Metastasis 3:234-242, 1983.
18. Weiss L: The Cell Periphery, Metastasis and Other Contact Phenomena. North Holland, Amsterdam, pp. 292-393, 1967.
19. Heppner GH, Dexter DL, Denocci T, Miller FR, Calabresi P: Heterogeneity in drug sensitivity among tumor cell subpopulations of a single mammary tumor. Cancer Res. 38:3758-3763, 1978.
20. Nicolson GL: Generation of phenotypic diversity and progression in metastatic tumor cells. Cancer Metastasis Rev. 3:25-42, 1984.
21. Weiss L: Metastasis: Differences between cancer cells in primary and secondary tumors. Pathobiol. Ann. 10:51-81, 1980.
22. Lotan R, Nicolson GL: Heterogeneity in growth inhibition by β-transretinoic acid of metastatic B16 melanoma clones and in vivo selected cell variant lines. Cancer Res. 39:4767-4771, 1979.
23. Tsuruo T, Fidler IJ: Differences in drug sensitivity among tumor cells from parental tumors, selected variants and spontaneous metastases. Cancer Res. 41:3058-3064, 1981.

38

24. Suh O, Weiss L: The development of a technique for the morphometric analysis of invasion in cancer. J. Theor. Biol. 108:547-562, 1984.
25. Weiss L: Tumor necrosis and cell detachment. Int. J. Cancer 20:87-92, 1977.
26. Weiss L: Sublethal autolysis. The Cell Periphery, Metastasis and Other Contact Phenomena. North-Holland, Amsterdam, pp. 92-99, 1967.
27. Biswas C: Host-tumor cell interactions and collagenase activity. IN: Liotta LA and Hart IR (eds.) Tumor Invasion and Metastasis. Martinus Nijhoff, The Hague, pp. 404-425, 1982.
28. Weiss L: Some mechanisms involved in cancer cell detachment by necrotic material. Int. J. Cancer 22:196-203, 1978.
29. Halaka AN, Bunning RAD, Bird CC, Gibson M, Reynolds JJ: Production of collagenase and inhibitor (TIMP) by intracranial tumors and dura in vitro. J. Neurosurg. 59:461-466, 1983.
30. Turner GA, Weiss L: Differential cell migration into stromal and protein-impregnated synthetic membranes and the effects of tumor necrotic extracts. Invasion Metastasis 2:361-368, 1982.
31. Kuettner KE, Pauli BU: Resistance of cartilage to invasion. IN: Weiss L and Gilbert HA (eds.) Bone Metastasis. G.K. Hall, Boston, pp. 131-165, 1981.
32. Wallace AC, Chew EC, Jones DS: Arrest and extravasation of cancer cells in the lung. IN: Weiss L and Gilbert HA (eds.) Pulmonary Metastasis. G.K. Hall, Boston, pp. 26-42, 1978.
33. Weiss L, Glaves D: Cancer cell damage at the vascular endothelium. Ann. NY Acad. Sci. 416:681-692, 1983.
34. Weiss L, Ward PM, Holmes JC: Liver-to-lung traffic of cancer cells. Int. J. Cancer 32:79-83, 1983.
35. Weiss L: Biophysical aspects of initial cell interactions with solid surfaces. Fed. Proc. Fed. Am. Soc. Exp. Biol. 30:1649-1657, 1971.
36. Varani J, Lovett EJ, McCoy JP, Shibata S, Maddox DE, Goldstein IJ, Wicha M: Differential expression of a laminin-like substance by high and low metastatic tumor cells. Am. J. Pathol. 111:27-34, 1983.
37. Weiss L, Dimitrov DS: A fluid mechanical analysis of the velocity, adhesion and destruction of cancer cells in capillaries during metastasis. Cell Biophys. 6:9-22, 1984.
38. Malik AB: Pulmonary microembolism. Physiol. Rev. 63:1114-1207, 1983.
39. Sundsmo JS, Fair DS: Relationships among the complement, kinin, coagulation and fibrinoltyic systems in the inflammatory reaction. Clin. Physiol. Biochem. 1:225-284, 1983.
40. Johnson WJ, Masmo PA, Schreiber RD, Adams DO: Sequential activation of murine mononuclear phagocytes for tumor cytolysis: Differential expression of markers by macrophages in several stages of development. J. Immunol. 131:1038-1043, 1983.
41. Adams DO, Nathan CF: Molecular mechanisms operative in cytolysis of tumor cells by activated macrophages. Immunol. Today 4:166-170, 1983.

42. Klebanoff SS: Oxygen-dependent cytotoxic mechanisms of phagocytes. IN: Gullin JI (ed.) Advances in Host Defense Mechanisms. Raven Press, New York, pp. 111-162, 1982.

43. Fridovich I: Superoxide radical: An endogenous toxicant. Ann. Rev. Pharmacol. Toxicol. 23:239-257, 1983.

44. Poste G, Fidler IJ: Therapeutic amplification of macrophage-mediated destruction of tumor cells. IN: Fidler IJ and White TRJ (eds.) Design of Models for Testing Cancer Therapeutic Agents. Van Nostrand Reinhold, New York, pp. 225-238, 1982.

45. Brem H, Folkman J: Inhibition of tumor angiogenesis mediated by cartilage. J. Exp. Med. 141:427-439, 1975.

46. Ziche M, Jones J, Guillino P: Role of prostaglandin E and copper in angiogenesis. J. Natl. Cancer Inst. 69:475-482, 1982.

47. Taylor S, Folkman J: Protamine is an inhibitor of angiogenesis. Nature (London) 297:307-308, 1982.

48. Peterson MI: Effects of prostaglandin synthesis inhibitors on tumor growth and vascularization. Invasion Metastasis 3:151-159, 1983.

49. Weiss L: Cancer cell traffic from the lungs to the liver: An example of metastatic inefficiency. Int. J. Cancer 25:385-392, 1980.

50. Goldmann EE: Anatomische untersuchungen ueber die verbreitungsweise geschwuelste. Beitr z Klin Chir (Tubingen) 18:595-612, 1897.

51. Iwasaki T: Histological and experimental observations on the destruction of tumour cells in the blood vessels. J. Pathol Bacteriol. 20:85-105, 1915.

52. Griffiths JD, Salsbury AJ: Circulating Cancer Cells. C.C. Thomas, Springfield, IL, pp. 54-56, 1965.

53. Tarin D, Vass ACR, Kettlewell MGW, Price JE: Absence of metastatic sequelae during long-term treatment of malignant ascites by peritoneo-venous shunting. Invasion Metastasis 4:1-12, 1984.

54. Weiss L, Ward PM, Harlos JP, Holmes JC: Target organ patterns of tumors in mice following the arterial dissemination of B16 melanoma cells. Int. J. Cancer (In press).

55. Weiss L, Haydock K, Pickren JW, Lane WW: Organ vascularity and metastatic frequency. Am. J. Pathol. 101:101-114, 1980.

56. Viadana E, Bross IDJ, Pickren JW: An autopsy study of some routes of dissemination of cancer of the breast. Br. J. Cancer 27:336-340, 1973.

57. Onuigbo WIB: Historical concepts of cancer metastasis with special reference to bone. IN: Weiss L and Gilbert HA (eds.) Bone Metastasis. G.K. Hall, Boston, pp. 1-10, 1981.

58. Weiss L, Bronk J, Pickren JW, Lane WW: Metastatic patterns and target organ blood flow. Invasion Metastasis 1:126-135, 1981.

59. Harlos JP, Weiss L: Differences in the peripheries of Lewis lung tumor cells growing in different sites in the mouse. Int. J. Cancer 32:745-750, 1983.

60. Weiss L, Harlos JP: Differences in the peripheries of Walker cancer cells growing in different sites in the rat. Cancer Res. 39:2481-2485, 1979.

61. Kinsey DL: An experimental study of preferential metastasis. Cancer 13:674-676, 1960.
62. Nicolson GL, Brunson KW, Fidler IJ: Specificity of arrest, survival and growth of selected metastatic variant cell lines. Cancer Res. 38:4105-4111, 1978.

CHAPTER 4. EXPERIMENTAL MODELS FOR STUDYING THE PATHOGENESIS AND THERAPY OF METASTATIC DISEASE

GEORGE POSTE AND RUSSELL GREIG

I. INTRODUCTION

The task of discussing models of disease, whether for cancer metastasis or any other disease, is fraught with danger. Opinions on this subject are at risk of being interpreted as either overly simplistic or as making unwarranted claims for relevance to human disease. Similarly, it is impossible to avoid the truism that man is the only suitable model for studying disease in man. In strict terms even this is incorrect. The individual cancer patient represents the only valid model for their own disease since the full historical interplay of host and tumor factors and the selection pressures that have shaped the course of tumor progression and response to therapy can never be duplicated exactly in another individual.

The use of tumor models has been of overwhelming importance in research on the pathogenesis of neoplastic disease and the search for new antitumor agents. This will not change in the foreseeable future. It is therefore essential that the criteria used in choosing a tumor model be reexamined at regular intervals to determine if the model should be discarded or refined to accommodate the new advances in cancer biology that are occurring at a rapid pace as a result of dramatic progress in cell biology, immunology and molecular genetics.

Animal tumor models exhibit many important differences from human neoplasms. These have been documented in numerous publications (1-7). Prominent among these are: differences in body size and lifespan; species variation in the anatomy and physiology of major organ systems; variation in the contribution of different elements of host immune and non-immune reactions in combating neoplasia; and significant species variation in the absorption, distribution, metabolism and excretion of therapeutic agents. The incidence of spontaneous tumors arising in specific cell types also varies significantly in man and animals. Similarly, the risk of tumor formation occurring in the same target organ after exposure to carcinogens varies among species and this is recognized as a serious limiting factor in using animals to predict the carcinogenic liability of food additives, chemicals or drugs.

The extensive reliance on transplantable established tumor cell lines, usually of rodent origin, as models for human tumors represents a major source of potential irrelevancies and artifacts. Most human solid malignancies grow relatively slowly and contain cells that retain many of the properties of the cell type from which they originated. In

42

contrast, many of the more widely used established tumor cell lines of human and animal origin contain rapidly growing, anaplastic cells. These may have little or no phenotypic relationship even to the cell type from which they arose originally, yet alone tumors originating in entirely different cell types. This problem will be emphasized throughout this article in urging the need to pay greater attention to the biological uniqueness of neoplasms arising in different cell lineages. The increasing attention given by many laboratories to the development of model systems using freshly isolated human tumor cells is particularly relevant and represents a major initiative in increasing the technical sophistication of current experimental approaches. However, irrespective of whether human or animal tumor cells are used, we must begin to give more attention to the nature and the extent of the phenotypic changes that may result from the selection and serial propagation of tumor cells in vitro or in vivo and how far such changes render the cells unsuitable for detecting the cellular alterations responsible for tumorigenicity and metastasis and for evaluating cellular responses to antitumor agents.

No attempt will be made in this article to debate the merits of one tumor model versus another. Rather our intention is to emphasize a number of general concepts that are emerging from recent research in tumor cell biology which we consider merit attention in the design of experimental approaches for studying the pathogenesis and therapy of metastatic disease. The more sophisticated and subtle requirements that must be considered in designing models to investigate particular problems concerning the cell biology, immunology, genetics or therapy of metastasis are discussed in other chapters in this volume.

II. EXPERIMENTAL APPLICATIONS OF METASTATIC TUMOR MODELS

The value of any experimental model depends on the question(s) being asked. For studies in metastasis, the questions fall into three broad categories.

The first embraces experimental efforts to understand the mechanisms of metastasis used by different types of malignant neoplasms and the role of specific host and tumor cell properties in promoting or inhibiting specific steps in the metastatic process. The rationale for such studies is that by expanding knowledge of pathogenesis of metastatic disease, and awareness of the events that determine the outcome of each step in this process, the information can be used in the rational design of antimetastatic therapies.

The second category of research on metastasis is a logical extension of the first and involves experimental efforts to identify the specific properties that endow malignant cells with metastatic capacity. An extensive body of research has shown that the metastatic properties of different subpopulations of tumor cells coexisting within the same tumor can vary substantially (for review see 1,8,9). Identification of the cellular and subcellular properties that distinguish metastatic tumor cell subpopulations from their non-metastatic (but tumorigenic) counterparts would create potential targets for the design of therapeutic agents that could act selectively against metastatic cells.

The third, and final, segment of research activities on metastasis concerns the use of tumor models in the search for new therapeutic agents. However, the use of metastatic models in screening programs for detecting new anticancer agents and in the preclinical testing of such agents for activity against established metastases has been extremely limited (10). The reasons for this are discussed in more detail in a later section of this chapter.

A. Desirable Features of Metastatic Tumor Models

Each different application of metastatic tumor models will almost certainly impose unique experimental requirements which must be fulfilled by the model selected. Every investigator who has selected a particular tumor model presumably can cite a reason(s) to justify its use. Such opinions will range from the objective to the subjective, with the latter category embracing, at least in private conversation, such reasons as "the model was available in the laboratory" or "my senior colleagues chose it and I'm not going to ruin my career by challenging them."

Some of the strengths and weaknesses of the transplantable animal tumors that are commonly used in metastasis research have been discussed at length elsewhere (1,11). We do not intend to debate the merits of tumor A versus tumors B or C, or the greater or lesser value of different species of experimental animals. Each may have merits for the purpose for which it was chosen. Similarly, every model will have shortcomings, and personal perspectives concerning the balance between the strengths and weaknesses of a model vary enormously. Some of the more obvious examples of this are reflected in the long standing, yet unresolved, debates regarding the value of using induced versus spontaneous tumors; the merits of transplantable tumors (whether of spontaneous origin or induced) versus autochthonous tumors; the use of highly antigenic immunogenic tumors versus weakly immunogenic or non-immunogenic (?) tumors in evaluating host immune responses to tumors; the validity of intravenous (i.v.) inoculation of tumor cells as an assay of the "metastatic" properties of tumor cells; and the merits of using rapidly growing poorly differentiated animal tumors, particularly those of lymphoid cell origin, as screening systems for detecting agents to destroy solid human tumors that are typically less anaplastic and have low growth fractions.

Radical shifts in the opinions of the supporters of particular viewpoints in these debates are unlikely to occur. Consequently, a large number of tumor models will continue to be used. Cancer research, in common with other aspects of human behavior, is not unaffected by "fashions" and certain tumor models may gain in popularity, and be accepted without critical scrutiny, because of their use by laboratories that are currently influential in a particular area of investigation. The next generation of tumor models to achieve popularity will not be exempt from such events and their success will also stem in part from similar patronage.

A number of legitimate scientific advances can be identified, however, that have contributed significantly to the conceptual and/or the technical evolution of metastatic tumor models. The first is that to understand the pathogenesis of metastatic disease, and its under- lying mechanisms, it is necessary to study metastatic tumors. This may seem to be stating the obvious to the point of absurdity yet it is still not uncommon, though far less frequent than a few years ago, to read papers in which the stated rationale is to study "malignancy" or "metastatic disease" yet a non-metastasizing tumor is being used.

Second, with the demonstration that the cellular composition of most, if not all, malignant tumors is highly heterogeneous and that only certain subpopulations of tumor cells express metastatic properties, perhaps even in a transient fashion, it now becomes almost obligatory to characterize the extent of cellular heterogeneity within a particular tumor and to isolate representative examples of the constituent cellular subpopulations for detailed comparison. This technically more demanding approach is essential if we are to gain any insight into the phenotypic traits that are responsible for metastatic behavior (see below).

Third, the demonstration in various animal tumors of heterogeneity in the metastatic capabilities of different tumor cell subpopulations present within the same tumor has led logically to experimental efforts to investigate whether similar metastatic heterogeneity is present in human neoplasms. Initial attempts to study this important question were frustrated by the unexpected failure of human tumor cells to metastasize when implanted as xenografts into nude mice. This problem has been partially resolved with the finding that certain human tumor cells injected into newborn, or very young, nude mice exhibit greater metastatic propensity than when implanted into older animals (for review see 12,13). In addition, metastasis of human tumor cells in adult nude mice appears to be slow and may require prolonged assays (for other references see 13). Also, the detection of metastatic human tumor cells xenografted into nude mice may be facilitated by "conditioning" them prior to implantation by growing them in organ cultures of mouse tissue (14) or by implantation into organs such as the spleen (15). Although these methods are technically demanding and require considerable time, effort and resources, further refinement of these methods, together with the development of other techniques for evaluating the metastatic capacity of human tumor cells, is of high priority. With the more routine availability of such methods every consideration should then be given to using these systems in preference to animal tumors, unless human and animal tumor cells can be reliably shown not to differ appreciably in the particular property that is to be studied.

Finally, improvements in methods for the cultivation of tumor cells from freshly excised human tumors (for review see 16-19) and their propagation in nude mice or other immune deficient animals (20) will also mean that experiments can now begin to define the extent of the phenotypic changes that occur in tumor cells as a consequence of prolonged passage in vitro or in vivo. Concern regarding this question is certainly not new (21). However, we consider it to be one of the most critical issues facing contemporary cancer research. Unless we can define the phenotypic similarity between tumor cell populations used in experiments and tumor cells existing in the major human malignancies we are at risk of continuing to identify and study phenotypic alterations and therapeutic responses in established cell lines that may have little or no relationship to the properties of tumor cells in situ or low passage tumor cells isolated from freshly excised neoplasms. Definition of the extent and nature of the pheno-typic "shift" occurring in tumor cells isolated from human tumors of defined histologic origin will require careful examination of a broad panel of phenotypic markers whose relevance to tumor cells in situ has been confirmed. Development of such panels is only in its infancy and the technical sophistication and relevance of this exercise will, of course, change with the validation and introduction of new phenotypic markers. As in so many aspects of modern research on metastasis, this task will be tedious and require considerable resources. Until this information is obtained, however, we will not be able to answer the fundamental question of whether the established tumor cell lines that presently dominate many aspects of cancer research have any meaningful relationship to tumor cells present in different types of human neoplasms.

Notwithstanding the issues discussed above, for a tumor model to accommodate the changing dimensions of current research on metastasis it must meet as many as possible of the following criteria.

First, but certainly no guarantee of functional relevance to clinical disease, the similarities with human neoplasms should be maximized, either by using human tumor cells isolated from the neoplasm of interest or by using an animal tumor arising in the same organ and the same cell type as the human tumor.

Second, it is desirable that the route(s) of tumor dissemination and the resulting anatomic distribution of metastases produced by the model should resemble the human disease. However, anatomic differences between species, and the need to use transplantable tumors in which large numbers of tumor cells are implanted at sites chosen for their convenience rather than biological relevance, will inevitably impose differences. In addition, provided that the ability of tumor cells to metastasize "spontaneously" from the implantation site has been confirmed, it is convenient if the cells being studied exhibit a similar ranking in their capacities to produce tumor colonies (so called "experimental metastases") in different organs when injected directly into the circulation. This assay, if validated by the stringent criteria discussed in a later section of this chapter, can be of considerable value in reducing the time and cost of assaying metastatic behavior of different cell populations isolations from the same tumor.

Third, it is almost impossible to conduct research on cancer metastasis today without having some appreciation of the extent of the cellular heterogeneity present in the tumor being studied. Since cell cloning offers the most direct and effective method for studying phenotypic variation among different cells residing in the same parent cell population, it is helpful if the tumor selected for study has a reasonably high cloning efficiency. Furthermore, the use of defined media to facilitate the cloning and the recovery of the more fastidious tumor cell clones merits attention. These requirements are of particular relevance to studies with human tumor cells. A substantial effort will be required to solve these problems before detailed analyses of the clonal composition of tumors of the kind already completed for a few animal tumors can become routine practice for human tumors. Identification of clonal variation among cells present in a specific tumor also demands that a panel of stable phenotypic markers is available to permit reliable detection of clones with different phenotypes. Ideally, the panel should include karyotypic, immunologic and biochemical markers which can be assayed in reproducible fashion in tumor cells in vitro and in vivo (for review see 22). As emphasized earlier, few panels of these kind are presently available. Also, for experimental purposes it is acceptable to engineer the introduction of specific markers into individual subpopulations using gene transfer methods, mutagenesis or treatments that induce significant phenotypic change such as treatment with drugs that alter DNA methylation patterns (for review see 22). Also, in creating a panel of phenotypic markers it is essential to determine the (in)stability of such markers in clonal tumor cell populations maintained under different conditions in vitro and in vivo (see below).

Finally, if a tumor model is to be used in screening potential therapeutic agents for antineoplastic activities, it is important that the response of the tumor to existing therapeutic agents/modalities resembles as far as possible the responses observed in human neoplasms of similar histologic origins.

These criteria are utopian and varying deficiencies will exist in any model. Nonetheless, unless diligent efforts are constantly made to refine model systems to maximize their similarities with the patho-genesis and the therapeutic responses of human tumors we cannot reasonably expect major progress in advancing our understanding of the mechanisms of metastasis or in the detection of new therapeutic agents with improved efficacy against specific human tumors.

B. Metastasis Assays

In man, metastatic disease is diagnosed routinely before death and
the growth of metastases and their responses to therapy can be
evaluated using a variety of imaging techniques. In laboratory animals
such tests are not used routinely and metastasis is usually assayed at
necropsy. For tumors that arise spontaneously in experimental or
domestic animals, analysis of necropsy data from large numbers of
animals, particularly rodents maintained in identical, carefully
controlled environments, can provide useful data on the incidence of
metastases, their distribution and the likely routes of tumor
dissemination (for review see 23-26). Also, by sacrificing tumor-
bearing animals at different times after the initial development of the
primary tumor, information can be obtained concerning the timing of the
onset of metastatic disease. Relatively few studies of this kind have
been reported, however, presumably because the resources needed to
conduct such studies under carefully controlled conditions are not
widely available. A little used, and certainly overlooked, source of
such information is the long-term chronic toxicity testing protocols
used routinely by pharmaceutical companies and certain chemical testing
laboratories in which large numbers of mice and rats are maintained for
18 to 24 months under stringent conditions in accordance with
regulations set by governmental regulatory agencies. This material
should not be overlooked either as a useful source of data for
statistical analyses of the comparative pathology of various tumors in
man and animals and also as a direct source of tumor tissue for
experimental studies.

The metastatic capacity of transplantable tumors is usually
assayed either by i.p., s.c., i.m. or intrasplenic injection of a bolus
of tumor cells followed by subsequent assessment of the dissemination
of tumor cells to establish metastases in other organs. This assay has
come to be known as the "spontaneous" metastasis assay. This is in
contrast to assays in which tumor cells are injected directly into the
circulation to measure their capacity to form tumor colonies or so
called "experimental metastases" in various organs (for review see 1).
A full description of these methods and the various technical factors
that can influence the outcome of metastasis assays has been provided
elsewhere (1,11).

In strict terms, neither of these assays mimic events in the
"spontaneous" metastasis of naturally occurring tumors in which tumor
cell dissemination occurs at variable stages during the progressive
evolution of a primary tumor which originated from either a single
tumor cell or, at most, a focus of a few cells (1). In the so-called
"spontaneous assay" for transplantable tumors, large numbers of tumor
cells, typically 10^4 to 10^6 cells, are injected into superficial body
tissues with accompanying mechanical trauma to the tissues that may
affect initial vascularization of the tumor implant and subsequent
delivery of test drugs to the growing implant. Such trauma may also
predispose to local invasion and metastasis by disrupting local tissue
fascia and other mechanical barriers to tumor spread. Nonetheless, few
would dispute that with the exception of tumor cells that inadvertently

enter the bloodstream during the initial injection (27), the ability of tumor cells implanted s.c. or at other body sites to generate metastases in distant organs indicates that the tumor cells are capable of completing all of the steps in the metastatic process (8). This contrasts with the "experimental metastasis" assay in which tumor cells are introduced into the circulation thereby circumventing the need for initial invasion of host tissues to penetrate the vasculature. This feature has caused some to question the value of this method as an assay of metastatic capacity (27-29). As with all aspects of cancer cell biology, generalizations about tumor cell behavior are difficult, if not impossible to make, and are fraught with the danger that exceptions will be reported quickly. The methods for assaying the metastatic behavior of different tumors are no exception and must be validated for the particular tumor cells being investigated. The capacity of tumor cells to form tumor colonies ("experimental" metastases) in different organs after i.v. or intraarterial injection should be accompanied by parallel assays to determine the ability of replicate samples of the same cells to form "spontaneous" metastases when implanted at various sites, with or without amputation of the primary implant (1). For cloned tumor cell populations, parallel assay of their organ colonizing and spontaneous metastatic capacities allows the clones to be ranked for their proficiency in either assay. For some tumors, clones may have identical or very similar rank order in both assays (RC in Table 1) but in other tumors a rank correlation does not exist (NC in Table 1), even though the clones tested may still express both organ colonizing and spontaneous metastatic abilities.

In our opinion, the routine use of the organ colonization assay to evaluate "metastatic" potential of clonal tumor cell populations is likely to be more informative if the clones selected for study have been shown to exhibit a similar rank order in both the organ colonizing and spontaneous metastasis assays. Clones that show organ colonization abilities but lack spontaneous metastatic capacity are of less utility in experiments designed to identify the cellular properties that correlate with metastatic proficiency. Such clones particularly those with high organ colonization potential are still useful, however, in analyzing the factors that affect tumor cell behavior and survival in the circulation, the arrest and extravasation of circulating tumor cells and the proliferation of tumor cells in the extravascular parenchyma of different organs (1,8,11,12).

The diverse patterns of organ colonizing and spontaneous metastatic behavior that can be exhibited by different clones isolated from the same tumor when assayed under different conditions are illustrated by the following data obtained in our laboratory over the last few years.

The proportion of tumor cell clones that exhibited organ colonizing capacity but were unable to form spontaneous metastases varied significantly among different tumors (Table 2). The data in Table 2 indicate that for three of the four tumors studied in detail, the majority of clones tested exhibited spontaneous metastatic behavior after s.c. implantation and also formed tumor colonies when injected i.v. However, for clones isolated from spontaneous mammary tumors arising in CBA strain mice a significant fraction of the clones tested lacked the ability to metastasize when implanted s.c. Ironically, parallel studies using the same clones revealed that the number of clones that could metastasize "spontaneously" when implanted in the mammary gland was even lower. The failure of many mammary tumor cell clones to produce spontaneous metastases does not mean, however, that these cells lack metastatic potential. Similar data have been reported by Tarin and his colleagues working with mammary tumors (31-34). In a series of elegant studies, they demonstrated that the rate of release of mammary tumor cells into the circulation is important in determining whether "spontaneous" metastasis occurs and that failure of cells with high organ colonization capacities to form spontaneous metastases is a consequence of limited release into the bloodstream and should not be interpreted as indicating that they lack metastatic capacity (31-34).

A detailed classification of the organ colonization potential and spontaneous metastatic abilities of an extensive series of B16 melanoma clones is shown in Table 3. Only a small percentage (18%) of the clones tested were unable to form spontaneous metastases when implanted in the footpad and this was followed by amputation of the footpad 14 da after tumor implantation. The majority of clones metastasized spontaneously from the footpad and formed lung colonies when injected i.v. However, the proficiency of different clones in producing lesions varied depending on the route of inoculation (Table 3).

The incidence of spontaneous metastases may differ, however, depending on the site at which tumor cells are implanted (30,35-37). This is illustrated by the data in Table 4 in which a series of B16 melanoma clones were implanted s.c. at different sites and the number of animals with metastases was measured at 45 da and at 80 da or on the death of the animal (whichever occurred earlier). The data indicate significant variation in the incidence of spontaneous metastases from different implantation sites and in addition that amputation of the primary implant can enhance the importance of using different time periods as endpoints for tumors implanted at different anatomic sites.

Table 1. A Comparison of Spontaneous and Experimental Metastatic Behavior of Malignant Tumor Cells[A].

Species	Strain	Tumor or Cell Line	Source	Polyclonal (P) And/or Clonal (C)	EM Dose/Endpoint
Mouse	DBA/2	MDAY–D2	in vitro	P/C	10^5 moribund
Mouse	C57BL/6	Lewis lung carcinoma	in vitro	P/C	$2 \times 10^4 – 2 \times 10^5$ (4)/ 15–43 days
Mouse	BALB/c	RAW117 lymphosarcoma	in vitro	P/C	5×10^3/14 days
Mouse	C57BL/6	M5076 reticulum cell sarcoma	in vitro	P	2×10^4/21 days
Mouse	C57BL/6x C3HeB/FeJ	T10 sarcoma	in vivo	P/C	10^6/14–21 days
Mouse	C57BL/6	MN/MCA1 sarcoma	in vitro	P	10^5/28 days
Mouse	C57BL/6	mFS6 sarcoma	in vitro	P	10^5/18 days
Mouse	C57BL/6	B16 melanoma	in vitro	P	10^5/18 days
Mouse	C57BL/6	B16–BL6/F10 $F10^{LR}$	in vitro	P	10^5/21 days
Mouse	BALB/c	mouse mammary tumor	in vitro	P/C	$10^3 – 3 \times 10^6$ (7)/ 14–16 days
Mouse	DBA/2	T1699 mammary adenocarcinoma	in vitro	P/C	$10^3 – 10^7$ (9)/ 14–16 days
Mouse	C3H	spontaneous mammary	in vivo	P	5×10^6/moribund or 90 days
Mouse	BALB/c	Colon 26 adenocarcinoma	in vitro	P/C	5×10^4/23 days
Mouse	C3H/HeN	UV2237 fibrosarcoma	in vitro	P/C	10^5/18 days 10^6 moribund
Mouse	C57BL/6	B16–BL6	in vitro	C	$5 \times 10^2 – 3 \times 10^5$ (6)/ 19 days post–amputation
Mouse	C3H/HeN	K1735 melanoma	in vitro	C	$2.5 \times 10^4 . 1 \times 10^5$/ 35 days
Mouse	C57BL/6	B16. F1. F10. BL/6	in vitro	P	5×10^4/21 days
Rat	WAG	9–4/0 rhabdo–myosarcoma	in vitro	P/C	10^5/10 weeks
Rat	F344	13762 adenocarcinoma	in vitro	P/C	5×10^4/23 days
Rat	BDX	BSp73 adenocarcinoma	in vitro	P	10^5/21–35 days

[A]EM=experimental metastasis; SM=spontaneous metastasis; AMP=amputation; sc=subcutaneous; im=intramusclar; ifp=intrafootpad; ND=not determined; RC=rank correlation; NC=no correlation.

[B]Tumor cells that displayed a similar rank in both SM and EM assays were designated RC. The dose provided in parentheses was the only cell inoculum that provided a RC when multiple doses were employed.

[C]Comparison performed by authors.

SM Dose/Site/Endpoint	Synchronous (S) or Asynchronous (A)	Correlation[B]	Reference
10^5/sc flank/moribund	S	RC	46
5×10^5/im/flank/ moribund or 26 days	A	RC (10^5)[C]	47
5×10^5/sc/flank/ 21–28 days	ND	RC	48
5×10^4/ifp/42 days	S	RC	49
10^5/ifp/21–28 days post-amputation	A	RC	50
10^5/im flank/moribund	S	NC[C]	51
10^5/im flank/moribund	S	NC[C]	51
10^5/im flank/moribund	S	NC[C]	51
10^5/im flank/21 days	A	NC	52
10^4/mammary fat pad/ AMP (12–15 mm)/21–42 days post-amputation	S	RC (10^4)	53
10^5/sc flank/23 days	ND	RC	54
10^5/im flank/ AMP 9 days/40 days post-amputation			
spontaneous/mammary gland/variable	A	NC	55
5×10^5, 1×10^6/sc flank/26–29 days	S	NC	56
2.5×10^5/ifp/AMP 17 days/23 days post-amputation			
10^6/sc flank/moribund	S	RC[C]	57
5×10^2–4.5×10^5 (7)/AMP 1 cm/14–16 days	S	NC[C]	58
10^5/ifp/57–84 days	S	RC	49
10^5, 2×10^5/sc flank 28 days	S	NC[C]	27
10^3–10^6 (4)/sc flank/ moribund	ND	NC	59
10^6/sc mammary fatpad/23 days	S	RC[C]	60
2×10^5/sc flank 35 days post-amputation	S	NC	61

Table 2. Organ Colonization and Metastatic Properties of Tumor Cell Clones from a Series of Experimental Animal Tumors[*].

Tumor	Organ Colonization Activity Only	Organ Colonization and Metastatic Capacity
B16 melanoma	35/187 (19%)[†]	152/187 (81%)[†]
K1735 melanoma	14/98 (14%)	84/98 (86%)
UV2237 fibrosarcoma	3/31 (10%)	26/31 (89%)
CBA mouse mammary carcinoma	33/64 (52%)	31/64 (48%) flank 23/64 (36%) mammary gland

[*]Replicate preparations of tumor cell clones were injected i.v. to evaluate organ colonization capacity or s.c. to monitor metastatic capacity. Organ colonization activity was assayed 21 da after i.v. injection of 5×10^3, 5×10^4 or 1×10^5 tumor cells in 0.2 ml (five mice per inoculum). Clones were scored as positive if tumor colonies were detected in any organ 21 da later. Metastatic capacity was assayed by implanting 5×10^5 tumor cells in the rear footpad (B16; K1735; UV2237) or in the flank or mammary gland (CBA mammary tumor) in syngeneic hosts. Groups of five mice were injected per clone. For tumors implanted in the rear footpad, the limb was amputated at mid-thigh after 21 da and animals examined for the presence of metastases in any organ four weeks later. Tumors in the flank and the mammary gland were not amputated and metastasis was assayed at autopsy 48 da after implantation.

[†]Number of clones displaying the indicated behavior/the total number of total clones tested. The numbers in parentheses indicate the percentage of clones tested with the indicated behavior.

Table 3.   Organ Colonization and Metastatic Properties of B16 Melanoma Clones[*].

Organ Colonization Activity (i.v.)[†]	Metastatic Capacity (s.c.)[‡]	Number of Clones with Indicated Behavior/ Total Clones Tested
low	0	27/187 (14%)
high	0	6/187 (4%)
low	low	41/187 (22%)
high	low	58/187 (31%)
low	high	18/187 (10%)
high	high	35/187 (19%)

[*]Clones were tested in parallel for their ability to produce organ colonies after i.v. injection or to metastasize spontaneously after implantation in the rear footpad as described in footnote * in Table 2.

[†]low = < 50 tumor colonies in all organs examined (lung, liver, ovary, heart, spleen, lymph nodes and brain); high = > 50 tumor colonies in the same organs.

[‡]low = < 20 metastases in the organs listed in †.   high = > 20 metastases in these organs.

For organ colonization assays it is essential that dose-response relationships be established for each cell population studied. The rationale for such experiments is shown in Figure 1 which summarizes the formation of lung tumor colonies by different doses of ten B16 melanoma clones injected i.v. into C57BL/6 mice. The data illustrate that if colonizing potentials are to be evaluated using only a single uniform inoculum, misleading conclusions could be drawn regarding the colonizing capacities of the clones. For example, at the lowest cell inoculum tested (5×10^2 cells) only three clones would be classified as able to form colonies.   In contrast, at the highest inoculum tested (10^5 cells) all ten clones are positive and the majority would be classified as being of "high" colonization potential because of the large number of colonies produced. However, if the data in Figure 1 are replotted in terms of the number of tumor cells injected that are needed to form a detectable lung tumor colony, the clones fall into three categories. For two of the three categories the number of tumor cells required to produce a lung colony is consistently greater than 1×10^3 and is considerably higher at lower cell inocula (5×10^3 and

Table 4. Metastatic Properties of B16 Melanoma Clones Implanted at Different Anatomic Sites in C57BL/6 Mice*.

Time (da post-implantation)	Implantation Site					
	Footpad		flank	nape	Ear	
	non-amp	amp			non-amp	amp
45 da	20/23 (87%)†	16/23 (70%)	18/23 (78%)	10/23 (44%)	7/23 (31%)	11/23 (48%)
death or 80 da	21/23 (91%)	19/23 (83%)	19/23 (83%)	18/23 (78%)	13/23 (57%)	18/23 (78%)

*Replicate samples of 23 clones were injected (5 x 10⁵ cells) into the indicated sites. Certain tumors growing in the rear footpad or the pinna of the ear were surgically amputated (amp) after 21 da for comparison with animals in which the tumors were not removed (non-amp). Clones were scored as positive if metastases were detected in any organ in mice autopsied at 45 da, at 80 da or at death if this occurred earlier. The data are derived from analyses of groups of ten mice for each clone at each injection site.

†Metastatic clones/total clones tested. The numbers in parentheses indicate the percentage of total clones tested exhibiting metastatic capacity.

2-5 x 10^4 cells). In contrast, the third category reveals a series of three clones that require the least number of tumor cells to form a tumor colony and is independent of cell dose. These clones thus exhibit a uniformly high colonizing potential and are of particular attraction for experimental studies.

These data emphasize the need to use a variety of assay methods to achieve a detailed and stringent classification of the complex behavioral properties exhibited by clonal subpopulations of tumor cells isolated from any given tumor. The organ colonizing and metastatic profiles assigned to an individual clone can vary substantially depending on the assay conditions used. The results indicate that for the murine B16 melanoma the overwhelming majority of the clones tested express both organ colonizing and spontaneous metastatic abilities. However, as emphasized earlier, before the organ colonization assay can be adopted for routine use it is necessary to validate for each tumor cell population that quantitative variation in cellular performance in this assay correlates with similar variation in ability to produce spontaneous metastases. Detailed analyses of this kind temper the criticism voiced by Weiss, both in this volume (Chapter 3) and else- where (28), that the organ colonization assay has no value in evaluating cellular metastatic potential. For some tumors it does and for others it does not (Table 1). The reality must be tested experimentally for each tumor used and for each subpopulation of cells isolated from the same tumor.

C. Phenotypic Analysis of Tumor Cell Populations and Identification of Cell Properties that Correlate with Metastatic Ability

The knowledge that all human and animal tumor cell populations studied to date have been found to contain phenotypically different subpopulations of cells has important implications for experimental efforts to define the cellular and subcellular properties that correlate with complex, multifactorial behavioral traits such as metastasis. As discussed at length elsewhere (1,22,38), the coexistence within the same tumor (or tumor cell line) of sub- populations of cells with different metastatic properties dictates that the use of heterogeneous populations containing both non-metastatic and metastatic cells cannot be interpreted as yielding information about the metastatic subpopulations per se. If, for example, the metastatic cell subpopulations are in the minority, analysis of the entire cell population may provide little or no insight into the properties that are unique to metastatic cells since the probability is high that these would be obscured or lost in the "background noise" imposed by the majority fraction of non-metastatic cells. Consequently, characterization of the properties of metastatic tumor cell sub- populations requires either that such subpopulations comprise the overwhelming majority in a heterogeneous cell population or that individual clonal subpopulations be isolated to generate homogenous cell preparations for comparison with non-metastatic clones isolated

56

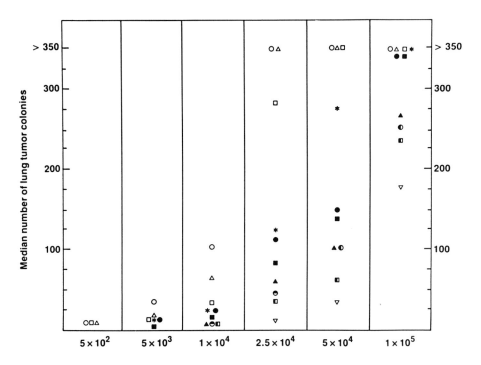

FIGURE 1. The Effect of Tumor Cell Dose on the Lung Colonizing Capacity of Ten B16 Melanoma Clones. Clones were injected i.v. into C57BL/6 mice at the indicated cell doses in 0.2 ml (38) and the number of lung colonies measured at autopsy 21 da later. The values for each clone are median values derived from ten mice.

from the same parent cell population. In the former strategy, selection pressures are imposed to favor the metastatic subpopulations with resulting enrichment of their contribution to the total cell population (for review see 1). Conversely, negative selection pressures can be applied to reduce selectively the fraction of metastatic cells (for references see 1). It is important to emphasize, however, that tumor cell preparations subjected to selection pressures to enrich or deplete specific subpopulations of cells are still heterogeneous and that non-metastatic subpopulations of cells are still likely to be present.

Also, the sublines of cells selected by such methods are still heterogeneous and contain a variable and unknown number of subpopulations. Examination of the literature indicates that some confusion exists on this point. For example, the B16F1 and B16F10 sublines of the B16 melanoma isolated by Fidler (39) are used by a large number of research laboratories and it is not uncommon to see publications in which such lines are described erroneously as being "clones." These sublines, or any subline selected by enrichment methods, are not clones. They are developed by exposing heterogeneous, polyclonal cell lines to a selection pressure(s) that favors the survival of cellular subpopulations with the greatest metastatic potential. Even though such subpopulations may be in the majority, heterogeneity is still present.

A more satisfactory approach for addressing the problems posed by tumor cell heterogeneity involves cloning of tumor cells from a heterogeneous cell population to generate a panel of clonal cell populations whose phenotypes can be compared (for review see 1). In this strategy the aim is to isolate a sufficient number of clones so that clones with the following properties can be compared to identify properties that are invariant features of metastatic clones but are absent from non-metastatic clones:

tumorigenic, non-invasive, non-metastatic clones ($T^+I^-M^-$)

versus

tumorigenic, invasive, non-metastatic clones ($T^+I^+M^-$)

versus

tumorigenic, invasive, metastatic clones ($T^+I^+M^+$).

Although this approach is conceptually straightforward, it is technically demanding and labor-intensive because of the need to isolate and examine a large number of clones from the same parent tumor cell population. Furthermore, as discussed in detail elswhere (1), reliable correlation of a specific phenotypic trait assayed in vitro with the metastatic properties of cells in vivo will require additional experiments to confirm that the same trait is expressed by the metastatic cells in vivo and in cells recovered from metastatic lesions and cultivated in vitro (1).

In comparing the phenotypes of metastatic and non-metastatic clones isolated from the same parent cell population it is necessary, however, to confirm that the metastatic properties of the clones are stable. This imposes the need for repeated subcloning at intervals of only a few weeks to examine whether the metastatic behavior of the original clone has been maintained or if variant subclones with signficiantly different metastatic properties from the original clones have emerged to create a heterogeneous cell population. Studies on several animal tumors have revealed that the metastatic properties of certain clones may be highly unstable and that subclones with altered metastatic behavior emerge rapidly, generating a heterogeneous cell population (1,9,38,40-42).

If clones from the tumor being studied undergo rapid phenotypic "drift", frequent subcloning will be needed to ensure that the clonal populations being compared are indeed homogeneous and that repeated experimental analyses are made using replicate subclones that display identical metastatic properties to the original clones. It is also informative to obtain data on the rate of phenotypic "drift." If no significant changes in metastatic behavior or other phenotypic properties occur or occur only over a period of several months rather than weeks, in vitro analyses of specific tumor cell properties can be undertaken with the reasonable belief that the metastatic properties of the cells being assayed are still comparable to samples of the same clones assayed a few weeks before or after the experiment. If, however, the rate of drift in metastatic properties is rapid, occurring within just a few weeks due to the rapid emergence of variant subclones with altered metastatic abilities, the experimental requirements for correlating cell properties assayed in vitro with metastatic behavior in vivo become far more stringent. For clones that show rapid drift in metastatic behavior (or other properties) the correlation of a specific cell property assayed in vitro with metastatic capacity in vivo will require that the in vitro and in vivo assays be conducted synchronously using replicate cell preparations and assayed at the shortest interval after cloning consistent with generating a sufficient number of cells for the assays (43). Unless such precautions are taken, a property assayed in vitro today cannot be correlated with the metastatic behavior of the same "clone" measured a few weeks earlier or later because rapid formation of variant subclones will render the "clone" heterogeneous. Consequently, for tumor cell clones that exhibit unstable metastatic properties during serial passage these more demanding synchronous assay protocols should be adopted routinely, unless experimental conditions can be developed to eliminate the drift in metastatic properties (1).

D.   The Use of Metastatic Tumor Models in the Identification and
     Preclinical Testing of New Antineoplastic Agents

     With the exception of primary tumors arising in anatomic sites in
which surgical excision of the tumor is extremely difficult, or at
sites in which early expansive tumor growth can quickly compromise
vital functions such as in the brain, the treatment of primary tumors,
usually by surgical removal, is successful. The major problem in
clinical oncology is metastatic disease. It is thus perhaps surprising
that until recently metastatic tumor models have not found extensive
use in the screening programs employed by companies or government
cancer agencies in searching for new antineoplastic agents. These
programs have relied primarily on a series of tests in which large
numbers of agents with diverse chemical properties are screened
initially for in vitro cytotoxic activity against one or more tumor
cell lines, typically of lymphoid origin. Then, if positive, they are
tested for in vivo activity against a panel of animal and human cell
lines growing as localized implants either in the peritoneal cavity,
s.c. or i.m. In most of the in vivo testing protocols, agents are
assayed only for their activity against a minimal tumor burden to allow
detection of positive cytotoxic activity. The issue of tumor burden is
less important in our opinion than the use of localized tumor implants
which cannot provide information as to whether the agent would have any
efficacy in treating disseminated disease in more than one target
organ. Our concern about the apparent reluctance to adopt metastatic
models in preclinical testing of putative antitumor agents is not based
on any belief that the responses of tumor cells in metastases will
differ in any significant manner from cells in the original implant
from which the metastases arose. Until metastatic proficiency can be
shown to correlate with an entirely different pattern of responses to
various therapeutic agents than that displayed by non-metastatic tumor
cells, initial testing of agents for activity against localized tumors
implanted i.p., s.c. or i.m. is acceptable for providing information on
the cytotoxic potential of a particular agent. However, such tests
will not determine whether the pharmacodisposition and pharmacokinetics
of the agent will be appropriate for the eradication of metastatic
disease in a variety of organs with differing vascularization patterns
and blood flow.

     Conceptually, the case for more widespread adoption of metastatic
tumor models in the screening and preclinical testing of new antineoplastic agents is persuasive. Technically, however, the choice of
models is more difficult and no satisfactory answer can be given. This
dilemma is created by a number of ambiguities.

     The first concerns the long debated question of how far the
responses of cells from rodent and other animal tumors mirror the
responses of human tumor cells of similar histologic origins to the
same agents. The logical corollary of this question is whether the
search for new antitumor agents should be conducted exclusively with
human tumor cells as targets. These questions are not new. They were
influential in the decision to include human tumor xenografts as part
of the test tumor panel for the evaluation of putative anticancer

agents used by the National Cancer Institute in the USA and by several pharmaceutical companies. Similarly, the recent introduction of the human tumor stem cell assay (HTSCA) is based on the rationale that the responses of freshly isolated human tumor cells to both current and new antineoplastic agents might more accurately predict the clinical responses of human tumors of similar histologic origins than cells from rodent tumors subjected to unknown selection pressures during serial passage over several months or years (44). Whether the HTSCA will be of greater predictive value than animal tumor cells in detecting agents with greater efficacy in the clinic remains to be established. Claims that this assay can be used in an analogous fashion to the use of antibiotic sensitivity testing in the design of clinical antimicrobial therapy (i.e., to identify the optimal therapeutic regimen for individual patients based on the responses of cells isolated from their own tumor to a panel of antitumor agents) cannot be justified. However, as in any emerging technique it would be unfortunate if excessive claims made by a few were to compromise a thorough and objective evaluation of the merits of this assay.

Efforts to culture human tumor cells, especially of epithelial origin, are still in their infancy. Isolation of cells from only one region of solid neoplasms that are known to exhibit zonal hetero-geneity (45), coupled with the low cloning efficiency of most human tumor cells (for review see 16-19), dictates that a substantial selection pressure has been imposed in obtaining any human tumor cell population and obvious ambiguities will exist as to how far the properties of such cells are representative of the complete spectrum of cells in the tumor. Even with further technical advances to enhance tumor cell recovery uncertainties will remain. We cannot, however, allow these to paralyze us from taking every opportunity to increase the similarities between the model systems and the human disease. The ability to isolate tumor cells from newly excised human tumors with reasonable success, together with continued progress in the development of methods for evaluating their metastatic properties in nude mice, are major technical advances that must be adopted increasingly in research on the mechanisms of metastasis and in the search for new agents for the therapy of metastatic disease. The next step in the evolution of these approaches must be to begin the slow and tedious task of examining a sufficiently large number of tumor cells recovered from newly excised tumors of comparable histology in different patients so that the phenotypic markers displayed by these cells can be cataloged and used to monitor the extent and rate of phenotypic change that accompanies their serial propagation in vitro and in vivo, and, equally important, the relationship of these changes to alterations in responsiveness to various classes of antineoplastic agents. For example, many established human tumor cell lines are highly susceptible to a broad range of cytotoxic drugs in vitro yet the same drugs frequently have little efficacy in the clinic. Notwithstanding the many complicating factors that can limit drug activity in vivo, we cannot reliably exclude the possibility that these cell lines have undergone significant biochemical alterations as a consequence of prolonged cultivation in vitro and thus may share few biochemical targets with the cells in a patient's tumor. In contrast, freshly isolated and/or low passage tumor cells might retain the "biochemical profile" of tumor cells growing in a patient and thus offer a more relevant test system for detecting new antitumor agents. Once again, there are no simple answers. However, the question is amenable to experimental analysis, even if the scale of the exercise is daunting.

The preceding remarks lead logically to the question of whether the search for improved anticancer agents might be more successful if the emphasis was shifted to seeking agents to treat specific neoplasms using screening methods in which antitumor activity is determined against the specific type of neoplastic cell of therapeutic interest. This contrasts with the current, albeit optimistic, strategy of attempting to develop agents that will be effective against a range of histologically diverse neoplasms. Unfortunately, the experience of the last thirty years suggests that this type of "panaceamycin" will not be easily found. With the exception of hormone analogs for therapy of endocrine-sensitive tumors, the dominant strategy in most cancer drug screening programs has been first to identify agents that display significant cytotoxic activity against a panel of transplantable tumor cell lines of diverse histologic origins and then to proceed to the clinic to evaluate their activity against a similarly diverse array of human neoplsms. For most agents entering the clinic there is no a priori reason to believe on the basis of their mode of action or their pharmacodisposition that they would be effective against the particular tumor(s) selected for study. It could also be argued, however, there is no reason to assume that they would not be active, since they were selected on the basis of their general cytotoxic activity against a range of tumors and might thus be similarly active against a broad spectrum of human tumors. Unfortunately, this has rarely been the case.

In short, the lack of effective therapy for many of the most important human solid tumors, together with the understandable desire of both oncologists and patients to seek every opportunity to treat an otherwise intractable disease, means that most putative anticancer agents entering clinical trials will be deployed initially against many different types of tumors in the hope that one or more tumor classes will show sufficient clinical responses to warrant the lengthy and expensive task of developing the drug for final regulatory approval.

By using preclinical tests to select antineoplastic agents that display a "broad spectrum" of cytotoxic activity against tumor cell lines of diverse origins is it possible that we are inadvertently selecting for agents that lack the ability to act against biochemical targets that may be more prominent in tumor cell populations in situ and which would be expected to vary significantly in tumor cells arising in different tissues? The same risk may also apply in over-looking agents that might be effective in circumventing the cellular mechanisms that account for intrinsic refractoriness to certain agents and/or acquired resistance to various antitumor agents. For example, the biochemical pathways responsible for refractoriness are presumably closely linked to the innate properties of the cell type in which the tumor arose. In common with other phenotypic traits unique to specific

62

cell lineages and/or particular states of cell differentiation, such properties might be lost relatively rapidly when the cells are removed from the tumors and grown as serially propagated cell lines in vitro or in vivo. For example, human colorectal adenocarcinomas are refractory to the cytotoxic action of a large number of the chemotherapeutic agents presently available yet most established human colon cell lines resemble cell lines from other tumors in being susceptible to these agents both in vitro and when implanted into nude mice. Could this discrepancy reflect the fact that the properties of neoplastic colon epithelial cells that render them refractory to drug action in situ are readily lost in culture?

The problem of acquired resistance is perhaps easier to address. A large number of tumor cells displaying enhanced resistance to destruction by antineoplastic drugs, hyperthermia and various humoral- and cell-mediated immune reactions have now been described and many of these phenotypes can be induced in cultured cell populations without undue difficulty. Resistant tumor cell populations of this kind merit consideration for greater use in screening for potential anticancer agents that can circumvent the resistant phenotype(s). This assumes, however, that the biochemical lesion(s) responsible for tumor cell resistance in vitro and in vivo is identical.

We believe that greater attention must be given to the biological uniqueness of histologically distinct classes of neoplasms and the cellular and molecular properties peculiar to the cell types in which different tumors arise. Certain properties will be unique to human tumor cells and can thus never be mimicked by animal tumor models. However, there may be a substantial number of tumor cell properties that are shared by human and animal tumors arising in cells with similar embryologic origins residing in organs with comparable anatomy and physiology. For example, there may be a greater relationship between the biochemical pathways that regulate the responses of both normal and neoplastic colonic epithelial cells in mouse and man than between human colon adenocarcinoma cells and human or animal tumor cells derived from a completely different cell lineage. From this perspective, the issue of species variation is less important than the need to screen potential antineoplastic agents for activity against test cell populations that display a demonstrably close phenotypic relationship to tumor cells from the specific class of tumor for which therapy is being sought. The feasibility of this approach will depend, however, on the ability to demonstrate such relatedness. As with many of the other questions posed in this chapter, the ability to define the questions often exceeds our capacity to convert them to technical realities. For the major human neoplasms there is presently little information available about the extent and nature of the phenotypic changes that occur in tumor cells relative to their normal counterparts. We are similarly ignorant of the nature and extent of phenotypic modulation that may occur in tumor cells when isolated and passaged for months or years in vitro and/or in vivo.

A long list of potential factors can be compiled to explain why cells removed from their microenvironment in vivo will undergo phenotypic alterations. Factors influential in inducing these alterations include, but are not limited to: growth in two-dimensional monolayer culture versus organized histotypic assemblies; loss of cell-to-cell communication; disruption of epithelial-mesenchymal cellular interactions; elimination of the complex patterns of autocrine, paracrine and endocrine regulation; and selection for cells with rapid and/or unlimited proliferative capacities. The inevitable outcome of such perturbations is that cell populations that are selected during serial cultivation in vitro or in vivo may represent subpopulations of cells that exhibit what might be called a "basal phenotype" for the original cell type from which they are derived. The "basal phenotype" represents the assembly of constitutive biochemical functions that are compatible with sustained proliferation and survival in an aberrant microenvironment devoid of the multiple inductive stimuli needed to maintain the more complex "differentiated phenotype" of the parent cell in its original location in vivo. The "basal phenotype" may include continued expression of a number of phenotypic traits unique to the cell of origin including such traits as tumorigenicity and metastatic ability. However, other phenotypic markers, including some which may be of great importance in determining cellular refractoriness or the susceptibility of tumor cells to therapy, may be lost at variable rates following removal from the in vivo microenvironment.

The technical challenge involved in examining these questions is formidable. A fundamental prerequisite will be to develop a suitably large panel of reliable phenotypic markers which can be used to compare human and animal tumor cells isolated from tumors of comparable histologic origins at similar stages in their progression in order to monitor possible changes in the expression of specific markers in tumor cells in vivo and in vitro. Since cultured tumor cell populations will continue to be used as a major research tool for the foreseeable future it will be equally important to establish the nature and the rate of phenotypic "drift" in specific markers occurring in tumor cells by comparing tumor cells in vivo, or as freshly isolated primary cultures, with low passage secondary cell strains and with established cell lines subjected to prolonged passage in vitro and in vivo. Only by undertaking this tedious and logistically demanding comparison can we gain insight into the extent of phenotypic modulation that may occur in the established cell lines that are used routinely in studying both the mechanism of metastasis and in screening new antineoplastic agents. Without this information we will have little guarantee that current experimental strategies are focusing on tumor cell properties that are relevant to the final goal of developing new and improved therapies for the eradication of metastatic disease.

If the answers to the questions posed in this chapter were easy they would have been identified long ago. The difficulties of discarding familiar and established experimental systems and retooling to test new models and paradigms that reflect advances in our understanding of tumor cell biology, immunology, genetics and the pathogenesis of different cancers will not be easy to overcome. The cost

64

in time, effort and resources will make many reluctant even to
contemplate the need for change, yet alone implement it. Also,
short-term cycles of grant funding, the pressure to maintain active
publication records, bureaucratic inertia, and for industrial
laboratories the need to continue to generate new drugs add further
barriers to shifts in experimental strategy. For those intrepid enough
to begin to discard some, or all, of the traditional approaches success
will not be rapid. Worse still, there is no guarantee that adoption of
some of the approaches described in this article will be any more
successful than the methods they replace.

In our opinion, however, the choice is clear. The search for new
therapeutic agents to combat metastatic disease must either continue
using models that have not, and probably cannot, yield the desired
outcome or we must now embark upon the slow process of developing new
models that attempt to integrate newer knowledge on the cellular and
molecular biology and the pathology of the tumor(s) of interest. A
decision to maintain the status quo, particularly in the search for
chemotherapeutic agents that act in the same way as existing agents and
which are identified and evaluated using non-metastatic tumor models,
carries the risk that in 10 to 20 years our success in treating the
major solid tumors of man will be no greater than today.

ACKNOWLEDGMENT

We are most grateful to our colleagues Drs. D. Trainer, T.
Koestler and S. Corwin for their comments and for contributing to the
data discussed in section B.

REFERENCES

1.   Poste G: Experimental systems for analysis of the malignant
     phenotype. Cancer Metastasis Rev. 1:141-199, 1982.
2.   Hewitt HB: Counterpoint: Animal tumor models and their relevance
     to human tumor immunology. J. Biol. Response Modifiers 1:107-119,
     1982.
3.   Herberman RB: Counterpoint: Animal tumor models and their
     relevance to human tumor immunology. J. Biol. Response Modifiers
     2:39-46, 1983.
4.   Donelli MG, D'Incalci M, Garattini S: Pharmacokinetic studies of
     anticancer drugs in tumor-bearing animals. Cancer Treat. Rep.
     68:381-400, 1984.
5.   Staquet MJ, Byar DP, Green SB, Rozencweig M: Clinical
     predictivity of transplantable tumor systems in the selection of
     new drugs for solid tumors: Rationale for a three-stage strategy.
     Cancer Treat. Rep. 67:753-765, 1983.
6.   Cancer Treatment Reports. 25th Anniversary Issue 68:1-356,
     1984.
7.   Goldin A: Animal models for cancer chemotherapy. In: Muggia FM
     (ed.) Cancer Chemotherapy. Martinus Nijhoff, The Hague, pp.
     65-102, 1983.

8. Poste G, Fidler IJ: The pathogenesis of cancer metastasis. Nature (London) 283:139-146, 1980.
9. Heppner GH: Tumor heterogeneity. Cancer Res. 44:2259-2265, 1984.
10. Poste G, Kirsh R: Site-specific drug delivery. Biotechnology 1:869-878, 1983.
11. Poste G, Nicolson GL: Experimental systems for analysis of the surface properties of metastatic tumor cells. In: Nowotny A (ed.) Biomembranes. Plenum Press, New York, Vol. 11, pp. 341-364, 1983.
12. Nicolson GL, Poste G: Tumor implantation and invasion at metastatic sites. Int. Rev. Exp. Pathol. 25:77-181, 1983.
13. Hanna N: Role of natural killer cells in the control of cancer metastasis. Cancer Metastasis Rev. 1:45-64, 1982.
14. Kerbel RS, Man MS, Dexter D: A model of human cancer metastasis: Extensive spontaneous and artificial metastasis of a human pigmented melanoma and derived variant sublines in nude mice. J. Natl. Cancer Inst. 72:93-108, 1984.
15. Kozlowski JM, Fidler IJ, Campbell D, Xu Z-L, Kaighn ME, Hart IR: Metastatic behavior of human tumor cell lines grown in the nude mouse. Cancer Res. 44:3522-3529, 1984.
16. Brattain MG: Short-term culture of cells from human solid tumors in semisolid medium. In: Cell Separation: Methods and Selected Applications. Vol. 2, pp. 235-246, 1983.
17. Agre P, Williams TE: The human tumor cloning assay in cancer drug development. A review. Invest. New Drugs 2:33-45, 1984.
18. Bertelsen CA, Sondak VK, Mann BD, Korn EL, Kern DH: Chemo-sensitivity testing of human solid tumors. A review of 1582 assays with 258 clinical correlations. Cancer 53:1240-1245, 1984.
19. Bradley EC, Issell BF, Hellman R: The human tumor colony-forming chemosensitivity assay: A biological and clinical review. Invest. New Drugs 2:59-70, 1984.
20. Sordat B: Editor. Immune-Deficient Animals. Karger, Basel, 1984.
21. New horizons for tissue culture in cancer research. J. Natl. Cancer Inst. 53:1429-1519, 1974.
22. Poste G, Greig R: Defining tumor cell properties that correlate with tumorigenicity and metastasis. Biochim. Biophys. Acta. In press.
23. Ilgren EB, Griner L, Benirschke K, Pang LSC: A comparative study of pulmonary tumors from the San Diego zoological gardens and the Tumor Reference Collection, Imperial Cancer Research Fund, London. Pathol. Ann. (Part 2) 17:331-351, 1982.
24. Sher SP: Tumors in control hamsters, rats, and mice: Literature tabulation. CRC Crit. Rev. Toxicol. 6:49-79, 1982.
25. Ward JM: Background data and variations in tumor rates of control rats and mice. In: Homburger F (ed.) Skin Painting Techniques and in Vivo Carcinogenesis Bioassays. S. Karger, Vol. 26, pp. 241-258, 1983.
26. Crotchin E: Veterinary oncology: A survey. J. Pathol. 142:101-127, 1984.

27. Stackpole CW: Distinct lung-colonizing and lung-metastasizing cell populations in B16 mouse melanoma. Nature (London) 289:798-800, 1981.

28. Weiss L, Mayhew E, Rapp DG, Holmes JC: Metastatic inefficiency in mice bearing B16 melanomas. Br. J. Cancer 45:44-53, 1982.

29. Neal GE, Manson MM, Legg RF: The production of carcinomas in vivo by the intravenous or subcutaneous injection of a hepatocellular tumour cell line. Cancer Lett. 19:325-332, 1983.

30. Gorelik G, Segal S, Shapiro J, Katzav S, Ron Y, Feldman M: Interactions between the local tumor and its metastases. Cancer Metastasis Rev. 1:83-94, 1982.

31. Price JE, Carr D, Jones LD, Messer P, Tarin D: Experimental analysis of factors affecting metastatic spread using naturally occurring tumours. Invasion Metastasis 2:77-112, 1982.

32. Unemori EN, Ways N, Pitelka DR: Metastasis of murine mammary tumour lines from the mammary gland and ectopic sites. Br. J. Cancer 49:603-614, 1984.

33. Juacaba SF, Jones LD, Tarin D: Organ preferences in metastatic colony formation by spontaneous mammary carcinomas after intra-arterial inoculation. Invasion Metastasis 3:208-220, 1983.

34. Potter KM, Juacaba SF, Price JE, Tarin D: Observations on organ distribution of fluorescein-labelled tumour cells released intra-vascularly. Invasion Metastasis 3:221-223, 1983.

35. Vaage J: Transplantation procedures in tumor immunology. Meth. Cancer Res. 8:33-58, 1973.

36. Auerbach R, Auerbach W: Regional differences in the growth of normal and neoplastic cells. Science 215:127-134, 1982.

37. Vaage J: Relationship between tumor growth characteristics and preferential sites of growth. J. Natl. Cancer Inst. 72:1199-1203, 1984.

38. Poste G, Greig R: The experimental and clinical implications of cellular heterogeneity in malignant tumors. J. Cancer Res. Clin. Oncol. 106:159-170, 1983.

39. Fidler IJ: Selection of successive tumor lines for metastasis. Nature (London) New Biol. 242:148-149, 1973.

40. Poste G, Tzeng J, Doll J, Greig R, Rieman D, Ziedman I: Evolution of tumor cell heterogeneity during progressive growth of individual lung metastases. Proc. Natl. Acad. Sci. USA 79:6574-6578, 1982.

41. Poste G, Doll J, Brown AG, Tzeng J, Ziedman I: Comparison of the metastatic properties of B16 melanoma clones isolated from cultured cell lines, subcutaneous tumors and individual lung metastases. Cancer Res. 42:2770-2778, 1982.

42. Poste G, Doll J, Fidler IJ: Interactions among clonal sub-populations affect the stability of the metastatic phenotype in polyclonal populations of B16 melanoma cells. Proc. Natl. Acad. Sci. USA 78:6226-6230, 1981.

43. Greig RG, Caltabiano L, Reid R, Jr., Feild J, Poste G: Hetero-geneity of protein phosphorylation in metastatic variants of B16 melanoma. Cancer Res. 43:6057-6065, 1983.

44. Salmon SE: Human tumor colony assay and chemosensitivity testing. Cancer Treat. Rep. 68:117-126, 1984.

45. Fidler IJ, Hart IR: Biological and experimental consequences of the zonal composition of solid tumors. Cancer Res. 41:3266-3267, 1981.
46. Lagarde AE, Donaghue TP, Dennis JW, Kerbel RS: Genotypic and phenotypic evolution of a murine tumor during its progression in vivo towards metastases. J. Natl. Cancer Inst. 71:183-191, 1983.
47. Van Lamsweerde A-L, Henry N, Vaes G: Metastatic heterogeneity of cells from Lewis lung carcinoma. Cancer Res. 43:5314-5320, 1983.
48. Reading CL, Brunson KW, Torrianni M, Nicolson GL: Malignancies of metastatic murine lymphosarcoma cell lines and clones correlate with decreased cell surface display of RNA tumor virus envelope glycoprotein gp70. Proc. Natl. Acad. Sci. USA 77:5943-5947, 1980.
49. Talmadge JE, Fidler IJ: Enhanced metastatic potential of tumor cells harvested from spontaneous metastases of heterogeneous murine tumors. J. Natl. Cancer Inst. 69:975-980, 1982.
50. Katzav S, DeBaetselier P, Tartakovsky B, Feldman M, Shraga S: Alterations in major histocompatibility complex phenotypes of mouse cloned T10 sarcoma cells: Association with shifts from nonmetastatic to metastatic cells. J. Natl. Cancer Inst. 71:317-324, 1983.
51. Giavazzi R, Alessandri G, Spreafico F, Garattini S, Mantovani A: Characterization of tumor lines derived from spontaneous metastases of a transplanted murine fibrosarcoma. Br. J. Cancer 42:462-472, 1980.
52. Weiss L, Mayhew E, Glaves D, Holmes JC: Metastatic inefficiency in mice bearing B16 melanomas. Br. J. Cancer 45:44-53, 1982.
53. Miller F, Miller B, Heppner G: Characterization of metastatic heterogeneity among subpopulations of a single mouse mammary tumor: Heterogeneity in phenotypic stability. Invasion Metastasis 3:22-31, 1983.
54. Yamamura Y, Fischer B, Harnaha J, Proctor J: Heterogeneity of murine mammary adenocarcinoma cell subpopulations. In vitro and in vivo resistance to macrophage cytotoxicity and its association with metastatic capacity. Int. J. Cancer 33:67-72, 1984.
55. Price JE, Carr D, Jones LD, Messer P, Tarin D: Experimental analysis of factors affecting metastatic spread using naturally occurring tumors. Invasion Metastasis 2:77-112, 1982.
56. Tsuro T, Yamori T, Naganuma K, Tsukagoshi S, Sakurai Y: Characterization of metastatic clones derived from a metastatic variant of mouse colon adenocarcinoma 26. Cancer Res. 43:5437-5442, 1983.
57. Kripke ML, Gruys E, Fidler IJ: Metastatic heterogeneity of cells from an ultraviolet light-induced murine fibrosarcoma of recent origin. Cancer Res. 38:2962-2967, 1978.
58. Trainer D, Corwin SP, Kline T: Smith Kline and French Laboratories. (Unpublished observations).
59. Sweeney F, Pot-Deprun J, Poupon M, Chouroulinkor I: Heterogeneity of the growth and metastatic behavior of cloned cell lines derived from a primary rhabdomyosarcoma. Cancer Res. 42:3776-3782, 1982.

68

60. Welch D, Neri A, Nicolson G: Comparison of spontaneous and
    experimetnal metastasis using rat 13762 mammary adenocarcinoma
    metastatic cell clones. Invasion Metastasis 3:65–80, 1983.
61. Matzku S, Komitowski D, Mildenberger M, Zoller M: Characterization
    of BSp73, a spontaneous rat tumor and its selected variants
    showing different metastasizing capacities. Invasion Metastasis
    3:109–123, 1983.

CHAPTER 5. PROBLEMS POSED FOR CANCER TREATMENT BY TUMOR CELL HETEROGENEITY

GLORIA H. HEPPNER

I. INTRODUCTION

The editors have not done me a favor by assigning such a dismal title to this article, one which focuses on the problems inherent in intra-tumor variability, although I suppose it would have been worse to be asked to discuss "Solutions Offered for Cancer Treatment by Tumor Cell Heterogeneity." Indeed, the presence of multiple tumor cell subpopulations within single cancers poses major problems to those who wish to understand and to treat neoplastic diseases. It can be argued that tumor cell heterogeneity, and the consequent "progression," over time, of the characteristics of any given cancer are major reasons for the treatment failure and ultimate recurrence so commonly experienced in the clinic. The purposes of this article are to outline the basic facts of tumor cell heterogeneity, to show how these facts impact on treatment selection and strategy, and to indicate various approaches to overcome the problems that result.

II. TUMOR HETEROGENEITY

The first problem is the definition of the problem. "Tumor heterogeneity" is a vague term. It can refer to differences between cancers of different hosts. Since both cancer and host factors can contribute to this variability, it is virtually impossible to analyze the basis for any particular differences without further definition. I will use the term "tumor heterogeneity" to refer only to variability within a single cancer, arising within a single host. It is still necessary, however, to further restrict the definition. Tumors can be heterogeneous in many ways. They are three-dimensional structures, and the cancer cell components are not distributed uniformly in regard to the host components, inflammatory infiltrates, supporting tissue, vasculature, etc. Tumors contain areas of necrosis and have discontinuities in pH, oxygen, nutrient and other gradients. These sources of variation, which I have elsewhere called "secular" heterogeneity (1), can affect both cancer cell replication and sensitivity to therapy.

In addition, but related, to the above sources of variation, are the kinetics of the cancer cells themselves. Not all cancer cells are cycling; some have ceased to be reproductively viable, others have temporarily dropped out of cycle and can rejoin the replication pool should circumstances warrant. The cells that are replicating are distributed throughout the cell cycle. This reproductive heterogeneity also impacts on response to therapy (2).

The definition of tumor heterogeneity that will be used throughout the rest of this article is: the simultaneous existence of multiple tumor cell subpopulations within the same cancer (and the extensions of that cancer). There are several points that need emphasis:

1. Strictly speaking, the existence of tumor heterogeneity is predicated on the demonstration of distinct, clonal populations that "breed true." The clones may be "unstable," that is give rise to new variants at high frequency (3-5), "stable," that is produce new variants at expected frequencies (5,6), or be somewhere in between (7). What seems certain is that new variants arise over the course of time, so that tumor heterogeneity is a dynamic process.

2. The generation of clonal subpopulations can be due to either genetic or epigenetic mechanisms.

3. Clonal subpopulations are themselves subject to both secular and cell cycle heterogeneity.

4. The relative importance to tumor behavior of clonal heterogeneity vs. cell cycle vs. secular heterogeneity is unknown for any phenotype, including sensitivity to therapy. A major difficulty is a lack of experimental methodology to quantitate, and thus compare, true variability, as opposed to statistical fluctuation.

III. INTRA-TUMOR HETEROGENEITY IN DRUG SENSITIVITY

Numerous investigators, starting with Law in 1952 (8), have demonstrated tumor cell heterogeneity in sensitivity to anti-neoplastic agents (see also Chapter 6). Tumor subpopulations from a wide variety of animal and human cancers have been shown to differ in sensitivity to chemotherapeutic drugs of virtually all the major classes used clinically, as well as to radiotherapy, hyperthermia, and immunotherapy (9). Sensitivity differences have been reported between subpopulations of primary cancers and their metastases (9,10) and among metastases from the same cancer (11). This diversity is demonstrable in subpopulations isolated prior to any treatment.

Table 1 presents a summary of results from my laboratory which are typical of those reported by others. We have used a series of subpopulations from a strain BALB/cfC3H mouse mammary cancer for our work (10,12). Subpopulations 66, 168 and 68H were isolated from the autochthonous tumor and line 410 was derived from a metastatic nodule growing in the lung of a syngeneic mouse transplanted, subcutaneously, with the tenth serial in vivo passage of the parent tumor. Line 410.4 is a variant of 410. It is clear that the subpopulations are differentially sensitive to the various drugs used. These subpopulations also differ in other properties, such as growth rate, immunogenicity and ability to metastasize, but there is no apparent correlation between these behavioral differences and sensitivity to chemotherapy.

In general, the data in Table 1 were obtained with a standardized regimen for each drug. Table 2 summarizes an experiment in which the response of two mammary tumor subpopulations was compared using two different times of administration of cyclophosphamide. In the first regimen, in which treatment was begun shortly after injection of the tumor cells, subpopulation 168 tumors were markedly more responsive than were 410 tumors. In the second regimen, in which tumor treatment was not initiated until palpable tumors were present, line 410 tumors responded at least as well, if not better, than did 168 tumors to the same dose of drug. These results illustrate that heterogeneity in drug response of different tumor subpopulations is not absolute, but depends upon the circumstances of administration. Different subpopulations from the same tumor differ in optimal regimens.

An important consideration in understanding the problems posed by tumor heterogeneity is the spatial relationship of tumor subpopulations in situ. One would imagine that variant clones would not be distributed randomly throughout a solid tumor, but would occupy more-or-less discrete foci or zones. Several investigators have demonstrated this to be so (13,14). Hakansson and Trope (15) showed that tumor cells from different quarters of the same tumor could be significantly different in sensitivity to drugs such as melphalan and cytosine arabinoside. These observations suggest that protocols to assess drug sensitivity of heterogeneous tumors by in vitro or nude mouse assays should contain methods to avoid the sampling errors inherent in the zonal distribution of tumor subpopulations. We are developing an in vitro assay in which pieces taken from different parts of a tumor are tested independently and a "heterogeneity index" is constructed that considers both the spectrum and the distribution of sensitivity to drugs (16). In this assay, pieces of tumor are embedded in a collagen gel matrix and bathed in culture medium with or without drug. (The collagen gel culture system is used because it optimizes growth of breast cells, which is the type of cancer we are using to validate the assay. Other tumor types might require different culture systems.) The tumor sample grows out in a three-dimensional array that is reminiscent of the in vivo tissue architecture. Drug effects are expressed as an inhibition of this growth, as measured by planimetry. By using tumor pieces rather than suspensions of tumor cells, we are able to maintain cell interactions that may be important in sensitivity to drugs (see below), as well as to estimate the heterogeneity of response to any given agent.

Table 1. Relative Sensitivity in vivo of Mammary Tumor Subpopulations to Anti-Cancer Drugs.

Subpopulations	Methotrexate	5-Fluorouracil	Cyclophosphamide	Melphalan	Adriamycin	PDl11815*
66	n.t.†	n.t.	n.t.	+	-	n.t.
168	-	-	++	+++	-	++
68H	+	+	+++	n.t.	n.t.	n.t.
410	-	-	-‡	n.t.	++	-
410.4	-	-	-	-	-	n.t.

*PDl11815 is an experimental anthrapyrazole (31)

†Not tested

‡See Table 2

Table 2. Effect of Regimen on Response of Mammary Tumor Subpopulation to Cyclophosphamide.

| | | Growth Rate Control/Growth Rate Treated[*] | |
Subpopulation	% "Cure"[†]	Regimen 1[‡]	Regimen 2[◊]
168	50	76/1 = 76	56/18 = 3.1
419	0	71/61 = 1.2	43/8 = 5.4

[*]Tumors were measured twice weekly with calipers. Growth rate = mm^2/wk.

[†]"Cure" is defined as inhibition of the development of a palpable tumor. There were 10 mice in the 168 and 9 in the 410 groups. 100% of control mice developed tumors in both groups.

[‡]Cyclophosphamide (100 mg/kg) was injected, intraperitoneally, once a week for 4 wk, beginning 2 da after subcutaneous tumor cell injection.

[◊]Same regimen as above, except treatment was withheld until the tumors were palpable.

IV. TUMOR HETEROGENEITY AND CHANGE

As mentioned previously, isolated tumor subpopulations and clones range in the degree to which they are stable phenotypically. Different phenotypes also are differentially stable; alterations in metastatic behavior are relatively common, whereas significant gain or loss of drug sensitivity is less often observed in the absence of any selection pressure (17). Regardless of the rate of change, however, change does occur. This is true whether or not selective agents (such as drugs) are present and can happen at any time during cancer growth and development. Although chance favors the homogeneity of smaller, earlier tumors (18), both theoretical and practical considerations dictate that each cancer be looked upon as heterogeneous and capable of continuous change. To the therapist, then, cancers are "moving targets," heterogeneous in time as well as space. The variability of cancer cell populations, and the random production of new variants, are the mechanisms underlying the concept of tumor progression, defined by Foulds (19) as the "acquisition of permanent, irreversible qualitative changes of one or more characteristics in a neoplasm." A pertinent example is the loss of responsiveness to a given drug over the course of treatment.

Foulds developed a number of "rules" that characterize progression. Rule 2 states that "progression occurs independently in different characters in the same tumor," in other words, that different cancer cell phenotypes, such as drug sensitivity and ability to metastasize, are independent variables. This rule has several practical consequences. The therapeutic sensitivities of metastases, may, or may not, be similar to the sensitivities of cells in the primary cancer. Thus, selection of drug treatment for metastatic disease on the basis of the assessment of the sensitivity of cells from the primary tumor may be futile. On the other hand, the suggestion that one should only attempt to use drugs with activity against metastatic cells ignores the fact that metastases are also heterogeneous, both within single foci (17), and, as has been mentioned, between different foci (11).

Application of probability theory to considerations of the clinical problems of cancer cell variability and change have led Goldie and colleagues to suggest a number of principles in the administration of chemotherapy (18). Firstly, the development of variant subpopulations is a stochastic process, and the relationship between 1) the probability that a drug-resistant cell has emerged and 2) the number of cells in a tumor, goes from essentially zero to virtual certainty over only a 2 log increase in tumor size. This indicates that adjuvant therapy should be started as early as possible, even prior to primary surgery. Since the probability that variants resistant to two or more independent agents, or modalities, will arise at any one time is much less than that for variants resistant to one agent, combination therapies should be more effective when given from the beginning and concurrently, rather than later and sequentially. Furthermore, since some phenotypes, including drug resistance, can be quite unstable and can revert to "wild type" at reasonably high rates, one might be able to induce remissions even with drugs that have not been able to prevent a prior relapse. Finally, it may be unwise to couple cytotoxic therapy with agents, such as hormones, that will stimulate tumor cell division since the chance of resistant variant development is proportional to the number of tumor cells.

V. CELLULAR INTERACTIONS IN TUMOR HETEROGENEITY

Many of our ideas about tumor heterogeneity have been developed on the basis of experiments that assess the characteristics of isolated tumor subpopulations. A number of investigators have shown, however, that the behavior of subpopulations when isolated may not be the same when the subpopulations are grown together. Poste et al. (17) have reported that tumor subpopulation interactions can result in a "stabilization," that is, a reduction in the rate at which clonal variants emerge. My laboratory has described interactions that modify growth rates, immunogenicity, ability to metastasize, and sensitivity to chemotherapy (20-23). A variety of mechanisms are responsible for these interactions. Depending upon the cellular phenotype and the circumstances under which the cells are grown, the interactions may be either host or tumor cell mediated and may either require, or proceed without, contact between the interacting cells (24). Tumors are societies of interacting subpopulations, "ecosystems," in which the properties of the whole transcend the properties of the individual components (24).

Tumor subpopulation interactions pose both problems and opportunities for cancer therapy. On the one hand they compromise accurate assessment of drug sensitivity by assays designed to predict the therapeutic response of individual cancers. An example is shown in Figure 1. The sensitivity of mammary tumor subpopulation line 66 cells to methotrexate and to adriamycin was tested in the presence or absence of line 410.4 cells in our in vitro collagen gel assay for drug sensitivity (see above). By themselves line 66 cells were only moderately sensitive to methotrexate and insensitive to adriamycin at the concentrations tested. Line 410.4 cells, however, reduced growth of 66 cells. When line 410.4 cells were present in the drug sensitivity assay, line 66 cells appeared sensitive to both drugs. Clearly such interactions could obscure the accurate assessment of drug sensitivity in fresh tumors where one is not only ignorant of the cellular composition of the test sample, but the assay conditions themselves are selective for only some of the subpopulations in the original tumor.

There is another side to the "problem" of subpopulation interactions in drug sensitivity, however. We have shown that such interactions can also occur in vivo. Thus, a subpopulation line that is by itself insensitive to cyclophosphamide responds to that drug in the presence of another, sensitive line (23). This suggests that the problem of tumor heterogeneity in drug sensitivity might not be as severe as once thought. So far we have never seen a situation in which subpopulation interactions decrease sensitivity, rather they have had the effect of rendering an insensitive population more sensitive to drug. The opportunity, then, lies in developing methods to assess and perhaps even exploit the tumor ecosystem to the benefit of the host.

VI. OVERCOMING TUMOR HETEROGENEITY

I have already mentioned several approaches to blunting the problems posed for effective cancer treatment by tumor heterogeneity. Goldie and colleagues are utilizing mathematical modeling to assess the impact of heterogeneity on treatment strategy (18). We are developing an in vitro assay of drug sensitivity that incorporates the requirement of zonal sampling and cellular interactions (16,25). Other approaches that have been suggested include the use of therapeutic modalities to which all, or at least most, tumor cells are sensitive (and, of course, normal cells are resistant). Such a modality may be nonspecific immunotherapy by activated macrophages (26). Although not all tumor cells are sensitive to macrophage-mediated inhibition (27), the range of tumor sensitivity is certainly greater than is seen with other immune effectors or with chemotherapy. The use of activated macrophages to treat heterogeneous tumors is discussed in detail in this volume by Schroit and Fidler (see Chapter 14).

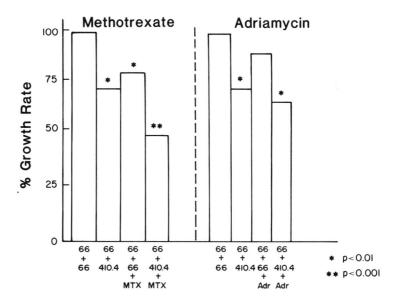

FIGURE 1. Cell boluses of 3×10^4 line 66 and line 410.4 cells were prepared from monolayer cultures and embedded in a collagen gel matrix in Dulbecco's Modified Eagle medium supplemented with nonessential amino acids and 5% calf serum. Two boluses (66 plus 66, or 66 plus 410.4) were embedded per dish. Methotrexate (MTX, 1 µM) or Adriamycin (0.03 µM) were added 24 hr later and colony size was measured by planimetry on da 1, 4 and 7. Growth rate was expressed as the slope of the line fitted by linear regression of time vs. square root of the colony area.

Another possibility is the neutralization of the mechanisms which are responsible for differential drug sensitivity between tumor subpopulations. Tsuruo et al. (28) have proposed using verapamil to neutralize the resistance to vincristine and other agents in cases where resistance is due to enhanced drug efflux. Although this specific approach is not applicable to all differentials in drug sensitivity, it suggests that a better knowledge of drug resistance mechanisms might lead to methods to blunt the impact of tumor heterogeneity on therapy.

Yet another approach is that of Leith and colleagues (29), namely, to eliminate tumor heterogeneity by inducing maturation or differentiation in the tumor subpopulations, presumably turning them into a more homogeneous target. This approach depends upon the basis of tumor heterogeneity being a difference in degree of differentiation among the subpopulations. There is evidence that this occurs in certain tumor systems, such as breast cancer (6) and small cell carcinoma of the lung (30). Tumor heterogeneity that results from mutational events (1) might not be amenable to maturational control.

An additional approach to circumventing the problems of tumor heterogeneity has been made possible by hybridoma technology. As described in this volume by Ceriani et al. (see Chapter16), monoclonal antibodies may be useful therapeutic, as well as diagnostic, reagents. If conjugated to a toxic substance, monoclonal antibodies against tumor antigens could concentrate the agent in the tumor mass and, if the toxin could act at a short distance (such as a radioactive emitter), result in the death of both the tumor cells that bear the specific antigen and non-antigen bearing "bystander" cancer cells as well. Alternatively, monoclonal antibodies to organ-specific, rather than "tumor-specific" antigens might be even more useful in neoplasms such as breast cancer, since organ specific antigens are expressed by a much greater range of tumor subpopulations than are tumor antigens (31).

Each of these approaches can be criticized on both theoretical and practical grounds. Their virtue, however, is the common attempt to utilize the concepts of cancer cell biology in the development of anti-cancer treatment. Hopefully, this orientation to experimental therapeutics will eventually turn our problems into solutions.

ACKNOWLEDGMENTS

I wish to thank Drs. Bonnie and Fred Miller for all their many contributions to the work described herein. The studies cited from my laboratory were supported by Grant Number CA-27419, awarded by the National Cancer Institute, Department of Health and Human Services, by the Warner-Lambert/Parke Davis Pharmaceutical Research Division, by the E. Walter Albachten bequest, and by the United Foundation of Metropolitan Detroit.

REFERENCES

1. Heppner GH: Tumor heterogeneity. Cancer Res. 44:2259-2275, 1984.
2. Valeriote F, van Putten L: Proliferation-dependent cytotoxicity of anticancer agents: A review. Cancer Res. 35:2619-2630, 1975.
3. Harris JF, Chambers AF, Hill RP, Ling V: Metastatic variants are generated spontaneously at a high rate in mouse KHT tumor. Proc. Natl. Acad. Sci. USA 79:5547-5551, 1982.
4. Bosslet K, Schirrmacher V: High frequency generation of new immunoresistant tumor variants during metastasis of a cloned murine tumor line (ES6). Int. J. Cancer 29:195-202, 1982.
5. Neri A, Nicolson GL: Phenotypic drift of metastatic and cell-surface properties of mammary adenocarcinoma cell clones during growth in vitro. Int. J. Cancer 28:731-738, 1981.
6. Hager J, Fligiel S, Stanley W, Richardson AM, Heppner GH: Characterization of a variant producing tumor cell line from a heterogeneous strain BALB/cfC3H mouse mammary tumor. Cancer Res. 41:1293-1300, 1981.
7. Miller FR, Miller BE, Heppner GH: Characterization of metastatic heterogeneity among subpopulations of a single mouse mammary tumor: Heterogeneity in phenotypic stability. Invasion Metastasis 3:22-31, 1983.
8. Law LW: Origin of the resistance of leukaemic cells to folic acid antagonists. Nature (London) 169:628-629, 1952.
9. Heppner GH, Miller BE: Tumor heterogeneity: Biological implications and therapeutic consequences. Cancer Metastasis Rev. 2:5-23, 1983.
10. Heppner GH, Dexter DL, DeNucci T, Miller FR, Calabresi P: Heterogeneity in drug sensitivity among tumor cell subpopulations of a single mammary tumor. Cancer Res. 38:3758-3763, 1978.
11. Tsuruo T, Fidler IJ: Differences in drug sensitivity among tumor cells from parental tumors, selected variants, and spontaneous metastases. Cancer Res. 41:3058-3064, 1981.
12. Dexter DL, Kowalski HM, Blazar BA, Fligiel Z, Vogel R, Heppner GH: Heterogeneity of tumor cells from a single mouse mammary tumor. Cancer Res. 38:3174-3181, 1978.
13. Prehn RT: Analysis of antigenic heterogeneity within individual 3-methylcholanthrene-induced mouse sarcomas. J. Natl. Cancer Inst. 45:1039-1045, 1970.
14. Fidler IJ, Hart IR: Biological and experimental consequences of the zonal composition of solid tumors. Cancer Res. 41:3266-3267, 1981.
15. Hakansson L, Trope C: On the presence within tumors of clones that differ in sensitivity to cytostatic drugs. Acta Pathol. Microbiol. Scand. Suppl. (Sect. A) 82:35-40, 1974.
16. Miller BE, Miller FR, Heppner GH: Development of a drug-sensitivity assay for heterogeneous tumors based on growth in 3-dimensional collagen gels. IN: Chabner BA (ed.) Rational Basis for Chemotherapy. Alan R. Liss, New York, pp. 107-118, 1983.

17. Poste G, Doll J, Fidler IJ: Interactions among clonal subpopulations affect stability of the metastatic phenotype in polyclonal populations of B16 melanoma cells. Proc. Natl. Acad. Sci. USA 78:6226-6230, 1981.

18. Goldie JH, Coldman AJ, Bruchovsky N: A quantitative model for drug resistance in cancer chemotherapy. IN: Chabner BA (ed.) Rational Basis for Chemotherapy. Alan R. Liss, New York, pp. 23-39, 1983.

19. Foulds L: Neoplastic Development. Vol. 1 and 2, Academic Press, New York, 1969, 1975.

20. Miller BE, Miller FR, Leith J, Heppner GH: Growth interaction in vivo between tumor subpopulations dervied from a single mouse mammary tumor. Cancer Res. 40:3977-3981, 1980.

21. Miller FR, Heppner GH: Immunologic interactions. Proc. Am. Assoc. Cancer Res. 21:201, 1980.

22. Miller FR: Tumor subpopulation interactions in metastasis. Invasion Metastasis 3:234-242, 1983.

23. Miller BE, Miller FR, Heppner GH: Interactions between tumor subpopulations affecting their sensitivity to the antineoplastic agents cyclophosphamide and methotrexate. Cancer Res. 41:4378-4381, 1981.

24. Heppner GH: Tumor subpopulation interactions. IN: Owens AH, Jr., Coffey DS, Baylin SB (eds.) Tumor Cell Heterogeneity Origins and Implications. Academic Press, New York, pp. 225-236, 1982.

25. Miller BE, Miller FR, Heppner GH: Assessing tumor drug sensitivity by a new in vitro assay which preserves tumor heterogeneity and subpopulation interactions. J. Cell. Physiol. (In press).

26. Fidler IJ, Hart IR: Biological diversity in metastatic neoplasms: Origins and implications. Science 217:998-1003, 1982.

27. Miner KM, Nicolson GL: Differences in the sensitivities of murine metastatic melanoma/lymphosarcoma variants to macrophage-mediated cytolysis and/or cytostasis. Cancer Res. 43:2063-2067, 1983.

28. Tsuruo T, Iida H, Naganuma K, Tsukagoshi S, Sakurai Y: Promotion by verapamil of vincristine responsiveness in tumor cell lines inherently resistant to the drug. Cancer Res. 43:808-813, 1983.

29. Leith JT, Gaskins LA, Dexter DL, Calabresi P, Glicksman AS: Alteration of the survival response of two human colon carcinoma subpopulations to x-irradiation by N,N-dimethylformamide. Cancer Res. 42:30-34, 1982.

30. Baylin SB, Weisburger WR, Eggleston JC, Mendelsohn G, Beaven MA, Abeloff MD, Ettinger DS: Variable content of histaminase, L-DOPA decarboxylase and calcitonin in small-cell carcinoma of the lung. N. Engl. J. Med. 299:105-110, 1978.

31. Miller BE, Jackson RC, Heppner GH: Comparison of the effect of PD111815, a substituted anthra [1,9-cd] pyrazole-6(2H)-one on mouse mammary tumor subpopulations differentially sensitive to doxorubicin. Proc. Am. Assoc. Cancer Res. 25:301, 1984.

CHAPTER 6. MULTIDRUG RESISTANCE AND METASTASIS

VICTOR LING

I. INTRODUCTION

Treatment of metastatic cancers often involves application of extensive chemotherapy. In many instances, an initial response is followed by relapse into a non-responsive disease. This non-response may extend to drugs or combination of drugs with which the patient had not been treated previously. The basis of this non-response is not well understood, although studies with model systems have provided insights to a number of possible factors. These may include: (a) insufficient delivery of drugs to metastatic tumors, (b) the presence of a tumor burden in excess of chemotherapeutic capacity, or (c) development of tumor cell variants resistant to the drugs applied.

A model invoking mechanism (c) requires that drug-resistant variants be generated at significant rates during malignant progression (1-5). Initially, such variants may only represent a minor proportion of the tumor cell population, but on application of chemotherapy, they may have a selective growth advantage, and eventually dominate the tumor. The validity of such a model has been demonstrated in tissue culture cell systems, and with transplantable animal tumors (1,6,7); however, it still needs to be verified at the clinical level. If proved correct, and shown to be a major factor in the non-response of advanced disseminated cancers, this model has major implications for our understanding of chemotherapy and tumor progression. For example, the presumptive drug-resistant cells that survive and become the dominant tumor cell population may present the therapist with a disease exhibiting properties quite different from the original one. In this context, mechanisms of drug resistance need to be delineated, and properties of drug-resistant cells characterized in order to design rational approaches towards more effective therapy.

This chapter focuses on mutations that result in the multidrug resistance phenotype. The outstanding feature of such mutants is the wide-ranging pleiotropic resistance to a variety of anticancer drugs that are structurally and functionally not related to each other. Malignant cells carrying such mutations obviously could be resistant even to treatment by combination chemotherapy. Aspects of the multidrug resistance phenotype studied in tissue culture cells will be reviewed. Preliminary evidence of such mutations occurring in human neoplasms will be described along with speculations on the implications of these findings for our understanding of tumor progression.

II. THE MULTIDRUG RESISTANCE (MDR) PHENOTYPE

A. Pleiotropic Drug-Resistance

In a number of human and animal cell lines selected for resistance
to a single cytotoxic agent, a concomitant pleiotropic resistance to
other *unrelated* compounds is often observed (8-10). This is called
the multidrug resistance (MDR) phenotype. Detailed characterization of
this phenotype indicates that it is highly complex and displays both
cross-resistance and collateral sensitivity. This is illustrated in
Table 1. Several features are noteworthy. First, it is seen that
although cross-resistance to unrelated drugs is a common feature among

Table 1. Relative Drug Resistance in Multidrug Resistance Cell Lines[1].

	Cell Lines		
Drugs	CH^RC5	UV-2237 ADM^R	CEM/VLB^R100
colchicine	180	–	45
daunomycin	76	50	124
adriamycin	25	140	112
vinblastine	30	44	420
vincristine	–	109	> 600
emetine	29	–	–
melphalan	4-15	–	–
mitomycin C	–	26	–
1-dehydrotestosterone	0.1	–	–
acronycine	< 0.06	–	–
Triton X-100	0.3	–	–
xylocaine	0.1	–	–

[1]Relative resistance was determined by the concentration of drug
required to inhibit growth or colony formation in the drug-resistant
line compared with the parental drug-sensitive line. A value greater
than 1 denotes cross-resistance and one less than 1 denotes collateral
sensitivity. Data from this table were compiled from previous studies
(1,11,40,47). A dash indicates that no value was reported for that
drug. Line CH^RC5 is a Chinese hamster ovary cell line selected for
resistance to colchicine, UV-2237 ADM^R is a mouse fibrosarcoma cell
line selected for resistance to adriamycin, and CEM/VLB^R100 is a human
leukemia line selected for resistance to vinblastine.

MDR lines, the degree of resistance to particular drugs may be quite different. In some cases clonal lines derived from a single selection for drug resistance display significantly different patterns of resistance (8,9). Second, although isolates are often most resistant to the drug initially used for selection, this need not necessarily be the case. In the CEM human line selected for resistance to vinblastine, for example, significantly higher resistance to vincristine is observed, a drug to which the cells have not been exposed previously. Third, collateral sensitivity (increased sensitivity) to a number of compounds is sometimes observed in highly MDR lines. Such compounds are hydrophobic and may have "membrane active" properties. This aspect, however, is not unique to the collateral sensitive compounds as some of the cross-resistant compounds also have similar properties.

A more detailed characterization of the MDR phenotype indicates that relatively subtle changes in the structure of the cytotoxic molecules can be discriminated. For example, a colchicine-resistant hamster line is observed to display responses ranging from cross-resistance to collateral sensitivity to a family of non-ionic detergents of the Triton series. The response is apparently dependent on the number of ethylene oxide residues present on the side chain of the detergent molecule (11). All these findings indicate that, at present, we cannot predict *a priori* the drug response profile of a particular MDR cell line.

B. Altered Drug Uptake

The basis of the MDR phenotype appears to be a reduced accumulation of the drugs involved (1,12-15). The mutant cells are able to maintain a lower intracellular drug level than the drug-sensitive parental cells. How this is accomplished is still not completely understood. In theory, a reduced drug accumulation could result from a decreased drug influx, or an increased efflux, or both. Practical experimental difficulties are associated with measuring initial rates of flux of complex amphipathic drug molecules into and out of cells (16). Given these limitations, studies have indicated that the influx process is via unmediated diffusion and is reduced in a number of MDR cell systems (1,16,17). Drug efflux is apparently an energy-dependent process, and an increased efflux has been observed in some systems as well (18,19). Whether a decreased drug influx and an increased drug efflux are mediated by a common mechanism is not known at present. It is possible that alteration in one process could pleiotropically affect the other.

C. Modulation of the MDR Phenotype

A number of agents are able to affect the reduced accumulation of different drugs associated with the MDR phenotype. These include local anesthetics, non-ionic detergents, some amphipathic drugs, inhibitors of calcium metabolism, and inhibitors of energy metabolism

(13,17,20-23). These agents all promote an increased accumulation of drugs such that under certain conditions, the stimulatory effect is greater in the MDR mutant cells than in the drug sensitive cells. Thus, the difference in drug accumulation between sensitive and resistant cells is reduced.

The cytotoxic activity of certain drugs on MDR cells can also be modulated by some of the above compounds. Tsuruo and his colleagues (21,22) have shown that verapamil and quinidine can overcome to a large extent the resistance observed in MDR vincristine-resistant and adriamycin-resistant P388 mouse transplantable tumors. Verapamil has also been reported to overcome resistance to adriamycin in human ovarian cell lines (24). A non-ionic detergent, Tween 80, at non-toxic doses is also able to reduce the relative resistance of MDR hamster cells (25).

III.   P-GLYCOPROTEIN OVER-EXPRESSION

Analyses of a variety of multidrug resistant animal and human cell lines have revealed the presence of an increase in a cell surface glycoprotein of approximately 150,000 to 180,000 daltons (1,9,13-16,26). This high molecular weight surface component has been extensively characterized in the MDR, colchicine-selected, Chinese hamster ovary (CHO) cell lines and found to be a 170,000 dalton glycoprotein (P-glycoprotein; 1,27-29). In a direct comparison, Kartner et al. (30) observed that different MDR lines all possess increased amounts of a surface component fractionating in a gel electrophoresis system with an apparent molecular weight identical to the P-glycoprotein of CHO cells. Moreover, an antiserum raised against the P-glycoprotein of MDR CHO cells crossreacts with a similar component in other MDR lines. It was concluded, therefore, that P-glycoprotein, initially characterized in CHO cells, is a membrane component whose structure is conserved across species and that over-expression of this component is a common feature of MDR cell lines.

Changes in other membrane components and in cytoplasmic components have been reported in MDR lines (16); however, none of these components is a consistent feature of the MDR phenotype. What role increased P-glycoprotein expression and other alterations play in the MDR phenotype is currently still not understood.

IV.   GENETIC ANALYSIS

Genetic studies of the MDR phenotype further confirmed the intimate association of the pleiotropic resistance to different drugs with the expression of P-glycoprotein. These include characterization of independent isolates, analyses of cell:cell hybrids, and characterization of revertants in a number of different systems (1). Moreover, in a DNA-mediated transfection study where genomic DNA from MDR colchicine-resistant CHO cells was used to transfect drug-sensitive mouse L cells, both pleiotropic drug resistance and increased

P-glycoprotein expression are observed in the transfectants (31). Unrelated or unlinked genes are apparently not co-transferred under the conditions used to select for the transfectants. All these results are consistent with the notion that the MDR phenotype is specified by a single gene or a single set of closely linked genes. Furthermore, the P-glycoprotein gene appears to be the gene or one of the genes involved.

Karyotypic analyses have provided information as to the genetic mechanism resulting in the MDR phenotype. Homogeneous staining regions (HSRs) and double minute (DM) chromosomes have been observed in a variety of MDR cell lines (13,32-35). These are features associated with gene amplification (36). That amplified DNA sequences are associated with multidrug resistance in hamster cells has been demonstrated directly by Roninson and coworkers (37) by renaturation of DNA fragments in agarose gels (38). Recently, a cDNA probe specific for P-glycoprotein has been isolated from CHO cells (Riordan et al., submitted). By Southern blot analysis, it was observed that the genomic sequences homologous to this probe were amplified in different MDR lines. Moreover, there was a correlation between the degree of amplification with P-glycoprotein expression, and with multidrug resistance. Remarkably, it appears from Southern blot analyses that P-glycoprotein is encoded by a family of genes, and they are amplified in the MDR cells. Whether or not all members of this family are functionally expressed at the protein level, and whether the members are structurally distinct are not yet known. These results, however, clearly indicate that over-expression of P-glycoprotein in the MDR cells results from amplification of the P-glycoprotein genes, and that these genes, along with possibly other amplified contiguous DNA sequences, code for the gene products that mediate the multidrug resistance phenotype. Isolation of different members of these amplified genes by molecular cloning and transfection into recipient cells to analyze function will provide insights into the molecular mechanism mediating the MDR phenotype.

V. MULTIDRUG RESISTANCE IN TUMOR CELLS

As alluded to above, the acquisition of the MDR phenotype in malignant stem cells could result in a neoplastic disease resistant to chemotherapeutic treatment. It was of interest, therefore, to determine if such mutations do occur in vivo and if tumor cells with MDR phenotype have a growth advantage during chemotherapeutic treatment. In addition, it would be of interest to determine if P-glycoprotein over-expression in such cells affects their malignant properties. In an actinomycin D-resistant MDR hamster tumor cell line, for example, Biedler and coworkers (39) observed that the drug-resistant cells are less tumorigenic than the parental drug-sensitive cells. This may have resulted from membrane changes in the resistant cells. However, in another study, Giavazzi et al. (40) isolated an adriamycin-resistant, MDR murine fibrosarcoma line (Table 1) which expresses increased amounts of P-glycoprotein. This line is tumorigenic and metastatic (41). This latter observation indicates that expression of the MDR phenotype per se does not preclude expression of malignant properties.

The question of whether MDR mutations can occur in vivo was investigated in the P388 murine transplantable tumor system. By treating animals carrying this tumor with adriamycin, vincristine or actinomycin D under conditions where the majority of the tumor cells were killed, a resistant population of tumor cells emerged. These cells displayed cross-resistance to unrelated drugs, and also over-expression of P-glycoprotein (Gerlach and Ling, unpublished). Recently, in a preliminary study of stages III and IV ovarian patients who have undergone extensive chemotherapy, over-expression of P-glycoprotein in tumor cells obtained from ascites fluid was observed in two of five cases (42). These studies provide strong evidence that multidrug resistance mutations in tumor cells, as detected by P-glycoprotein over-expression, do occur in vivo, and that such cells have a selective advantage during chemotherapeutic treatment so that they become enriched in the tumor population.

VI. CONCLUSIONS

Combination chemotherapy is often the treatment of choice for metastatic cancers. An understanding of mechanisms which could render malignant cells refractory to a combination of anticancer drugs should allow for rational approaches towards more effective therapy. Thus, the study of the multidrug resistance phenotype, as outlined in this chapter, has particular relevance to our understanding of the development and therapy of metastatic neoplastic diseases.

A number of conclusions can be drawn from the studies outlined here. It seems clear that multidrug resistance mutations can arise in patients with metastatic cancers, although the frequency of their occurrence is not known. Nor is it known at present, whether such mutations generally play a major role in a patient's response to combination chemotherapy. From the study with advanced ovarian carcinomas (42) where, in a few specific instances, the tumor population is apparently greatly enriched for MDR cells, it would be surprising if such cells were not a critical factor since they apparently have some selective growth advantage. Presumably, drug-sensitive tumor cells have been largely eradicated by chemotherapy. Further studies will be required to determine what properties of such MDR malignant cells may be exploited for therapy. In this context, the observations that some MDR cells are collaterally sensitive to some agents and that certain compounds such as verapamil are able to modulate MDR phenotype are areas that deserve further investigation.

The finding that amplification of the P-glycoprotein genes is involved in the MDR phenotype provides additional support for the notion that gene amplification may be an important mechanism in tumor progression. Gene amplification has been implicated in the development of resistance to chemotherapeutic drugs different from the MDR mutation. These include variants resistant to drugs such as methotrexate, ara A, hydroxyurea, PALA, asparaginase (1,43). Amplification of cellular oncogenes is also thought to be a major mechanism of carcinogenesis (43,44). In addition, it has been suggested that gene amplification may play a role in certain dynamic properties of metastatic cells (45,46). What factors affect the rate of gene amplification, or what regulates the size of the genome amplified, or whether certain genes are more prone to amplification is not known. Studies of model systems such as those involving P-glycoprotein over-expression may provide further insights to these questions.

ACKNOWLEDGMENTS

This work was supported by grants from the Medical Research Council of Canada, the National Cancer Institute of Canada, and from the National Institutes of Health, USA, grant number CA37130. I thank my colleagues who have contributed to the work described here.

REFERENCES

1. Ling V: Genetic basis of drug resistance in mammalian cells. IN: Brukchovsky N and Goldie JH (eds.) Drug and Hormone Resistance in Neoplasia. CRC Press, Boca Raton, Vol. I, pp. 1-19, 1982.
2. Goldie JH, Coldman AJ: A mathematical model for relating the drug sensitivity of tumors to their spontaneous mutation rate. Cancer Treat. Rep. 63:1727-1733, 1979.
3. Goldie JH, Coldman AJ: Clinical implications of the phenomenon of drug resistance. IN: Bruchovsky N and Goldie JH (eds.) Drug and Hormone Resistance in Neoplasia. CRC Press, Boca Raton, Vol. I, pp. 111-127, 1982.
4. DeVita VT, Jr.: Principles of chemotherapy. IN: DeVita VT, Jr., Hellman S and Rosenberg SA (eds.) Cancer: Principles and Practice of Oncology. J.B. Lippincott Co., Philadelphia-Toronto, pp. 132-155, 1982.
5. Brockman RW: Pharmacological Basis of Cancer Chemotherapy. Williams and Wilkins, Baltimore, 691 p., 1975.
6. Schable FM, Jr., Skipper HE, Trader MW, Laster, WR, Jr., Corbett TH, Griswold DP, JR.: Concepts for controlling drug-resistant tumor cells. IN: Mouridsen HT and Palshof T (eds.) Breast Cancer: Experimental and Clinical Aspects. Pergamon Press, Oxford, pp. 199-211, 1980.
7. Curt GA, Clendeninn NJ, Chabner BA: Drug resistance in cancer. Cancer Treat. Rep. 68:87-99, 1984.
8. Ling V, Gerlach J, Kartner N: Multidrug resistance. Breast Cancer Res. Treat. 4:89-94, 1984.
9. Ling V, Kartner N, Sudo T, Siminovitch L, Riordan JR: The multidrug resistance phenotype. Cancer Treat. Rep. 67:869-874, 1983.

88

10. Skipper HE, Hutchison DJ, Shabel FM, Schmidt LH, Goldin A, Brockman RW, Venditt JM, Wodinsky I: A quick reference chart on cross resistance between anti-cancer agents. Cancer Chemo. Rep. Part 1. 56:493-498, 1972.
11. Bech-Hansen NT, Till JE, Ling V: Pleiotropic phenotype of colchicine-resistant CHO cells: Cross-resistance and collateral sensitivity. J. Cell. Physiol. 88:23-31, 1976.
12. Ling V, Thompson LH: Reduced permeability in CHO cells as a mechanism of resistance to colchicine. J. Cell. Physiol. 83:103-116, 1974.
13. Biedler JL, Peterson RHF: Altered plasma membrane glycocongugates of Chinese hamster cells with acquired resistance to actinomycin D, daunorubicin, and vincristine. IN: Sartorelli AC, Lazo JS and Bertino JR (eds.) Molecular Actions and Target for Cancer Chemotherapeutic Agents. Academic Press, New York, pp. 453-482, 1981.
14. Beck WT: Vinca alkaloid-resistant phenotype in cultured human leukemic lymphoblasts. Cancer Treat. Rep. 67:875-882, 1983.
15. Kartner N, Shales M, Riordan JR, Ling V: Daunorubicin-resistant Chinese hamster ovary cells expressing multidrug resistance and a cell surface P-glycoprotein. Cancer Res. 43:4413-4419, 1983.
16. Riordan JR, Ling V: Genetic and biochemical characterization of multidrug resistance. IN: Goldman ID (ed.) International Encyclopedia of Pharmacology and Therapeutics. Pergamon Press, Oxford, in press.
17. Carlsen SA, Till JE, Ling V: Modulation of membrane drug permeability in Chinese hamster ovary cells. Biochim. Biophys. Acta 455:900-912, 1976.
18. Inaba M, Kobayashi H, Sakurai Y, Johnson RK: Active efflux of daunorubicin and adriamycin in sensitive and resistant sublines of P388 leukemia. Cancer Res. 39:2200-2203, 1974.
19. Danø K: Active outward transport of daunomycin in resistant Ehrlich ascites tumour cells. Biochim. Biophys. Acta 323:466-483, 1973.
20. See YP, Carlsen SA, Till JE, Ling V: Increased drug permeability in Chinese hamster ovary cells in the presence of cyanide. Biochim. Biophys. Acta 373:242-252, 1974.
21. Tsuruo T, Iida H, Tsukagoshi S, Sakurai Y: Overcoming of vincristine resistance in P388 leukemia in vivo and in vitro through enhanced cytotoxicity of vincristine and vinblastine by verapamil. Cancer Res. 41:1967-1972, 1981.
22. Tsuruo T, Iida H, Kitatani Y, Yokota K, Tsukagoshi S, Sakurai Y: Effects of quinidine and related compounds on cytotoxicity and cellular accumulation of vincristine and adriamycin in drug-resistant tumor cells. Cancer Res. 44:4303-4307, 1984.
23. Ganapathi R, Grabowski D, Rouse W, Riegler F: Differential effect of the calmodulin inhibitor trifluoperazine on cellular accumulation, retention, and cytotoxicity of anthracyclines in doxorubicin (adriamycin)-resistant P388 mouse leukemia cells. Cancer Res. 44:5056-5061, 1984.
24. Rogan AM, Hamilton TC, Young RC, Klecker RW, Jr., Ozols RF: Reversal of adriamycin resistance by verapamil in human ovarian cancer. Science 224:994-996, 1984.

25. Ling V, Aubin JE, Chase A, Sarangi F: Mutants of Chinese hamster ovary (CHO) cells with altered colcemid-binding affinity. Cell 18:423-430, 1979.
26. Garman D, Center MS: Alterations in cell surface membranes in Chinese hamster lung cells resistant to adriamycin. Biochem. Biophys. Res. Commun. 105:157-163, 1982.
27. Ling V, Thompson LH: Reduced permeability in CHO cells as a mechanism of resistance to colchicine. J. Cell. Physiol. 83:103-116, 1974.
28. Juliano RL, Ling V: A surface glcoprotein modulating drug permeability in Chinese hamster ovary cell mutant. Biochim. Biophys. Acta 455:152-162, 1976.
29. Riordan JR, Ling V: Purification of P-glycoprotein from plasma membrane vesicles of Chinese hamster ovary cell mutants with reduced colchicine permeability. J. Biol. Chem. 254:12701-12705, 1979.
30. Kartner N, Riordan JR, Ling V: Cell surface P-glycoprotein associated with multidrug resistance in mammalian cell lines. Science 221:1285-1288, 1983.
31. Debenham PG, Kartner N, Siminovitch L, Riordan JR, Ling V: DNA-mediated transfer of multiple drug resistance and plasma membrane glycoprotein expression. Mol. Cell Biol. 2:881-889, 1982.
32. Baskin F, Rosenberg RN, Dev V: Correlation of double-minute chromosomes with unstable multidrug cross-resistance in uptake mutants of neuroblastoma cells. Proc. Natl. Acad. Sci USA 78:3654-3658, 1981.
33. Kopnin BP: Specific karyotypic alterations in colchicine-resistant cells. Cytogenet. Cell. Genet. 30:11-14, 1981.
34. Howell N, Belli TA, Zaczkiewica LT, Belli JA: High-level unstable adriamycin resistance in a Chinese hamster mutant cell line with double minute chromosomes. Cancer Res. 44:4023-4029, 1984.
35. Robertson SM, Ling V, Stanners CP: Co-amplification of double minute chromosomes, multidrug-resistance, and cell surface P-glycoprotein in DNA-mediated transformants of mouse cells. Mol. Cell. Biol. 4:500-506, 1984.
36. Cowell JK: Double minutes and homogeneously staining regions: Gene amplification in mammalian cells. Annu. Rev. Genet. 16:21-59, 1982.
37. Roninson IB, Abelson HT, Housman DE, Howell N, Varshavsky A: Amplification of specific DNA sequences correlates with multidrug resistance in Chinese hamster cells. Nature (London) 309:626-628, 1984.
38. Roninson IB: Detection and mapping of homologous, repeated, and amplified DNA sequences by DNA renaturation in agarose gels. Nucleic Acids Res. 11:5413-5431, 1983.
39. Biedler JL, Riehm H, Peterson RHF, Spengler BC: Membrane-mediated drug-resistance and phenotypic reversion to normal growth behavior of Chinese hamster cells. J. Natl. Cancer Inst. 55:671-680, 1975.
40. Giavazzi R, Kartner N, Hart IR: Expression of cell surface P-glycoprotein by an adriamycin-resistant murine fibrosarcoma. Cancer Chemother. Pharmacol. 13:145-147, 1984.

90

41. Giavazzi R, Scholar E, Hart I: Isolation and preliminary characterization of an adriamycin-resistant murine fibrosarcoma line. Cancer Res. 43:2216-2222, 1983.
42. Bell DR, Gerlach JH, Kartner N, Buick RN, Ling V: Detection of P-glycoprotein in ovarian cancer: A molecular marker associated with multidrug resistance. J. Clin. Oncol. (In press).
43. Stark GR, Wahl GM: Gene amplification. Annu. Rev. Biochem. 53:447-491, 1984.
44. Pall ML: Gene-amplification model of carcinogenesis. Proc. Natl. Acad. Sci. USA 78:2465-2468, 1981.
45. Harris JF, Chambers AF, Hill RP, Ling V: Metastatic variants are generated spontaneously at a high rate in mouse KHT tumor. Proc. Natl. Acad. Sci. USA 79:5547-5551, 1982.
46. Ling V, Chambers AF, Harris JF, Hill RP: Dynamic heterogeneity and metastasis. J. Cell. Physiol. Suppl. 3:99-103, 1984.
47. Beck WT: Cellular pharmacology of vinca alkaloid resistance and its circumvention. Adv. Enzyme Regulation 22:207-227, 1984.

CHAPTER 7. POLYAMINE BIOSYNTHESIS: A TARGET FOR ANTIMETASTATIC THERAPY

PRASAD S. SUNKARA AND NELLIKUNJA J. PRAKASH

I. INTRODUCTION

The naturally occurring polyamines, putrescine, spermidine, and spermine, are ubiquitous in eukaryotic organisms. The structural formulae for these physiological cations are shown in Figure 1. Although Leeuwenhoek's discovery of spermine as precipitating crystals in human semen dates back to 1677 (1), a critical role for these amines has been recognized only since specific inhibitors of polyamine biosynthetic enzymes became available in the last decade (2,3). A number of studies have suggested that polyamines play an important role in cell proliferation and differentiation (4-7).

In this review we will examine the role of polyamines in tumor metastasis. In addition, the biochemical and pharmacological consequences of inhibiting polyamine biosynthesis by DL-α-difluoromethylornithine (DFMO), a specific inhibitor of ornithine decarboxylase, and the potential therapeutic use of this inhibitor as an antimetastatic agent is also described in some detail.

II. POLYAMINE BIOSYNTHESIS

The biosynthetic pathways leading to polyamines have been reviewed extensively in recent years (8,9). The following overview is intended to give the reader a necessary basis to understand the rationale behind the biological activities of specific inhibitors of polyamine biosynthesis.

L-ornithine and S-adenosyl L-methionine are the primary precursors of polyamines in mammalian cells. Arginase, a widely distributed extra-hepatic enzyme of the urea cycle, converts arginine to ornithine. Arginine can, therefore, be thought of as a precursor in the polyamine biosynthetic pathway. The biosynthetic pathway of polyamines in animal cells is summarized in Figure 2.

Ornithine decarboxylase (ODC), a pyridoxal phosphate-dependent enzyme catalyzes the formation of putrescine from ornithine. This reaction appears to be an important step in the polyamine biosynthetic pathway. ODC is present in very small amounts in quiescent normal cells and tissues. A dramatic increase in enzyme activity occurs during the early phase of cell growth as a result of exposure to trophic stimuli such as hormones, drugs and growth factors (10,11). Mammalian ODC turns over rapidly with an apparent half life of 15-20 min and has the shortest half life of any mammalian enzyme known so far.

$$H_2N-CH_2-CH_2-CH_2-CH_2-NH_2$$

putrescine

$$H_2N-CH_2-CH_2-CH_2-NH-CH_2-CH_2-CH_2-CH_2-NH_2$$

spermidine

$$H_2N-CH_2-CH_2-CH_2-NH-CH_2-CH_2-CH_2-CH_2-NH-CH_2-CH_2-CH_2-NH_2$$

spermine

FIGURE 1. The Structural Formulae of Naturally Occurring Polyamines.

93

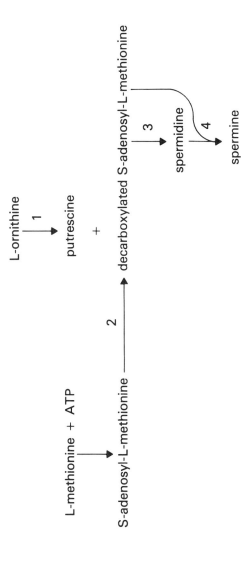

FIGURE 2. Biosynthetic Pathway of Polyamines in Mammalian Tissues. The enzymes involved in the biosynthesis are (1) ornithine decarboxylase, (2) S-adenosylmethionine decarboxylase, (3) spermidine synthase, and (4) spermine synthase.

The synthesis of higher polyamines spermidine and spermine, is catalyzed by spermidine synthase and spermine synthase, respectively. These enzymes catalyze the transfer of a propylamine group from decarboxylated S-adenosyl L-methionine to putrescine and spermidine, respectively. Decarboxylation of S-adenosylmethionine is carried out by the enzyme S-adenosyl L-methionine decarboxylase (SAMDC). Mammalian SAMDC has pyruvate covalently linked to the enzyme as a prosthetic group. SAMDC activity also fluctuates rapidly upon growth stimulation by hormones or growth factors.

III. DL-α-DIFLUOROMETHYLORNITHINE

Dl-α-difluoromethylornithine (DFMO) is a potent and specific irreversible inhibitor of ornithine decarboxylase (3,12). The inhibition is irreversible because no enzyme activity can be recovered after extensive dialysis. This inactivation of ODC by DMFO can be protected by L-ornithine suggesting that the action of the inhibitor is active site-directed.

DFMO has been shown to inhibit ODC and decrease intracellular putrescine and spermidine concentrations and inhibit cell growth in a number of cells in culture (13-16) and in animal tumors in vivo (17-21). DFMO also exhibits contragestational activity (22) and antiprotozoal activity (23-25) because of its interference with polyamine metabolism.

DFMO has been generally well tolerated by experimental animals. Single oral doses of 5 g/kg have no apparent adverse effects on mice. Administration of a total daily dose of 4 g/kg for 4 wk to mice and rats does not slow their normal weight gain and no organ toxicity is found. The only side effect seen is diarrhea in rats which is easily reversible when administration of the drug is stopped (26).

IV. EFFECT ON TUMOR METASTASIS OF INHIBITION OF POLYAMINE BIOSYNTHESIS BY DFMO

Although a vast amount of literature indicates an important role for polyamines in tumor cell growth, there is no available information on the role of these cations in the process of tumor metastasis. Recently the effect of DFMO on the growth and pulmonary metastasis of Lewis lung (3LL) tumors in mice was examined (20,27).

The results of our study (20) show that administration of DFMO starting 1 da after tumor inoculation results in a 69% and 75% decrease in the intracellular levels of putrescine and spermidine in the primary tumor, respectively, without any change in spermine concentrations (Figure 3). The decreased polyamine levels are also associated a 43% inhibition of tumor growth. Inhibition of polyamine biosynthesis as a result of DFMO administration not only inhibits growth of the primary tumor but also dramatically decreases secondary pulmonary metastases by 79% with 25% of the animals showing no visible metastases (Table 1). Further, this

Table 1. Effect of DFMO on the Inhibition of Growth and Pulmonary Metastases of Lewis Lung Carcinoma in Mice[*].

Treatment	Tumor weight (g) (Mean ± SEM; n = 20)	% Inhibition	No. animals showing no visible metastases	Metastatic foci (Mean ± SEM; n = 20)	% Inhibition
Control	7.01 ± 0.39		0/20	21.38 ± 5.8	
DFMO	4.01 ± 0.46[†]	43	5/20	4.60 ± 1.43	79
DFMO + Put	6.54 ± 0.78[‡]	7	0/20	24.80 ± 5.10[‡]	0

[*]1×10^6 3LL tumor cells/animal were injected subcutaneously at the intrascapular region. DFMO was administered as a 2% aqueous solution as the sole drinking fluid (~3 g/kg/da). Putrescine (100 mg/kg) was given intraperitoneally daily, starting on da 1 and continuing through da 18. At the end of 18 da the animals were sacrificed, tumors were excised and weighed.

[†]significant at $p < 0.01$

[‡]not significant

inhibition of tumor growth and metastases could be reversed by simultaneous administration of putrescine to the animals (Figure 3 and Table 1). Administration of putrescine to animals receiving DFMO does not result in any significant elevation of tumor putrescine concentrations although spermidine concentrations are substantially elevated compared to tumors from animals which received DFMO alone. The lack of any effect on tumor putrescine concentration following exogenous putrescine administration to DFMO-treated animals is most likely due to its rapid conversion to spermidine. Since polyamine depletion in tumor cells leads to an increase of SAMDC (S-adenosyl-L-methionine decarboxylase), the rate-limiting enzyme involved in the conversion of putrescine to spermidine, DFMO treatment is likely to facilitate the conversion of exogenous putrescine to spermidine in the solid tumor employed in the study. Essentially similar results were obtained by Bartholeyns (27); DFMO treatment, started 8 da after tumor inoculation when a palpable tumor is seen, also shows an 82% reduction in lung metastases.

Our recent studies (Sunkara et al., unpublished data) with another malignant tumor, B16 amelanotic melanoma (B16a), in mice also showed a dose response effect of DFMO on the inhibition of polyamine levels on both tumor growth and pulmonary metastases. DFMO when administered as 0.5, 1 and 2% solutions in drinking water resulted in 0, 24.5 and 60 percent inhibition of tumor growth, respectively. In addition, metastasis was inhibited 55, 83 and 96 percent, respectively; 30 and 65% of the animals were free of metastases in the animals treated with 1 and 2% DFMO (Table 2). DFMO treatment resulted in a significant reduction of putrescine levels and a dose dependent inhibition of spermidine levels with an increase in spermine concentration in the tumor tissue (Table 3). A good correlation of the inhibition of tumor growth and decrease in the spermidine levels by DFMO was observed suggesting that threshold levels of spermidine are required for tumor growth.

The data presented in these studies indicate that inhibition of polyamine biosynthesis by DFMO results in a decrease in the spread of tumor cells to lungs. The fact that the inhibition of metastasis could be reversed by simultaneous administration of putrescine suggests that polyamines may play a role not only in tumor growth (18,19,21,28) but also in the process of tumor metastasis. Although the mechanism by which DFMO inhibits tumor metastasis is not yet clear, one can envisage that the depletion of cellular polyamines in the primary tumor could have affected: 1) the invasation of the tumor cells into the lymphatics or blood vessels, 2) their transport into distant organs, and 3) the establishment of a microenvironment unfavorable to the growth of pulmonary metastases (29).

Table 2. Effect of DFMO on the Growth and Pulmonary Metastases of B16 Amelanotic Melanoma (B16a) in Mice*.

Treatment	Tumor weight (g) (Mean ± SEM; n = 20)	% Inhibition	No. animals showing no visible metastases	Metastatic foci (Mean ± SEM; n = 20)	% Inhibition
Control (n = 20)	4.99 ± 0.29		0/20	48.3 ± 5.3	
DFMO (0.5%) (n = 12)	5.13 ± 0.50†	0	0/12	21.5 ± 5.6‡	55
DFMO (1%) (n = 23)	3.77 ± 0.32‡	24.5	7/23	8.4 ± 2.1†	83
DFMO (2%) (n = 17)	2.03 ± 0.18‡	60.0	11/17	2.2 ± 0.9‡	96

*B16a cells (1 x 10⁵) were injected s.c.in the intrascapular region of C57BL/6J mice on da 0. Animals were divided into 4 groups. One group was put on normal drinking water and served as control. The other 3 groups were allowed to drink water containing 0.5, 1 or 2% DFMO starting on da 1. At the end of 25 da the animals were sacrificed, tumors were dissected and weighed. A portion of the tumor was frozen at -70°C for polyamine determinations. The lungs were fixed in Bouin's fixative for determining the extent of pulmonary metastases.

†not significant compared to control

‡p < 0.01 compared to control

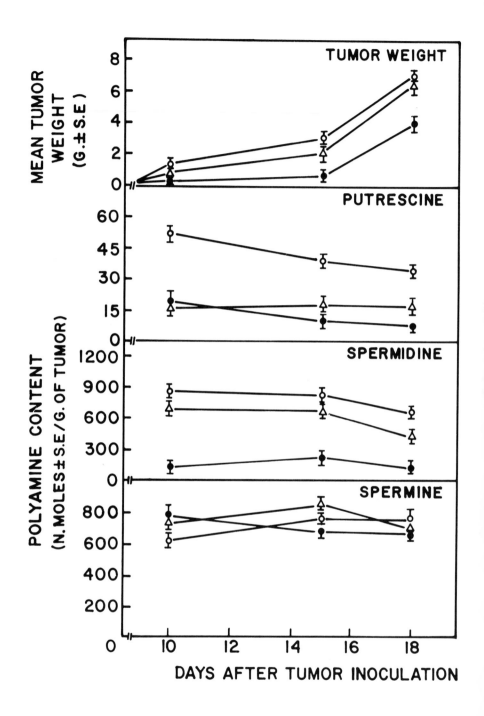

FIGURE 3. Effect of DFMO on the Growth and Polyamine Levels of Lewis Lung Tumor (3LL) in Mice. Tumors were induced in C57BL/6J mice by s.c. injection of 1 x 10^6 viable 3LL cells/mouse in the intrascapular region. DFMO was administered in the drinking water as a 2% aqueous solution (approximately 3 g/kg/da). Putrescine was administered i.p. at a dose of 100 mg/kg/da. This experimental protocol is the same as in Table 1. Points represent mean ± S.E.M. (n = 20). open circle, untreated animals; closed circle, DFMO treated; triangle, DFMO + putrescine treated animals. [From Sunkara et al. (20) with permission.]

Table 3. Effect of DFMO on the Polyamine Levels of B16 Amelanotic Melanoma in Mice[*].

Treatment	Polyamine Concentration (nmoles/g) Mean ± SD; n = 6		
	Putrescine	Spermidine	Spermine
Control	26.2 ± 4.6	398 ± 8.2	298 ± 46
DFMO (0.5%)	8.9 ± 4.1	164 ± 69	427 ± 139
DFMO (1%)	7.1 ± 4.1	109 ± 24	420 ± 73
DFMO (2%)	9.5 ± 2.3	103 ± 21	354 ± 90

[*]The experimental details are as described in Table 2.

Recent data suggest that DFMO might affect the second phase in the metastatic process. We found that administration of DFMO did not inhibit the spread of metastatic cells from the primary tumor. However, their transportation to the distant organs and establishment into pulmonary metastases was inhibited (Sunkara et al., unpublished data). These results indicate that polyamines play an important role in tumor metastasis, and specific inhibitors of polyamine synthesis, such as DFMO, merit consideration as potential therapeutic agents in clinical management of metastasis.

ACKNOWLEDGMENTS

The authors would like to thank Mrs. Andrea L. Rosenberger and Mr. Philip J. Lackmann for their technical assistance and Ms. B.J. Hunt for her expert secretarial assistance.

REFERENCES

1. Mann T: The Biochemistry of Semen and of the Male Reproductive
    Tract. Methuen, London, 1964.
2. Abdel-Monem MM, Newton NE, Weeks CE: Inhibitors of polyamine
    biosynthesis.   I.   α-methyl-(+)-ornithine, an inhibitor of
    ornithine decarboxylase. J. Med. Chem. 17:447-451, 1974.
3. Metcalf BW, Bey P, Danzin C, Jung MJ, Casara P, Vevert JP:
    Catalytic irreversible inhibition of mammalian ornithine
    decarboxylase (E.C.4.1.1.17) by substrate and product analogues.
    J. Am. Chem. Soc. 100:2551-2553, 1978.
4. Sunkara PS, Rao PN: Differential cell cycle response of normal
    and transformed cells to polyamine limitation.   Adv. Polyamine
    Res. 3:347-356, 1981.
5. Heby O: Role of polyamines in the control of cell proliferation
    and differentiation. Differentiation 19:1-20, 1981.
6. Pegg AE, McCann PP: Polyamine metabolism and function: A review.
    Am. J. Physiol. 243:C212-C221, 1982.
7. Sunkara PS, Prakash NJ: Inhibitors of polyamine biosynthesis as
    antitumor and antimetastatic agents.   IN: Sunkara PS (ed.) Novel
    Approaches to Cancer Chemotherapy. Academic Press, New York, (In
    press).
8. Tabor CW, Tabor H: 1,4-Diaminobutane (putrescine), spermidine and
    spermine. Ann. Rev. Biochem. 45:285-306, 1976.
9. Pegg AE, Williams-Ashman HG: Biosynthesis of putrescine.   IN:
    Morris DR and Marton LJ (eds.), Polyamines in Biology and
    Medicine. Marcel Dekker, New York, pp. 3-42, 1981.
10. Janne J, Poso H, Raina A: Polyamines in rapid growth and cancer.
    Biochim. Biophys. Acta: 473:241-293, 1978.
11. Russell DH: Ornithine decarboxylase: Transcriptional induction
    by trophic hormones via a cAMP and cAMP dependent protein kinase
    pathway.   IN: Morris DR, Marton LJ (eds.), Polyamines in Biology
    and Medicine. Marcel Dekker, New York. pp. 109-125, 1981.
12. Bey P: Substrate-induced irreversible inhibition of α-amino acid
    decarboxylases. Application to glutamate, aromatic L-α-amino acid and
    ornithine decarboxylases.   IN: Seiler N, Jung MJ, Koch-Weser J
    (eds.), Enzyme-Activated Irreversible Inhibitors. Elsevier/North
    Holland, Amsterdam, pp. 27-41, 1978.
13. Mamont PS, Duchesne MC, Grove J, Bey P: Antiproliferative
    properties of DL-α-difluoromethyl ornithine in cultured cells. A
    consequence   of   the   irreversible   inhibition   of   ornithine
    decarboxylase. Biochem. Biophys. Res. Commun. 81:58-66, 1978.
14. Sunkara PS, Fowler SK, Nishioka K, Rao PN: Inhibition of
    polyamine biosynthesis by α-difluoromethyl ornithine potentiates
    the   cytotoxic   effects   of   arabinosylcytosine   in   HeLa   cells.
    Biochem. Biophys. Res. Commun. 95:423-430, 1980.
15. Sidenfield J, Gray JW, Marton LJ: Depletion of 9L rat brain tumor
    cell polyamine content by treatment with DL-α-difluoromethyl
    ornithine inhibits proliferation and the Gl to S transition. Exp.
    Cell. Res. 131:209-216, 1981.
16. Luk GD, Goodwin G, Marton LJ, Baylin SB: Polyamines are necessary
    for the survival of human small-cell lung carcinoma in culture.
    Proc. Natl. Acad. Sci. USA 78:2355-2358, 1981.

17. Prakash NJ, Schecter PJ, Grove J, Koch-Weser J: Effect of α-difluoromethylornithine, an enzyme-activated irreversible inhibitor of ornithine decarboxylase, on L1210 leukemia in mice. Cancer Res. 38:3059-3062, 1978.

18. Prakash NJ, Schechter PJ, Mamont PS, Grove J, Koch-Weser J, Sjoerdsma A: Inhibition of EMT6 tumor growth by interference with polyamine biosynthesis; effects of α-difluoromethylornithine, an irreversible inhibitor of ornithine decarboxylase. Life Sci. 26:181-194, 1980.

19. Marton LJ, Levin VA, Hervatin SJ, Koch-Weser J, McCann PP, Sjoerdsma A: Potentiation of the antitumor therapeutic effects of 1,3-bis(2-chloroethyl)-1-nitrosourea by α-difluoromethyl ornithine, an ornithine decarboxylase inhibitor. Cancer Res. 41:4426-4431, 1981.

20. Sunkara PS, Prakash NJ, Rosenberger AL: An essential role for polyamines in tumor metastases. FEBS Lett. 150:397-399, 1982.

21. Sunkara PS, Prakash NJ, Chang CC, Sjoerdsma A: Cytotoxicity of methylglyoxal bis(guanyl hydrazone) in combination with α-difluoromethylornithine against HeLa cells and mouse L1210 leukemia. J. Natl. Cancer Inst. 40:505-509, 1983.

22. Fozard JR, Part ML, Prakash NJ, Grove J, Schechter PJ, Sjoerdsma A, Koch-Weser J: L-ornithine decarboxylase: An essential role in early mammalian embryogenesis. Science 208:505-508, 1980.

23. Bacchi CJ, Nathan HN, Hutner SH, McCann PP, Sjoerdsma A: Polyamine metabolism: A potential therapeutic target in trypanosomes. Science 210:332-334, 1980.

24. McCann PP, Bacchi CJ, Clarkson AB, Seed JR, Nathan HC, Amole BO, Hutner SH, Sjoerdsma A: Further studies on dirluoromethyl-ornithine in African trypanosomes. Med. Biol. 59:434-440, 1981.

25. Sjoerdsma A, Schechter PJ: Chemotherapeutic implications of polyamine biosynthesis inhibition. Clin. Pharmacol. Ther. 35:287-300, 1983.

26. Merrell Dow Research Center. Investigational Brochure, 1982.

27. Bartholeyns J: Treatment of metastatic Lewis lung carcinoma with DL-α-difluoromethyl ornithine. Eur. J. Cancer Clin. Oncol. 19:567-572, 1983.

28. Sunkara PS, Prakash NJ, Mayer GD, Sjoerdsma A: Tumor suppression with a combination of α-difluoromethyl ornithine and interferon. Science 219:851-853, 1983.

29. Poste G, Fidler J: The pathogenesis of cancer metastasis. Nature 283:139-146, 1980.

CHAPTER 8. CHEMICAL MECHANISMS OF MODULATION OF TUMOR GROWTH AND METASTASIS BY PROSTAGLANDINS

LAWRENCE J. MARNETT AND KENNETH V. HONN

I. GROWTH AND DIFFERENTIATION

Prostaglandins are powerful local hormones that are biosynthesized from unsaturated fatty acids, in particular arachidonic acid. Their actions appear to be mediated by receptors and in some cases via stimulation of adenylate cyclase (1-4). Numerous reports indicate that they can modulate tumor initiation, promotion and progression (5,6). This chapter discusses mechanisms by which prostaglandins inhibit tumor cell proliferation and mechanisms by which pharmacological agents inhibit metastasis by modulating prostaglandin biosynthesis.

Prostaglandin E_1 is a potent stimulator of adenylate cyclase in peritoneal macrophages, thyroid, neuroblastoma, diaphragm, lung , pancreatic islets, uterus and spleen (1). The hallmark of the activity of PGE_1 is the presence of oxygen functionalities in the cyclopentane ring and the S absolute configuration of the hydroxyl group at carbon 15; PGE_2 contains an additional double bond at the 5,6 position. These various functionalities are important determinants of receptor-mediated activities. Santoro et al. (7,8) first reported that the long-lived PGE_2 analogue, 16,16-dimethyl-PGE_2, inhibits replication of cultured B16 melanoma cells. Honn et al. (9) subsequently showed that the dehydration product PGA_2 inhibits the proliferation of B16 amelanotic melanoma (B16a) cells (9). The present data on proliferation were obtained with secondary cultures of B16a cells.

PGA differs from PGE in that the water molecule at the 11 position has been eliminated (eq. 1). PGA can isomerize to PGB via an inter-

eq. 1

104

mediate PGC (eq. 2). Figure 1 shows the effects of several

eq. 2

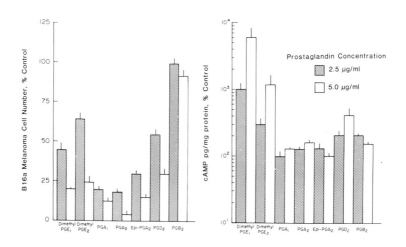

prostaglandins on proliferation of B16a cells. PGA type compounds are
potent inhibitors of proliferation (10). The presence of the double
bond at the 5,6 position has essentially no effect on activity and the
absolute configuration of the hydroxyl group at carbon 15 is also
unimportant in that the 15-epi isomer is nearly equipotent to PGAs. In
fact, the 15-keto metabolites of PGA's are nearly as active as PGA's
themselves (data not shown), which rules out any sort of receptor-
mediated mechanism because 15-keto-prostaglandins are normally
inactive. Figure 1 also shows that PGD$_2$, an isomer of PGE$_2$, was active
as an inhibitor of proliferation. PGB$_2$, the isomer of PGA in which the
double bond has moved to the 8,12 position is inactive.

FIGURE 1. Comparision of the Effects of Various Prostaglandins on
Proliferation and cAMP Generation by B16a Cells.

Further support for the unimportance of receptor-mediated mechanisms in the PGA effects are provided by the data in Figure 1. The ability to stimulate adenylate cyclase in the melanoma cells is exhibited by PGE's but not exhibited by PGA's, epi-PGA$_2$ or PGD$_2$, all of which are inhibitory of tumor cell proliferation. These data indicate that inhibition of proliferation is not a cyclic nucleotide-mediated event.

What then is the mechanism of this effect? Simple α,β-unsaturated carbonyl compounds are known to inhibit bacterial and viral growth by chemically reacting with sulfhydryl groups of critical cellular proteins and enzymes (11). As shown in eq. 3 a sulfhydryl protein (in this case glutathione) could add to the α,β-unsaturated double bond and

eq. 3

perhaps cause inhibition of proliferation. If so, glutathione should antagonize the anti-proliferative activity of PGA-like compounds. As one can see from the data in Figure 2, increasing the amount of glutathione in the incubation mixture in the culture flask antagonizes and eventually completely abolishes the inhibitory effects of PGA on tumor cell DNA synthesis. This is consistent with an addition to the α,β-unsaturated carbonyl group being a critical determinant of the anti-proliferative activity of prostaglandins.

A critical test for this theory is based on the observation that PGD$_2$ is a good inhibitor of tumor cell proliferation. PGD$_2$ is quite active against a broad range of human tumors (12). These prostaglandins are as potent in vitro as any commonly employed chemotherapeutic agent for inhibition of proliferation. PGD$_2$ is an isomer of PGE$_2$ and if our theory is correct elimination of the hydroxyl group at the 9 position should geneate an enone that is a potent inhibitor of tumor cell proliferation (eq. 4). The dehydration product is called PGJ$_2$ and has been synthesized (13). It is extremely unstable due to

106

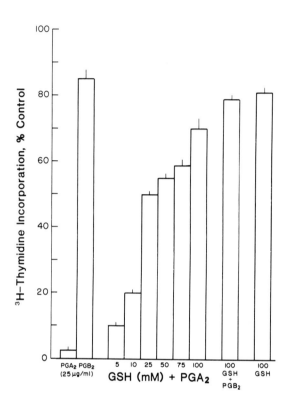

FIGURE 2. Inhibition of B16a Cell DNA Synthesis by PGA₂ and PGB₂
Following Preincubation with Reduced Glutathione.

eq. 4

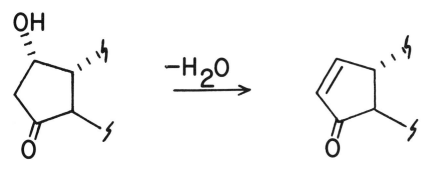

isomerization to a $\Delta^{12,13}$ isomer. Figure 3 compares the effects of PGD$_2$ and PGJ$_2$ on B16a proliferation. As predicted, PGJ$_2$ was a more potent inhibitor. Similar results have recently been reported by Narumiya and Fukushima (14) for inhibition of proliferation of L-1210 leukemia cells by Δ^{12}-prostaglandin J$_2$.

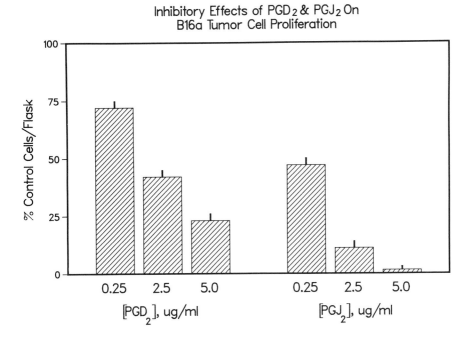

FIGURE 3. Comparison of the Effects of PGD$_2$ and PGJ$_2$ on Proliferation of B16a Cells.

It appears that our hypothesis, if not correct, is at least useful for predicting structures that can inhibit proliferation and, of course, there are a number of obvious modifications of the molecule which can be synthesized. Our results with the NP-2 neuroblastoma cell line suggests that the same analysis can be applied to the induction of differentiation by prostaglandins (Figure 4; 10). PGA_2, PGA_1 and epi-PGA_2 are about equipotent at induction of differentiation of a mouse neuroblastoma line. PGE_2 is less active and PGB_2 is inactive.

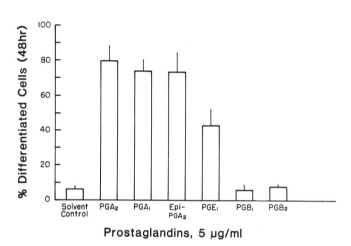

Effects of Prostaglandins on Neuroblastoma Cell Differentiation

FIGURE 4. Effects of Prostaglandins on Neuroblastoma Cell Differentiation.

II. METASTASIS

Nafazatrom was originally developed by Bayer Pharmaceuticals as an antithrombotic agent (15). Vermylen and co-workers (16) reported that nafazatrom stimulates prostacyclin (PGI_2) biosynthesis and that this might be the mechanism by which it exerts an antithrombotic effect . Based on this hypothesis and the known antimetastatic activity of PGI_2 (17-19), Honn et al. (20) tested nafazatrom as an antimetastatic agent and found that it demonstrated efficacy against spontaneous metastasis from subcutaneous B16 amelanotic melanoma and Lewis lung carcinoma tumors. An apparent lack of toxicity makes nafazatrom an ideal candidate for chronic administration in humans for the prevention of metastasis. There have been three mechanisms proposed in the literature for nafazatrom's activity. Nafazatrom 1) may protect the enzymes of PGI$_2$ biosynthesis from inactivation (21), 2) inhibit lipoxygenase activity (22) or 3) inhibit 15-hydroxy prostaglandin dehydrogenase, an enzyme that inactivates PGI$_2$ (23).

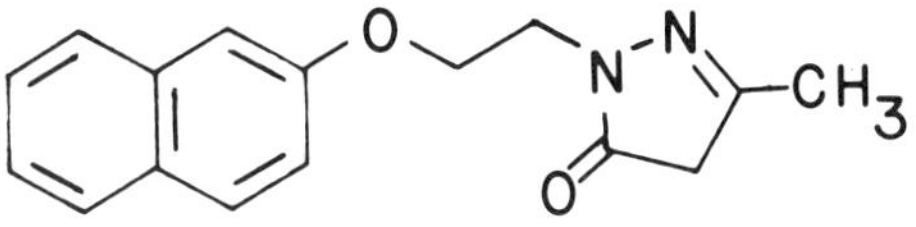

Nafazatrom

(Bay g 6575)

Antithrombotic, antimetastatic, elevates PGI$_2$ levels in vivo.

There are two major pathways (lipoxygenase and cyclooxygenase) of oxygenation of unsaturated fatty acids in mammalian tissue; both generate hydroperoxides as intermediates. The lipoxygenases introduce one molecule of molecular oxygen to form fatty acid hydroperoxides whereas cyclooxygenase introduces two molecules of oxygen to make a hydroperoxy endoperoxide PGG$_2$ (Figure 5). The hydroperoxide group is then reduced by peroxidases to PGH$_2$.

Several of the enzymes of prostaglandin biosynthesis are heme proteins; heme proteins are very sensitive to irreversible inactivation by hydroperoxy fatty acids. The hydroperoxide PGG$_2$ inactivates the cyclooxygenase component of PGH synthase and PGI$_2$ synthase irreversibly (24,25). In contrast, it has very little effect on thromboxane synthase or the isomerases that convert PGH$_2$ to PGE$_2$ and PGD$_2$. Molecules that are reducing substrates for the peroxidase reduce PGG$_2$ to PGH$_2$ (26). PGH$_2$ has an alcohol at carbon 15 instead of a hydroperoxide and does not irreversibly inactivate any of these proteins. It was our hypothesis that molecules like nafazatrom might act by being peroxidase substrates, lowering the steady state level of hydroperoxide and protecting the various enzymes of PGI$_2$ biosynthesis from inactivation.

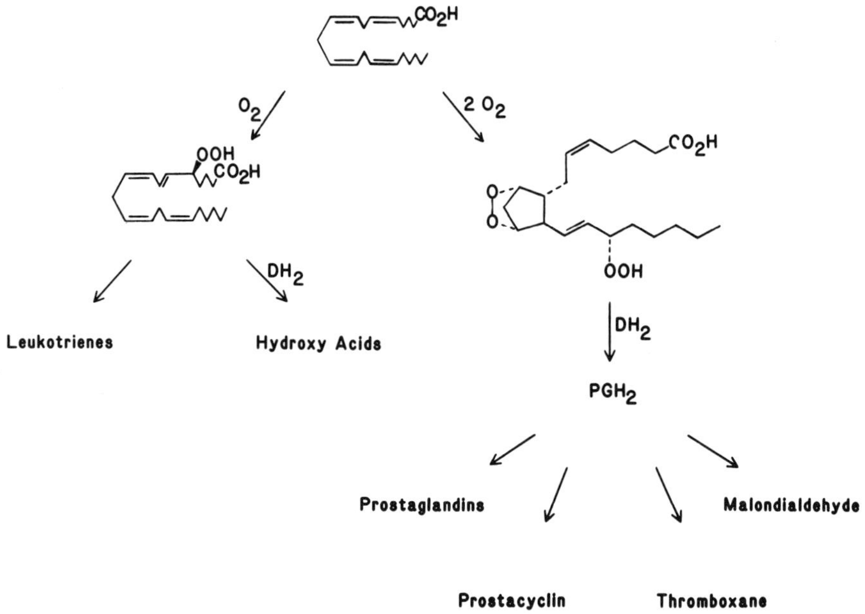

FIGURE 5. Pathways of Arachidonic Acid Oxygenation in Animal Tissue.

We developed a new assay to determine the ability of molecules to act as peroxidase reducing substrates (Figure 6). 5-Hydroperoxide-1-phenyl-1-pentene was incubated with a peroxidase in the presence or absence of a reducing substrate. If the molecule is a reducing substrate it triggers many catalytic turnovers and there is a net reduction of the hydroperoxide to the alcohol. Of the three examples depicted in Figure 6, nafazatrom was the best. The data in Figure 7 demonstrates the ability of nafazatrom to stimulate the cyclooxygenase activity of purified PGH synthase when incubated in increasing concentrations. Nafazatrom caused about a twofold stimulation of cyclooxygenase activity, which may be due to its ability to protect the cyclooxygenase from hydroperoxide-induced inactivation.

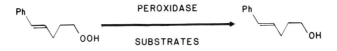

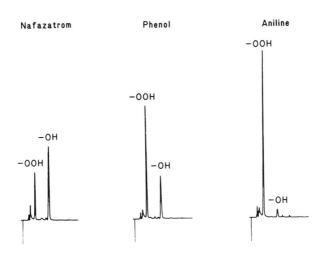

FIGURE 6. HPLC Analysis of Incubations of 5-Phenyl-4-pentenyl-hydro-
peroxide with PGH Synthase and Reducing Substrates. -OOH is
5-phenyl-4-pentenyl-hydroperoxide and -OH is the reduction product
5-phenyl-4-pentenyl-alcohol.

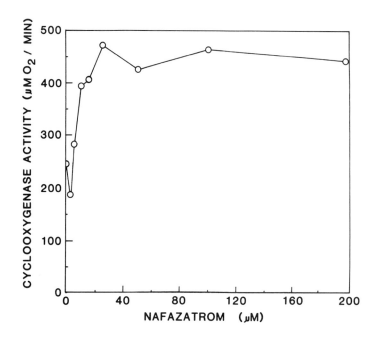

FIGURE 7. Effect of Increasing Nafazatrom Concentrations on Arachidonate Oxygenation by Purified and Hematin-Reconstituted PGH Synthase.

Previous work from our laboratory has demonstrated that nafazatrom can protect PGI_2 synthase from inactivation by fatty acid hydro-peroxides (21). Incubation of increasing amounts of 15-HPETE with PGI_2 synthase preparations diminishes their ability to convert PGH_2 to PGI_2. Inactivation is nearly completely prevented by nafazatrom. Under similar conditions we can show in vitro that nafazatrom stimulates prostacyclin biosynthesis about 10-fold (21). The ability of nafazatrom to act as a lipoxygenase inhibitor may also contribute to its protection or enhancement of PGI_2 biosynthesis in vivo because hydroperoxy fatty acid products of lipoxygenase are also potent irreversible inactivators of heme proteins.

Does inactivation of cyclooxygenase and PGI_2 synthase by hydro-peroxides occur in vivo and are molecules like nafazatrom protective? Brotherton and Hoak (27) have shown that repeated stimulation of cultured vascular endothelial cells by A23187, arachidonic acid, and thrombin inactivates cyclooxygenase but not PGI_2 synthase. Kent et al. (28) have reported that arachidonate oxygenation by perfused aorta leads to more extensive inactivation of cyclooxygenase than PGI_2 synthase. Deckmyn et al. (29) have demonstrated that stimulation of vascular arachidonate oxygenation in vivo leads to local "exhaustion" of PGI_2 biosynthesis within 5 hr. Nafazatrom substantially protects against this exhaustion (29). Thus, it appears that the enzymes of PGI_2 biosynthesis are labile to peroxide-induced inactivation during arachidonate oxygenation. Surprisingly, though, cyclooxygenase is apparently more sensitive than PGI_2 synthase. This may be due to a proximity effect (the hydroperoxide inactivates more extensively near the site of its generation) or to inactivation by an oxidant generated during the oxygenation of arachidonate to PGG_2 (30). Regardless, the ability to protect enzymes of PGI_2 biosynthesis from suicide inactivation appears to be a new mechanism of drug action and assays of the protective ability of different compounds may constitute a rapid in vitro screen for the development of a novel class of antimetastatic agents.

ACKNOWLEDGMENTS:

LJM is a recipient of a Faculty Research Award from the American Cancer Society (FRA 243). Original work in the authors' laboratories have been generously supported by the Williams International Corporation.

REFERENCES

1. Gorman RR: Prostaglandin endoperoxides: Possible new regulators of cyclic nucleotide metabolism. J. Cycl. Nucleotide Res. 1:1-9, 1975.
2. Mills DCB, Smith JB: Influence on platelet aggregation of drugs that affect accumulation of adenosine 3'-5-cyclic monophosphate in platelets. Biochem. J. 121:185-196, 1971.
3. Harris RH, Ramwell PW, Gilmer PJ: Cellular mechanisms of prostaglandin action. Ann. Rev. Physiol. 41:653-668, 1979.
4. Gorman RR, Bunting S, Miller OV: Modulation of human platelet adenylate cyclase by prostacyclin (PGX). Prostaglandins 13:377-388, 1977.
5. Powles TJ, Bockman RS, Honn KV, Ramwell P (eds.) Prostaglandins and Cancer: First International Conference. Alan R. Liss, New York, 1982.
6. Thaler-Dao H, Crastes de Paulet A, Paoletti R (eds.) Icosanoids and Cancer , Raven Press, New York, 1984.
7. Santoro MG, Philpott GW, Jaffe BM: Inhibition of tumor-growth in vivo and in vitro by prostaglandin-E. Nature 263:777-779, 1976.
8. Santoro MG, Philpott GW, Jaffe BM: Inhibition of B-16 Melanoma growth in vivo by a synthetic analog of prostaglandin-E2. Cancer Res. 37:3774-3779, 1977.
9. Honn KV, Dunn JR, Morgan LR, Bienkowski M, Marnett LJ: Inhibition of DNA synthesis in Harding-Passey melanoma cells by prostaglandins A_1 and A_2: comparison with chemotherapeutic agents. Biochem. Biophys. Res. Comm. 87:795-801, 1979.

114

10. Honn KV, Marnett LJ: Requirement of a reactive α,β-unsaturated carbonyl for inhibition of tumor growth and induction of differentiation by "A" series prostaglandins. Biochem. Biophys. Res. Comm. 129:34-40, 1985.
11. Schauenstein E, Esterbauer H, Zollner H (eds): Aldehydes in Biological Systems. Their Natural Occurrence and Biological Activities. Pion Limited, London, 1977.
12. Fukushima M, Kato T, Ueds R, Ota K, Narumiya S, Hayaishi O: Prostaglandin D-2: A potential anti-neoplastic agent. Biochem. Biophys. Res. Comm. 105:956-964, 1982.
13. Fukushima M, Kato T, Ota K, Arai Y, Narumiya S, Hayaishi O: 9-Deoxy-delta-9-prostaglandin-D2: A prostaglandin-D2 derivative with potent anti-neoplastic and weak smooth muscle contracting activities. Biochem. Biophys. Res. Comm. 109:626-633, 1982.
14. Narumiya S, Fukushima M: Δ^{12}-Prostaglandin J$_2$, an ultimate metabolite of prostaglandin D$_2$ exerting cell growth inhibition. Biochem. Biophys. Res. Comm. 127:739-745, 1985.
15. Seuter F, Busse W-D, Meng K, Hoffmeister F, Moller E, Horstman H: The antithrombotic activity of Bay g6575. Arzneim. Forsch. 29:54-59, 1979.
16. Vermylen J, Chamone DAF, Verstraete M: Stimulation of prostacyclin release from vessel wall by Bay g6575: an antithrombotic compound. Lancet 1:518-520, 1979.
17. Honn KV, Cicone B, Skoff A: Prostacyclin: A potent anti-metastatic agent. Science 212:1270-1272, 1981.
18. Gorelik E, Bere WW, Herberman RB: Role of NK cells in the antimetastatic effects of anticoagulant drugs. Int. J. Cancer 33:87-94,1984.
19. Gasic TB, Gasic GJ, McEntee C, Viner ED, Gorelik E: Role of immune cells in lung tumor colony (LTC) inhibition by leech salivary gland extracts (SGE) and anticoagulants. Proc. Am. Assoc. Cancer Res. 26:51, 1985.
20. Honn KV: Control of tumor growth and metastasis with prostacyclin and thromboxane synthetase inhibitors: Evidence for a new anti-tumor and anti-metastatic agent (Bay g 6575). In: Interaction of Platelets and Tumor Cells. (Jamieson GA, ed.) Alan R. Liss, New York, pp. 295-331, 1982.
21. Marnett LJ, Siedlik PH, Ochs RC, Pagels WR, Das M, Honn KV, Warnock RH, Tainer BE, Eling TE: Mechanism of the stimulation of prostaglandin H synthase and prostacyclin synthase by the antithrombotic and antimetastatic agent, nafazatrom. Mol. Pharmacol. 26:328-335, 1984.
22. Honn KV, Dunn JR: Nafazatrom (Bay g6575) inhibition of tumor cell lipoxygenase activity and cellular proliferation. FEBS Letts. 139:65-68, 1982.
23. Wong PY-K, Chao PH-W, McGiff JC: Nafazatrom (Bay g 6575), an antithrombotic and antimetastatic agent, inhibits 15-hydroxy-prostaglandin dehydrogenase. J. Pharmacol. Exp. Ther. 223:757-760, 1982.
24. Egan RW, Paxton J, Kuehl FA,Jr.: Mechanism for irreversible self-deactivation of prostaglandin synthetase. J. Biol. Chem. 251:7329-7335, 1976.

25. Moncada S, Gryglewski RJ, Bunting S, Vane JR: A lipid peroxide inhibits the enzyme in blood vessel microsomes that generates from prostaglandin endoperoxides the substance (prostaglandin X) which prevents platelet aggregation. Prostaglandins 12:715-737, 1976.
26. Ohki S, Ogino N, Yamamoto S, Hayaishi O: Prostaglandin hydroperoxidase, an integral part of prostaglandin endoperoxide synthetase from bovine vesicular gland microsomes. J. Biol. Chem. 254:829-836, 1979.
27. Brotherton AF, Hoak JC: Prostacyclin biosynthesis in cultured vascular endothelium is limited by deactivation of cyclooxygenase. J. Clin. Invest. 72:1255-1261, 1983.
28. Kent RS, Diedrich SL, Whorton AR: Regulation of vascular prostaglandin synthesis by metabolites of arachidonic acid in perfused rabbit aorta. J. Clin. Invest. 72:455-465, 1983.
29. Deckmyn H, Van Houte E, Verstraete M, Vermylen J: Manipulation of the local thromboxane and prostacyclin balance in vivo by the antithrombotic compounds dazoxiben, acetylsalicylic acids, and nafazatrom. Biochem. Pharmacol. 32:2757-2762, 1983.
30. Hemler ME, Graff G, Lands WEM: Accelerative autoinactivation of prostaglandin biosynthesis by PGG_2. Biochem. Biophys. Res. Comm. 85: 1325-1331, 1978.

CHAPTER 9. PLATELET-TUMOR CELL INTERACTIONS AS A TARGET FOR ANTIMETASTATIC THERAPY

K.V. HONN, J.M. ONODA, D.G. MENTER, P.G. CAVANAUGH, J.D. CRISSMAN, J.D. TAYLOR AND B.F. SLOANE

I. INTRODUCTION

The capacity for metastatic spread can be reasonably regarded as the single most important characteristic of malignant tumors. Metastasis as simply defined is the loss of contiguity between a tumor cell or clumps of tumor cells and the primary lesion followed by successful transfer to and growth at a site spatially separate from the original tumor. The overall process can be viewed as a series of sequential events representing complex interactions between the tumor cell and the host (Figure 1). Following the release of tumor cells from the primary tumor they are transported passively (dissemination) in the circulatory system. In order to successfully colonize the distant metastatic site the tumor cell must first arrest (implantation) and then invade (extravasation) through the vessel wall. The process of arrest and extravasation are the most critical steps in the metastatic cascade for circulating tumor cells.

Several studies report large numbers of circulating cancer cells in tumor bearing animals. Butler and Gullino (1) determined that 3-4,000,000 cells/24 hr/g of tumor are shed from subcutaneous MTWG mammary carcinomas. Glaves (2) has recently demonstrated large numbers of Lewis lung carcinoma cells released into circulation from primary subcutaneous tumors. The above mentioned studies report large numbers of circulating cancer cells in tumor-bearing animals. The actual number of metastases found in these animals is orders of magnitude lower than would be predicted by the number of circulating cells, suggesting that metastasis is an inefficient process (3). In our laboratory we found that B16 amelanotic melanoma (B16a) tumor cells were temporarily arrested in the pulmonary microvasculature following intravenous injection into the tail vein of mice. These cells were then slowly released so that less than 5% of the original inoculum remained in the lung after 20 hr (4). Weiss and co-workers demonstrated that the majority of tumor cells initially arrested in the lung (5) of mice following tail vein injection, or arrested in the liver (6) following portal vein injection, are subsequently released as non-viable cells. They have suggested that metastatic inefficiency is due to the death of most circulating cancer cells in the first organ encountered after leaving the primary tumor (6). For example, bioassay data indicated that of 80,000 B16 cells released from the liver after portal vein injection of 100,000 cells, only 1% were delivered to the lung in a viable state (6). This suggests that metastasis to these

118

"secondary organs" might be the result of cells released from
metastases in the "first organ" as opposed to direct seeding from the
primary tumor (metastasis from metastases, see Chapter 23).

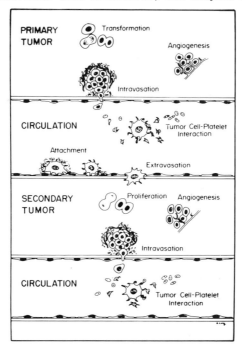

FIGURE 1. Overview of the Metastatic Cascade. The primary tumor is
believed to be initiated by transformation (i.e., chemical, radiation
or viral) of a normal cell which then proliferates until limited by
blood supply and invasive properties of the tumor. As the tumor grows,
the tumor cells release angiogenesis factors which induce neovascularization. To move to a secondary site, the tumor cells must be
able to detach from the primary tumor and invade into the circulatory
system (intravasate), wherein the tumor cells may interact with host
cells during transport. Tumor cells can induce platelet aggregation
and this in turn is thought to facilitate attachment of tumor cells to
the endothelium. Endothelial cell retraction followed by dissolution
of the basement membrane by proteolytic enzymes released from the tumor
cell then may enable the cells to extravasate at a secondary site, at
which the processes of proliferation, angiogenesis, invasion and
metastasis (from a metastasis) can reoccur.

The mechanism for the killing of tumor cells following arrest in
the first organ is unclear. Gabor and Weiss (7) have suggested that
mechanically induced trauma to cancer cells passing through the
microcirculation may decrease their ability to successfully
metastasize. Using an in vitro model of tumor cells passing through
polycarbonate membranes these authors have categorized damage to L1210

and Ehrlich ascites tumor cells which includes loss of viability. A detailed fluid mechanical analysis suggests that the friction generated between cancer cell membranes and the intraluminal surface of capillaries could cause membrane rupture (8). Circulating tumor cells may be also destroyed by effectors of the host cytotoxic immune system (natural killer cells, see Chapter 15; monocytes, see Chapter 14). In addition, neutrophils may accelerate the clearance of arrested tumor cells (9). Inflammatory neutrophils are capable of effecting the lysis of tumor cells in vitro (10). In contrast, Starkey et al. (11) have demonstrated that polymorphonuclear leukocytes (PMN) and activated macrophages lead to a considerable increase in the number of tumor cells attaching to endothelial cell monolayers in vitro. Mixed spheroids containing tumor cells and PMN's led to increased tumor cell retention in the lungs following i.v. injection when compared to tumor cells alone (11).

Once a tumor cell is in circulation it can undergo a variety of cell-cell interactions. Some of these interactions may be deleterious as suggested above. Others may facilitate tumor cell metastasis. One type of cell-cell interaction which may facilitate metastasis is the interaction between the circulating tumor cells and the host platelet. This interaction may be mediated via the activation of elements of the host's coagulation cascade as described below.

II. PLATELETS, COAGULATION AND METASTASIS

Patients with malignant neoplasms often demonstrate abnormalities in their blood coagulability (12-15). These abnormalities include hyperaggregability of platelets (12), with resultant thrombocytopenia (16), and a reduction in fibrinogen concomitant with an increase in fibrin-fibrinogen degradation products (13,17,18). Tumor cells have been reported to possess both a platelet-activating material (19-22 and see below) and a procoagulant activity responsible for alterations in the fibrin-fibrinogen system (23-25, Chapter 11 and see below) and possibly platelet aggregation (26). The incidence of thromboembolic disease (TED) in cancer patients is not peculiar to any single tumor type. However, some tumor types have an increased frequency. For example, a recent review of the literature revealed TED frequencies of 25.6%, 17.5% and 15.2% in lung, pancreas and colon cancer patients respectively (15). In contrast, the frequency in breast and kidney cancer patients were 2% and 0.4% respectively (15). The incidence of TED may be related to the hemostatic parameter being measured and the extent of disease.

Measurement of fibrinopeptide A in a series of patients with various malignancies revealed elevated levels in 95% of the patients with metastatic disease and 27% of the patients with local disease (15). Ferriere et al. (27) measured β-thromboglobulin levels in a series of breast cancer patients. β-thromboglobulin is normally found in platelet α granules and its presence in serum is an indication of platelet activation. In this series all patients demonstrated elevated β-thromboglobulin levels compared to age matched controls. No correlation with stage of disease was observed.

The interaction of tumor cells with host platelets is believed to facilitate metastasis; however, the exact mechanism is, at this time, unknown. It is generally accepted that tumor cells become damaged during circulatory transport. This circulatory trauma may be due to humoral factors (i.e., macrophages, natural killer cells and antibody-mediated complement lysis) and physical factors (i.e., shear forces and mechanical trauma due to passage through the microvasculature). Tumor cells shielded within platelet thrombi may be protected from some or all of the above. In addition, platelets may enhance tumor cell adhesion to endothelial or de-endothelialized surfaces via platelet bridges. Finally, tumor cell survival and multiplication may be enhanced due to the release of platelet mitogenic factors [i.e., platelet-derived growth factor (28)]. It is generally accepted that platelets enhance metastasis by facilitating processes that occur during tumor cell arrest and adhesion (29,30); whether that includes direct facilitation of adhesion and/or protection of arrested tumor cells from cellular immune destruction (31) is not certain. Injection of tumor cells i.v. has been observed to induce platelet aggregation (32). Thrombocytopenia induced by neuraminidase or antiplatelet antiserum results in decreased lung colony formation from tail vein-injected tumor cells (33) and spontaneous metastasis from s.c. tumors (34).

III.   TUMOR CELL PLATELET AGGREGATING ACTIVITY/PROCOAGULANT ACTIVITY (PAA/PCA)

A. Purification from Rodent Tumors

The factor(s) responsible for the induction of platelet aggregation by tumor cells have not been purified by other laboratories. Partial purification of platelet aggregating activity from cultured tumor cells has been accomplished by urea (1 M) extraction (35,36). Plasma membrane fragments (37) and plasma membrane-derived vesicles (38) from tumor cells have also been shown to possess platelet aggregating activities.

O'Meara and his associates were the first to study a tumor-derived procoagulant (39). In the past ten years two separate factors have been identified as responsible for the initiation of blood coagulation by tumor cells. The first of these is named cancer procoagulant and is a cysteine proteinase that directly activates factor X (see Chapter 11). The second of these is tissue factor which is a lipo-protein procoagulant also associated with normal tissue. Gordon and co-workers (40-43) purified cancer procoagulant from a soluble extract of rabbit V_2 carcinoma cells, extracted at alkaline pH (7.8). The factor X activating activity of cancer procoagulant can be inhibited with cysteine proteinase inhibitors, however, cancer procoagulant appears to differ in amino acid composition from other known cysteine proteinases.

Many investigators who have examined the mechanism of tumor cell accelerated coagulation have suggested thromboplastin (tissue factor) as the tumor cell procoagulant. However, tissue factor has not been purified to homogeneity from any tumor sources. The activity of thromboplastin is dependent on the presence of coagulation factor VII in the assay system (44). The absence of tumor procoagulant activity in factor VII deficient plasma has been used as the criterion for identifying tumor procoagulant activity as thromboplastin. Based on this criterion Kinjo et al. (45) found that the procoagulant activity of 14 lines of human cultured tumor cells is due to the presence of thromboplastin in the cells themselves. Hudij and Bajaj (46) have reported that the human monocytic tumor line U-937 coagulates plasma through the action of thromboplastin. Khato et al. (47) concluded that the procoagulant activity in 8 strains of Yoshida ascites hepatoma cells is due to thromboplastin. Dvorak et al. (48) have found that plasma membrane vesicles shed from 13 different lines of guinea pig mouse and human origin coagulate plasma through a thromboplastin dependent mechanism. All of the above mentioned studies are suspect because of the possibility that the tumor cells themselves adsorbed factor VII on their surface, i.e., the source of the factor VII could have been the serum used as a growth supplement in the tissue culture media. To eliminate this possibility cells must be grown in a chemically defined medium. In another study, Gouault-Heilmann et al. (49) found that antibodies to normal human brain thromboplastin neutralize the procoagulant activity of human leukemic promyelocytes. The latter work is the most convincing evidence for thromboplastin's role as a tumor procoagulant. However, the presence of thromboplastin in leukemia cells may have no relevance to solid tumor metastasis. Thromboplastin has not been purified to homogeneity from any tumor source.

We have recently purified to homogeneity from two rodent tumors a membrane bound protein that possesses both platelet aggregatory and procoagulant activities (PAA/PCA). PAA/PCA from 15091A and W256 tumor cells has a protein component, based on the fact that activity was precipitated by ammonium sulfate, was not dialyzable and was sensitive to trypsinization. This component was insoluble in an aqueous solution, however, it was readily solubilized by CHAPS, indicating that the protein involved may be hydrophobic. Like many hydrophobic enzymes and receptors (51,52), PAA/PCA required reconstitution with lipids for activity. Other investigators working with semipurified material have also found that tumor cell platelet aggregating activity is dependent on protein (53-55) and lipid (53,54,56) constituents Murine PAA/PCA (15091A) has a molecular weight of 51,000 ± 2,000 and rat PAA/PCA (W256) a molecular weight of 58,000 ± 2,000 (Figure 2).

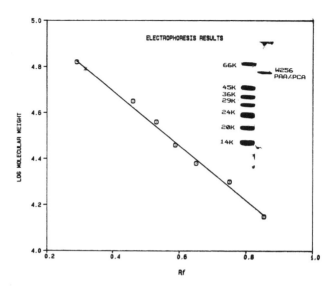

FIGURE 2. SDS-PAGE of W256 PAA/PCA. □ = M_r standards. * = PAA/PCA.

PAA/PCA induced platelet aggregation was inhibited by the thrombin inhibitors DAPA and PPACK and the coagulation inhibitor heparin; this indicates that thrombin and perhaps some other elements of the coagulation system may be involved in the aggregation process. Platelet aggregating activity copurified with procoagulant activity. Since exposure of PAA/PCA to trypsin, pH's from 5.5-10.0, different reconstitution lipids and proteinase inhibitors equally affected procoagulant and platelet aggregating activity, the cell components responsible for these two activities may be the same. Initially, PAA/PCA may be reacting in the washed platelet system, with calcium and plasma, to activate the coagulation cascade and produce thrombin. The thrombin formed could then induce platelet aggregation. Washed platelets are activated and will aggregate in response to low levels of thrombin (56).

Some investigators have found proteinases in tumor cells which can activate coagulation cascade zymogens (39,57,58). Pretreatment of PAA/PCA with high levels of phenanthroline, PMSF, TLCK, iodoacetamide or Z-Phe-Ala-CHN$_2$ did not significantly inhibit PAA/PCA's ability to induce platelet aggregation or to cause coagulation, indicating that PAA/PCA was probably not a metalloproteinase, a serine proteinase or a cysteine proteinase. These results are in disagreement with our previously published reports which hypothesized that a tumor cathepsin B-like cysteine proteinase is involved in tumor cell induced platelet aggregation (59,60). Low concentrations of the cysteine proteinase inhibitors, leupeptin, iodoacetamide and antipain, inhibit cathepsin B-like activity in B16a and 15091A tumor cells in parallel with their inhibition of platelet aggregation induced by these cells, whereas two serine proteinase inhibitors, aprotinin and SBTI, have no effect on either tumor cell cathepsin B-like activity or platelet aggregation (59,60). However, we have since determined that leupeptin (100 μM) was also able to prolong the recalcification time of human and rat plasmas (unpublished results). In our previous studies, the proteinase inhibitors may have been acting on coagulation factors activated during platelet aggregation and not on a tumor cell cathepsin B-like cysteine proteinase. However, we have not excluded the possibility that tumor cells possess more than one platelet aggregating and/or procoagulant activity.

B. Purification of Procoagulant from Normal Rat Lungs

As discussed above two procoagulants have been previously reported: a cysteine proteinase and tissue factor. We have demonstrated that PAA/PCA is devoid of cysteine and all other proteinase activities (50) and is, therefore, not the factor isolated by Gordon and co-workers (see Chapter 11). In order to demonstrate that PAA/PCA is distinct from normal cell procoagulant we purified the procoagulant material from normal rat lungs. Like tumor PAA/PCA, lung procoagulant was particulate associated, was solubilized with CHAPS and was separated on DEAE cellulose. There seem to be differences between the procoagulant nature of normal lung tissue and that of tumor tissue. Normal rat lung procoagulant appeared to possess less of a negative charge at pH 7.5 or 8.5 than rat tumor PAA/PCA does. The lung procoagulant eluted from DEAE cellulose at low (0.05 - 0.1 M) KCl concentrations and eluted from octylamine agarose with detergent only; tumor PAA/PCA required both detergent and KCl for elution from this gel.

C. Mechanistic Studies

We have recently performed mechanistic studies with PAA/PCA isolated from rat Walker 256 carcinosarcoma (W256) tumor cells and procoagulant isolated from normal rat lungs. Purified material from W256 tumor cells was tested in factor deficient human plasma for coagulation time and the ability of plasma to support tumor cell induced platelet aggregation (TCIPA). The data in Table 1 demonstrates a lack of PAA/PCA dependence on factors V, VII, IX and XII for induction of coagulation. However, PAA/PCA was found to be dependent on factor X (Table 1). PAA/PCA induced platelet aggregation was independent of factors I, V, VII X and XII (Table 2). As observed with PAA/PCA induced coagulation, platelet aggregation was dependent upon Factor X in addition to Factor II (prothrombin). In contrast to the above studies with PAA/PCA, normal rat lung procoagulant was dependent on the presence of Factor VII suggesting that this material may be tissue factor (Table 3).

Table 1. W256 PAA/PCA Induced Coagulation of Factor Deficient Human Plasmas.

Plasma	Coagulation Time (min)	
	Without W256 PAA/PCA	With W256 PAA/PCA
Normal	4.30 ± .05	2.27 ± .04
V Deficient	4.55 ± .10	2.26
VII Deficient	4.40 ± .15	1.96 ± .05
IX Deficient	5.00 ± .10	2.40 ± .10
X Deficient	7.70 ± .20	6.20 ± .10*
XII Deficient	6.82 ± .23	1.94 ± .05

Table 2. W256 PAA/PCA Induced Platelet Aggregation Supported by Factor Deficient Human Plasmas.

Plasma added to System	Aggregation Lag Time (min)	
	Without W256 PAA/PCA	With 256 PAA/PCA
Normal	> 11.0	2.5
I Deficient	9.2	2.3
II Deficient	> 12.0	6.8*
V Deficient	7.0	2.3
VII Deficient	> 10.0	2.3
IX Deficient	> 10.0	2.1
X Deficient	> 10.0	6.3*
XII Deficient	> 10.0	2.1

Table 3.   Coagulation of Normal and Factor VII Deficient Human Plasmas
by Normal Rat Lung Procoagulant.

Plasma	Coagulation Time (min)	
	Without Rat Lung PCA	With Rat Lung PCA
Normal	4.70	1.33
VII Deficient	4.50	3.27

IV.   IN VITRO OBSERVATIONS OF TUMOR CELL-PLATELET INTERACTIONS AND
THEIR INHIBITION BY PROSTACYCLIN (PGI$_2$)

A. Aggregometry Studies

Numerous investigators have demonstrated that a variety of human
and animal tumor cells induce platelet aggregation (for review see 61).
All of these studies have utilized whole dispersates (mechanical or
enzymatic) of solid tumors or tissue-cultured cells. We have utilized
tumor cells purified by centrifugal elutriation from a collagenase-
derived dispersate of a solid tumor or from an ascites tumor (62).
Elutriated B16a, Lewis lung carcinoma (3LL), 15091A mammary adenocarcinoma, and W256 carcinosarcoma cells induced aggregation of human
platelet-rich plasma (PRP) following a short lag time (63).   The
aggregation of human PRP by tumor cells occurred concomitantly with the
generation of thromboxane A$_2$ (TXA$_2$; 64,65). Tumor cells do not cause
the aggregation of washed platelets. Calcium ($>$ 1.2 mM) and a small
amount ($>$ 0.5% v/v) of platelet poor plasma are absolute requirements.

B. Ultrastructural Studies

We have recently examined by electron microscopy, tumor cell
platelet interactions in vitro and in vivo. For the in vitro studies
rat (Sprague Dawley) platelet rich plasma was placed in an aggregometry
cuvette and challenged with elutriated rat W256 carcinosarcoma cells.
Samples were removed, fixed at timed intervals (0.5 - 10 min) and
examined via SEM or TEM to evaluate the extent of tumor cell-platelet
interactions.

Tumor cell-platelet interactions begin with the association of
individual platelets and platelet chains with the surface of tumor
cells (Figure 3). Homotypic aggregates of platelets form which remain
associated with tumor cells in a polar arrangement (Figure 4).   Tumor
cell-platelet interactions become progressively more extensive with
tumor cells enmeshed within platelet aggregates (Figure 5).   Tumor
cells formed large processes during the later stages of aggregation
which extend deep into the aggregate core (Figure 6). Platelet shape

126

change, granule release, and surface interactions increased with each
successive time interval until the bond between the two cell types was
irreversible.

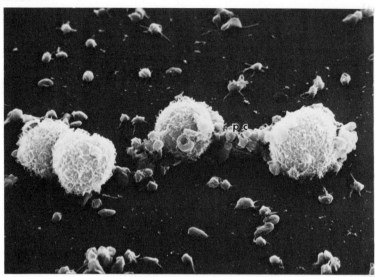

FIGURE 3.   Samples Fixed at 30 Seconds Following W256 Tumor Cell
Addition Show Activated Platelets and Platelet Chains (pc) Associated
with Tumor Cell Surfaces (magnification = 2,300).

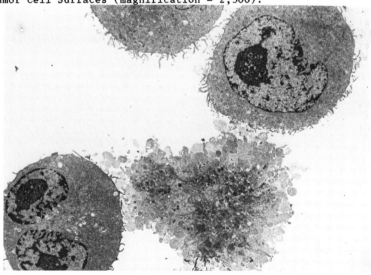

FIGURE 4.   Samples Fixed at the Midphase (2-3 min) of Aggregation
(magnification = 3,200).

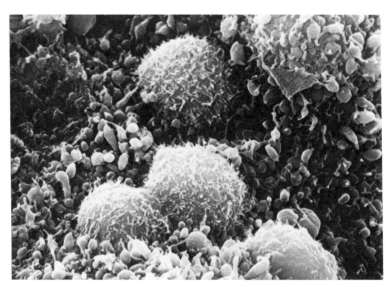

FIGURE 5. Samples Fixed Between 6-10 min Following W256 Tumor Cell
Addition Displayed Gradual Integration of Tumor Cells Deeper into the
Growing Aggregate (magnification = 4,400).

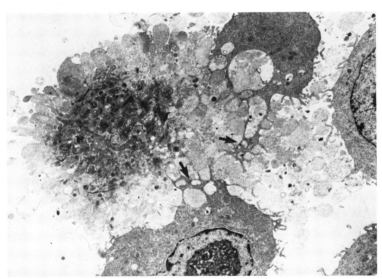

FIGURE 6. Samples Fixed at 10 min Revealed Cellular Processes which
Interdigitate with Platelets and Penetrate Toward the Center of the
Aggregate (arrows; magnification = 6,400).

128

C.   Prostacyclin Effects on Tumor Cell-Induced Platelet
      Aggregation (TCIPA) and Tumor Cell Induced Platelet Release
      Reaction (TCIPR)

1. Aggregometry studies. Menter et al. (63) studied the effectiveness
of PGI$_2$ for inhibition of TCIPA using four histologically distinct
rodent tumors (amelanotic melanoma, carcinoma, adenocarcinoma and
carcinosarcoma).   Complete inhibition of TCIPA is achieved with PGI$_2$
(10 ng/ml) despite differences in the abilities of the various tumor
lines to induce aggregation (Figure 7).   Lerner et al. (66) have also
found that PGI$_2$ inhibits platelet aggregation induced by a variety of
human tumor cell lines in vitro.   These results suggest that the
inhibitory effect of PGI$_2$ on TCIPA is not peculiar to tumor type.   In
contrast, inhibitors of TCIPA thought to be induced by ADP (67) or
thrombin (68) do not exhibit generalized inhibition.

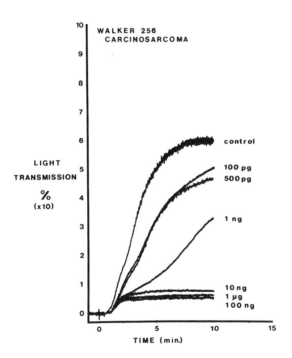

FIGURE 7.   Prostacyclin Inhibition of W256 Carcinosarcoma Induced
Platelet Aggregation.

Comparison of the inhibitory effects of PGI$_2$ on TCIPA with that of other icosanoids reveals that the stable hydrolysis product of PGI$_2$ (6-keto-PGF$_{1\alpha}$) is essentially ineffective in inhibiting TCIPA, whereas PGE$_1$ and PGD$_2$ are 100-fold less potent than PGI$_2$ (63). Prostacyclin is also ten times more potent than 6-keto-PGE$_1$ or dibutyryl cAMP for inhibition of TCIPA (66).

One characteristic feature of platelet aggregation is the release reaction. During the release reaction, materials stored in platelet granules (dense granules, α granules and lysosomes) are released from the platelet. Not all stimuli provoke release from all three granule compartments. The dense granules contain high concentrations of amines (serotonin), adenine nucleotides and divalent cations. The α granules contain a variety of proteins, among which are heparin-neutralizing protein (PF4), β-thromboglobulin, fibrinogen, fibronectin, thrombo-spondin and platelet-derived growth factors. Lysosomes contain acid phosphatase, β-N-acetylglucosaminidase (β-NAG), β-glucuronidase, cathepsins D and B, collagenase and others. Several of the platelet-derived factors could conceivably aid in tumor metastasis. Dense-granule serotonin is a potent vascoconstrictor and can stimulate further platelet aggregation. α Granule-derived β-thromboglobulin inhibits production of PGI$_2$, which has demonstrated antimetastatic activity (see below), by the vascular endothelium, whereas platelet-derived fibronectin could coat tumor cells and increase adhesiveness. In addition, platelet-derived fibrinogen could contribute to tumor cell-associated fibrin. Finally, platelet-derived growth factors have been demonstrated to be mitogenic for several animal and human tumor cells (28).

A variety of human and animal tumor cells have been demonstrated to evoke the release of platelet dense granules. We have previously demonstrated that prostacyclin inhibits the release of platelet dense granules measured by the release of ^{14}C serotonin (69). In addition, we have found that PGI$_2$ caused a dose-dependent decrease in platelet α granule release (measured as β-thromboglobulin release) induced by W256 cells (Table 4).

Table 4. W256 Carcinosarcoma-Induced β-Thromboglobulin Release.

Dose of Prostacyclin	% Control β-thromboglobulin release	% Control platelet aggregation
100 ng	3.5 ± 3.5[*]	10.7 ± 1.7
10 ng	8.5 ± 4.3	12.5 ± 2.7
1 ng	58.9 ± 36.6	64.2 ± 14.2
100 pg	87.2 ± 19.3	92.5 ± 16.0

[*]Mean ± SEM; n = 3.

2. Ultrastructural studies. Platelets were treated with PGI_2 prior to the addition of elutriated W256 cells. Samples were removed, fixed at 0.5 and 10 min and examined ultrastructurally. Prostacyclin effectively inhibited tumor cell induced platelet aggregation at a dose of 10 ng/ml. Ultrastructural studies revealed that most platelets retained their normal discoid appearance. A few platelets demonstrated pseudopod formation and an occasional platelet was found attached to a tumor cell (Figure 8). Platelets found in association with the tumor cell plasma membrane had undergone the release reaction (Figure 9). Higher doses of prostacyclin (> 10 ng/ml) completely inhibited pseudopod formation and platelet association with the tumor cell plasma membrane (Figure 10).

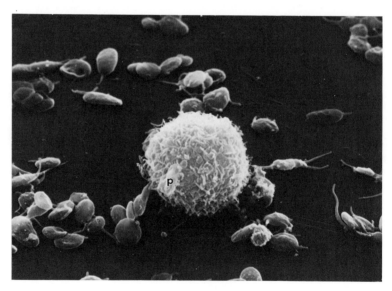

FIGURE 8. In Prostacyclin Treated Samples (10 ng/ml) the Majority of Platelets Were Not Activated and Only Small Numbers of Platelets (p) Were Associated with Tumor Cell Surfaces (magnification = 3,700).

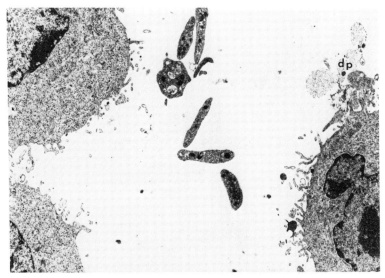

FIGURE 9. Prostacyclin Treated Samples (10 ng/ml) Revealed Only a Few Degranulated Platelets (dp) Associated with Tumor Cell Surfaces (magnification = 6,800).

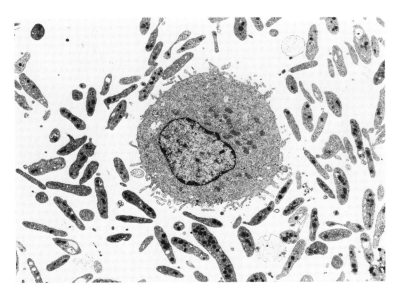

FIGURE 10. Higher Doses of Prostacyclin Completely Prevented Platelet Shape Change, Granule Release, or Association with Tumor Cell Plasma Membrane (magnification = 6,800).

Table 5. Summary of the Various In vivo Morphological Studies.

Reference	Tumor	Route of Injection	Time at Which Platelets Appear	Time of Platelet Dissolution	Time at Which Endothelium Breached With Basal Lamina Contact Established	Time at Which Tumor Cells Perivascular
Sindelar et al. (70)	Murine Fibrosarcoma	IV	Immediately	18 hr	1 da	< 3 da
Jones et al. (71)	Walker 256	IV	Immediately	8 hr	78 hr	< 2 da
Chew et al. (72)	Walker 256	IV	Immediately	12 hr	6 hr	< 36 hr
Kinjo (73)	Ascites hepatoma cell AH130	IV	Immediately	N/D	1 hr	> 2 da
Kinjo (73)	Ascites hepatoma cell AH130 F(N)	IV	Not involved	N/D	did not invade	> 10 da
Warren (74)	Walker 256	IV	Immediately	6 hr	6 hr	3 da
Wood (75)	V2 squamous cell carcinoma	IV	Immediately	N/D	30 min	3-48 hr
Crissman et al. (76)	B16 amelanotic melanoma	IV	< 10 min	24 hr	4 hr	> 5 da
Crissman et al.*	Lewis lung carcinoma	IV	< 2 min	24 hr	4 hr	> 2 da

*unpublished

V.   IN VIVO OBSERVATIONS OF TUMOR CELL-PLATELET-VESSEL WALL
     INTERACTIONS

During the past 20 years there have been several in vivo
morphological studies which have examined the role of platelets in
tumor cell arrest (Table 5).   In general platelets are found in
association with arrested tumor cells at the earliest times examined
(10 min - 1 hr).   The time to dissolution of the platelet thrombi and
eventual extravasation of the tumor cell is variable (Table 5).   None
of these earlier studies quantitated the extent of platelet involvement
in tumor cell arrest or adequately examined the temporal nature of the
association between platelets and tumor cells.   We have performed a
quantitative study of platelet involvement in the pulmonary arrest and
retention of i.v. injected B16a (76) and 3LL cells.

Elutriated tumor cells (B16a and 3LL) were injected into the
lateral tail vein of unanesthesized C57BL/6J mice.   Each animal
received 1×10^6 tumor cells in a volume of 100 µl.   The mice were
sacrificed by cervical dislocation at time intervals from 10 min to
120 hr after tumor cell injection (5 mice per time interval).   The
lungs were excised immediately and processed for light and transmission
electron microscopy.

At the earliest time interval (10 min) examined in the B16a study
platelet thrombi were observed in association with less than half of
the tumor cells (Figure 11B), increasing to a maximum association of
84% at 4 hr (Table 6).   The percentage of tumor cells in association
with platelets subsequently declined to 22% at 24 hr and 2% at 48 hr
(Table 6).   The initial arrest of circulating tumor cells was not
always associated with platelets; during the first 10 min some of the
cells appeared to have lodged in the small pulmonary capillaries.   At
later time intervals, platelet aggregates were usually identified,
often in the vascular space behind or ahead of the arrested tumor cell
(76).   At the light microscopic level, no distinction could be made
between unactivated and activated platelets, but on ultrastructural
examination platelet aggregation and degranulation could be easily
identified.   Although fibrin could be recognized by light microscopy
due to its homogeneously darker staining properties, polymerized fibrin
was more definitively observed by ultrastructural evaluation (76).
Ultrastructural observations included: association of platelets and/or
fibrin with the tumor cells, association of these cells to the
endothelium and basal lamina of the blood vessels, penetration of the
vessel walls by the tumor cells or their processes, location of the
tumor cells in an extravascular position, mitotic figures, and the
number and distribution of cytoplasmic organelles.   Platelet
activation was identified in two ways: 1) the presence of pseudopods in
platelets associated with tumor cells indicating that shape change had
occurred and 2) platelet aggregates devoid of cytoplasmic granules
indicating that the release reaction had occurred.

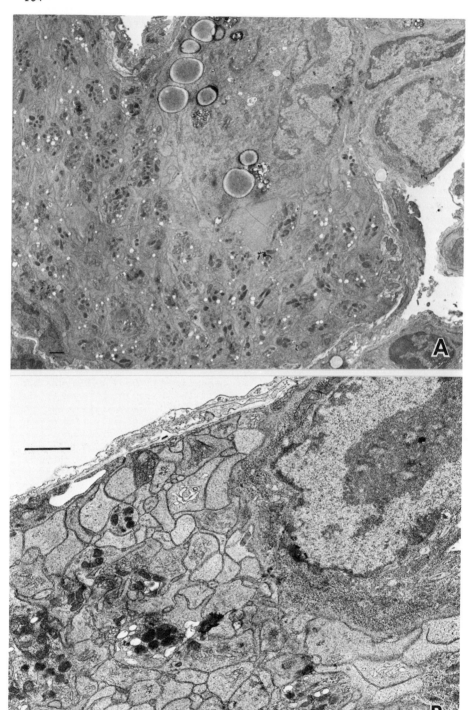

FIGURE 11. A: Lewis Lung Tumor Cell in Association with Platelets within a Pulmonary Blood Vessel at 10 min after Tail Vein Injection. Micron bar = 10 μm. B: B16a Cell in Association with Platelets within a Pulmonary Blood Vessel at 10 min after Tail Vein Injection. Micron bar = 10 μm.

Platelets were commonly adherent to the arrested B16a cells at 20 min post injection. Even at this earliest time interval numerous platelet aggregates showed evidence of degranulation indicating activation. The number of tumor cells in association with activated platelets continued to increase during the first 8 hr of observation. Similarly, the number of tumor cells with associated fibrin also increased to a maximum at 8 hr. Association between platelets/fibrin and tumor cells was defined as contact by either component with an arrested tumor cell. Every arrested B16a cell exhibited contact between the tumor cell plasma membrane and the endothelial cell plasma membrane. In no instance was the contact limited to a "bridge" of platelets or fibrin interposed between the tumor cell/endothelial cell plasma membrane. The platelet/fibrin thrombi were found on both the arterial and venous sides of the arrested tumor cell generally resulting in total occlusion of the vessel as judged by the absence of a lumen or erythrocytes in the area of the thrombi. Tumor cell associated thrombi rapidly disappeared after 24 hr. No denudation of endothelial cells with exposure of basal lamina, could be identified adjacent to arrested tumor cells and associated thrombi. Occasionally neutrophils, monocytes and lymphocytes were observed to be in contact with B16a tumor cells or to be trapped in associated thrombi. The number of these blood cells in association with B16a cells remained constant over the time intervals studied. No degeneration, necrosis or other evidence of tumoricidal interaction between leukocytes, monocytes or lymphocytes and tumor cell was observed.

Table 6. B16a Tumor Cells Observed in Pulmonary Microvasculature by Electron Microscopy.

Time after Injection	Tumor Cells With Platelets (% of Total Observed)
10 min	37%
30 min	50%
1 hr	75%
2 hr	53%
4 hr	84%
8 hr	88%
24 hr	22%
48 hr	2%
72 hr	0%
120 hr	0%

One of the most striking ultrastructural observations was the gradual displacement of the endothelial cells resulting in contact between the tumor cells and the vascular basal lamina. This phenomenon was first noted at 4 hr and by 72 hr up to 100% of the tumor cell circumference was in contact with the basal lamina. Endothelial cell displacement by tumor cells appeared to occur at endothelial-endothelial junctions with gradual "retraction" of the endothelial cells as the B16a cells progressively increased their area of basal lamina contact. The initial contact between B16a cells and basal lamina was established when thrombi were present, but this association continued to increase to 100% after the dissolution of platelet/fibrin thrombi. In many instances, after the dissipation of thrombi re-establishment of blood flow around attached tumor cells was suggested by the appearance of an identifiable lumen containing circulating erythrocytes (76). Although platelets were found near the attached tumor cells, thrombus formation or platelet activation was not identified after 48 hr (76). At this point even though tumor cells were exposed to the adjacent blood circulation no evidence of inflammatory cell, NK cell or monocyte killing of attached tumor cells could be detected.

Once contact with the basal lamina had been established, the arrested B16a cells appeared to flourish. By 24 hr, mitotic figrues could be identified in the tumor cells attached to the basal lamina. The percentage of tumor cells with mitotic figures increased with numerous examples evident at both 48 and 72 hr.

The pattern of platelet association with arrested 3LL cells was remarkably similar to that observed with B16a cells. At 2 min post injection 21% of the arrested tumor cells were associated with platelets (Table 7). This association increased to a maximum of 94% at 8 hrs and declined to zero at 48 hr. An arrested 3LL cell with associated platelets is depicted in Figure 11A.

Table 7. 3LL Tumor Cells Observed in Pulmonary Microvasculature by Electron Microscopy.

Time after Injection	Tumor Cells with Platelets (% of Total Observed)
2 min	21%
10 min	45%
30 min	74%
1 hr	72%
2 hr	75%
4 hr	72%
8 hr	94%
16 hr	38%
24 hr	20%
48 hr	0%

VI. PROSTACYCLIN, THROMBOXANES AND TUMOR CELL METASTASIS

Honn and co-workers (77-79) proposed the working hypothesis that
the primary tumor, tumor cell-shed vesicles, and/or circulating tumor
cells disrupt the intravascular balance between PGI_2 and TXA_2 in favor
of platelet aggregation. Based on the assumptions that platelet-tumor
cell and/or platelet-tumor cell-vessel wall interactions are important
for tumor cell metastasis, we proposed that (1) PGI_2 and TXA_2 synthase
inhibitors would inhibit tumor cell-induced platelet aggregation
(TCIPA) and platelet release reaction (TCIPR); (2) the exogenous
administration of PGI_2 should reduce lung colony formation by tail
vein-injected tumor cells; (3) a therapeutic synergism should result
from the use of PGI_2 with a phosphodiesterase inhibitor (since the
effect of PGI_2 is mediated by increasing concentrations of cAMP in
platelets, it follows that phosphodiesterase inhibitors, by slowing the
breakdown of cAMP, should potentiate the antithrombogenic action of
PGI_2 and thus its antimetastatic action); (4) prostacyclin acts as a
natural deterrent to tumor cell metastasis, therefore, an inhibitor of
endogenous PGI_2 biosynthesis should enhance metastasis; (5) agents
that augment PGI_2 biosynthesis or activity in vivo should function as
antimetastatic agents; and (6) thromboxane synthase inhibitors should
also possess antimetastatic activity. Evidence for the above has been
previously published (77-79).

We have previously reported that bolus i.v. injection of PGI_2 into
mice reduced lung colony formation from tail vein-injected B16a cells
by greater than 70% (77). The combination of PGI_2 with a phosphodiesterase inhibitor (theophylline) inhibited metastasis by > 93% (77).
Prostaglandins E_2, $F_{2\alpha}$ and the stable hydrolysis product of PGI_2,
6-keto-$PGF_{1\alpha}$, were ineffective (77). Prostaglandin D_2 is also antimetastatic (80), however, we found PGD_2 to be less than one-third as
effective as PGI_2 (77). The antimetastatic effects of PGI_2 are not due
to its pulmonary vasodilatory effects (78). In this regard, PGI_2 does
not significantly alter tumor cell distribution patterns. Using
$[^{125}I]$deoxyuridine-labeled tumor cells, we demonstrated (78) that,
although some alteration of cell distribution may occur, these cells
once released from the lung are not retained in the organ of secondary
arrest (liver, spleen, etc.). In addition, there is no effect of PGI_2
on the initial entrapment of tumor cells in the lung following i.v.
injection (78), which might be expected if the PGI_2 effect were due to
vasodilation. The lack of a PGI_2 effect on inititial tumor cell arrest
raises the question whether TCIPA occurs while the tumor cell is in
circulation or, alternatively, whether the critical aggregation event
occurs on arrest and attachment to the endothelium. It is clear from
our studies that PGI_2 significantly increases organ clearance of tumor
cells (78). Marcum et al. (81) utilized rabbit aortic segments in a
standard Baumgartner perfrusion chamber to study tumor cell (HUT
20)-platelet-endothelial interactions. Tumor cells and platelets were
perfused in the presence of PGE_1 (30 μg/ml) or PGI_2 (50 ng/ml). Both
agents totally inhibited TCIPA and the deposition of both tumor cells
and platelets on the vascular surface.

138

Gorelik et al. (82) have recently confirmed our initial observation that PGI_2 inhibits lung colony formation. These authors observed that the PGI_2 effect could be abrogated if the animals were pretreated with anti-asialo GM_1 serum. This antiserum inhibits natural killer (NK) cell activity. This observation led to the suggestion that platelets protect arrested tumor cells from cytotoxic immune destruction. Prostacyclin could inhibit or limit platelet association with arrested tumor cells and facilitate their destruction by NK cells. Gasic et al. (83) also observed that the antimetastatic effects of PGI_2 could be abrogated in mice rendered NK cell deficient. Despite the attractiveness of the NK cell hypothesis, we have not observed these cell-cell (NK, monocyte and tumor cell) associations in our ultra-structural studies with the B16a melanoma. There is, however, a significant association of neutrophils with arrested 3LL tumor cells (unpublished observation).

VII. CONCLUSION

The above results with PGI_2 are only representative of the antimetastatic effects which can be achieved with antiplatelet agents. Prostacyclin can only be administered parentally and, therefore, is not suited for long term antimetastatic therapy. However other anti-platelet agents, i.e., prostacyclin enhancing agents (84,85) thromboxane synthase inhibitors (84,85), adenylate cyclase stimulating agents (86), phosphodiesterase inhibitors (87) and calcium channel blockers (88) have all proved to be effective antimetastatic agents. The ideal agent should possess the following characteristics:

1. Orally active
2. Long biological half-life
3. Low chronic toxicity
4. Synergy with conventional chemotherapy
5. Absence of down-regulation in the target cell (e.g., platelets, endothelial cells).

Several of the agents described above comply with most of these characteristics and await clinical trial.

ACKNOWLEDGMENT

Original work in the authors' laboratories were supported in part by NIH/NCI grants CA29997 and CA29405 and a grant from Harper-Grace Hospitals. BFS is the recipient of a Research Career Development Award (CA00921) from the National Cancer Institute.

REFERENCES

1. Butler TP, Gullino PM: Quantitation of cell shedding into efferent blood of mammary adenocarcinoma. Cancer Res. 35:512-516, 1975.
2. Glaves D: Correlation between circulating cancer cells and incidence of metastases. Br. J. Cancer 48:665-673, 1983.
3. Weiss L: Metastatic inefficiency. In: Tumor Invasion and Metastasis. (Liotta LA and Hart IR, eds.) Martinus Nijhoff, The Hague, pp. 81-98, 1982.
4. Honn KV, Onoda JM, Menter JD, Taylor JD, Sloane BF: Prostacyclin/thromboxanes and tumor cell metastasis. In: Hemostatic Mechanisms and Metastasis. (Honn KV and Sloane BF, eds.) Martinus Nijhoff, The Hague, pp. 207-231, 1985.
5. Weiss L: Cancer cell traffic from the lungs to the liver: An example of metastatic inefficiency. Int. J. Cancer 25:385-392, 1980.
6. Weiss L, Ward PM, Holmes JC: Liver-to-lung traffic of cancer cells. Int. J. Cancer 32:79-83, 1983.
7. Gabor H, Weiss L: Mechanically induced trauma suffered by cancer cells passing through pores in polycarbonate membranes. Invasion Metastasis 5:71-83, 1985.
8. Weiss L, Dimitrou DS: A fluid mechanical analysis of the velocity, adhesion and destruction of cancer cells in capillaries during metastasis. Cell Biophys. 6:9-22, 1984.
9. Glaves P: Role of polymorphonuclear leukocytes in the pulmonary clearance of arrested cancer cells. Invasion Metastasis 3:160-173, 1983.
10. Lichtenstein A, Kahle J: Anti-tumor effect of inflammatory neutrophils: Characteristics of in vivo generation and in vitro tumor cell Lysis. Int. J. Cancer 35:121-127, 1985.
11. Starkey JR, Liggitt HD, Jones W, Hosick HL: Influence of migratory cells on the attachment of tumor cells to vascular endothelium. Int. J. Cancer 34:535-543, 1984.
12. Zacharski LR, Rickles FR, Henderson WG, Martin JF, Forman WB, van Eeckhoust JP, Cornell CJ, Forcier RJ: Platelets and malignancy. Rationale and experimental design for the VA Cooperative Study of RA-233 in the treatment of cancer. Am. J. Clin. Oncol. 5:593-609, 1982.
13. Rickles FR, Edwards RL: Activation of blood coagulation in cancer: Trousseau's syndrome revisited. Blood 62:14-31, 1983.
14. Laghi F, DiRoberto PF, Panici PB, Margariti PA, Scribano D, Cudillo L, Villani L, Bizzi B: Coagulation disorders in patients with tumors of the uterus. Tumori 69:349-353, 1983.
15. Edwards RL, Rickles FR: Hemostatic alterations in cancer patients. In: Hemostatic Mechanisms of Metastasis. (Honn KV and Sloane BF, eds.) Martinus Nijhoff, The Hague, pp. 342-354, 1984.
16. Brain MC, Azzopardi JG, Baker LRI, Pinco GF, Roberts PD, Dacic JV: Microangiopathic haemolytic anemia: The possible role of vascular lesions in pathogenesis. Br. J. Haematol. 18:183-190, 1970.
17. Donati MB, Poggi A: Malignancy and haemostasis. Br. J. Haematol. 44:173-182, 1980.

140

18. Harker LA, Slichter SJ: Platelet and fibrinogen consumption in man. N. Eng. J. Med. 287:999-1005, 1972.
19. Gasic GJ, Boettiger D, Catalfamo JL, Gasic TB, Stewart GJ: Aggregation of platelets and cell membrane vesiculation by rat cells transformed in vitro by Rous sarcoma virus. Cancer Res. 38:2950-2955, 1978.
20. Karpatkin S, Smerling A, Pearlstein E: Plasma requirement for the aggregation of rabbit platelets by an aggregating material derived from SV40-transformed 3T3 fibroblasts. J. Lab. Clin. Med. 96:994-1001, 1980.
21. Pearlstein E, Cooper LB, Karpatkin S: Extraction and characterization of a platelet-aggregating material from SV-40 transformed mouse 3T3 fibroblasts. J. Lab. Clin. Med. 93:332-344, 1979.
22. Pearlstein E, Salk PL, Yogeeswaran G, Karpatkin S: Correlation between spontaneous metastatic potential, platelet-aggregating activity of cell surface extracts, and cell surface sialylation in 10 metastatic-variant derivatives of a rat renal sarcoma cell line. Proc. Natl. Acad. Sci. USA 77:4336-4339, 1980.
23. Curatolo L, Colucci M, Cambini AL, Poggi A, Morasca L, Donati MB, Semararo N: Evidence that cells from experimental tumours can activate coagulation factor X. Br. J. Cancer 40:228-233, 1979.
24. Gordon SG, Cross BA: A factor X-activating cysteine protease from malignant tissue. J. Clin. Invest. 67:1665-1671, 1981.
25. Gordon SG, Franks JJ, Lewis B: Cancer procoagulant A: A factor X activating procoagulant from malignant tissue. Thromb. Res. 6:127-137, 1975.
26. Cavanaugh PG, Sloane BF, Bajkowski AS, Gasic TB, Gasic GJ, Honn KV: Involvement of a cathepsin B-like cysteine proteinase in platelet aggregation induced by tumor cells and their shed membrane vesicles. Clin. Exp. Metastasis 4:297-307, 1983.
27. Ferriere JP, Legros BM, Chassagne J, Chollet P, Guillard G, Plange R: β-thromboglobulin in patients with breast cancer. Am. J. Hematology 19:47-53, 1985.
28. Lipton A, Cano C, Leitzel K: Mitogenic stimulation of tumor cells by platelet derived growth factors. In: Hemostatic Mechanisms and Metastasis. (Honn KV and Sloane BF, eds.) Martinus Nijhoff, The Hague, pp. 266-281, 1984.
29. Fidler IJ: The relationship of embolic homogeneity, number, size and viability to the incidence of experimental metastasis. Eur. J. Cancer 9:223-227, 1973.
30. Liotta LA, Kleinerman J, Saidel GM: The significance of hematogenous tumor cell clumps in the metastatic process. Cancer Res. 36:889-894, 1976.
31. Gorelik E, Berc WW, Herberman RB: Role of NK cells in the antimetastatic effect of anticoagulant drugs. Int. J. Cancer 33:87-94, 1984.
32. Gastpar H: Platelet-cancer cell interaction in metastasis formation: A possible therapeutic approach to metastasis prophylaxis. J. Med. 8:103-114, 1977.
33. Gasic GJ, Gasic TB, Stewart CC: Antimetastatic effects associated with platelet reduction. Proc. Natl. Acad. Sci. USA 61:46-52, 1968.

34. Sindelar WR, Tralka TS, Ketcham AS: Electron microscopic observations on formation of pulmonary metastases. J. Surg. Res. 18:137-161, 1975.

35. Karpatkin S, Smerlin A, Pearlstein E: Plasma requirement for the aggregation of rabbit platelets by an aggregating material derived from SV40-transformed 3T3 fibroblasts. J. Lab. Clin. Med. 96:994-1001, 1980.

36. Pearlstein E, Salk P, Yogeeswaran G, Karpatkin S: Correlation between spontaneous metastatic potential, platelet aggregating activity of cell surface extracts, and cell surface sialylation in 10 metastatic-variant derivatives of a rat renal sarcoma cell line. Proc. Natl. Acad. Sci. USA 77:4336-4339, 1980.

37. Karpatkin S, Pearlstein E: Heterogenous mechanisms of tumor cell-induced platelet aggregation with possible pharmacologic strategy toward prevention of metastasis. In: Hemostatic Mechanisms of Metastasis. (Honn KV and Sloane BF, eds.) Martinus Nijhoff, The Hague, pp. 137-169, 1984.

38. Gasic GJ, Catalfamo JL, Gasic TB, Avdalovic N: In vitro mechanism of platelet aggregation by purified plasma membrane vesicles shed by mouse 15091A tumor cells. In: Malignancy and the Hemostatic System. (Donati MB, Davidson JF and Garratini S, eds.) Martinus Nijhoff, The Hague, pp. 27-35, 1981.

39. O'Meara RAQ: Coagulative properties of cancers. Irish J. Med. Sci. 394:474-479, 1958.

40. Gordon S, Cross B: A factor X-activating cysteine protease from malignant tissue. J. Clin. Invest. 67:1665-1671, 1981.

41. Gilbert LC, Gordon S: Relationship between cellular procoagulant activity and metastatic capacity of B16 mouse melanoma variants. Cancer Res. 43:536-540, 1983.

42. Gordon SG, Lewis B: Comparison of procoagulant activity in tissue culture medium from normal and transformed fibroblasts. Cancer Res. 38:2467-2472, 1978.

43. Gordon SG: A proteolytic procoagulant associated with malignant transformation. J. Histochem. Cytochem. 29:457-463, 1981.

44. Lorand L: Introduction to clotting and lysis in blood plasma. Meth. Enzymol. 45:31-37, 1976.

45. Kinjo M, Oka K, Naito S, Kohga S, Tanaka K, Oboshi S, Hayata Y, Yasumoto K: Thromboplastic and fibrinolytic activities of cultured human cancer cells. Br. J. Cancer 39:15-23, 1979.

46. Hudig D, Bajaj SP: Tissue factor-like activity of the human monocytic tumor cell line U937. Thromb. Res. 27:321-332, 1982.

47. Khato J, Suzuki M, Sato H: Quantitative study on thromboplastin in various strains of Yoshida ascites hepatoma cells of rat. GANN 65:289-294, 1974.

48. Dvorak HF, Livingston V, Bitzer AM, Dvorak AM, Anderson D, Harvey VS, Bach R, Davis GL, Dewolf W, Carvalho CA: Procoagulant activity associated with plasma membrane vesicles shed by cultured tumor cells. Cancer Res. 43:4334-4342, 1983.

49. Gouault-Heilmann M, Chardon E, Sultan C, Josso F: The pro-coagulant factor of leukaemic promyelocytes: Demonstration of immunologic cross reactivity with human brain tissue factor. Br. J. Haematol. 30:151-157, 1975.

142

50. Cavanaugh PG, Sloane BF, Bajkowski AS, Taylor JD, Honn KV: Purification and characterization of platelet aggregating activity from tumor cells: Copurification with procoagulant activity. Thromb. Res. 37:309-326, 1985.

51. Razin S: Reconstitution of biological membranes. Biochim. Biophys. Acta 265:241-296, 1972.

52. Racker E: Reconstitution of membrane processes. Meth. Enzymol. 55:699-711, 1979.

53. Hara Y, Steiner M, Baldini MG: Characterization of the platelet aggregating activity of tumor cells. Cancer Res. 40:1217-1222, 1980.

54. Karpatkin S, Pearlstein E, Salk PL, Ganesa Y: Platelet aggregating material (PAM) of two virally transformed tumors: SV3T3 mouse fibroblast and PW20 rat renal sarcoma. Role of cell surface sialylation. In: Interaction of Platelets and Tumor Cells. (Jamieson GA, ed.) Alan R. Liss, Inc., New York, pp. 445-475, 1982.

55. Gasic GJ, Gasic TB, Gasic MS, Jimenez SA: Platelet aggregating material in mouse tumor cells - removal and regeneration. Lab. Invest. 36:413-419, 1977.

56. Berndt MC, Philips DR: Platelet membrane proteins: Composition and receptor function. In: Platelets in Biology and Pathology - 2. (Gordon JL, ed.) Elsevier North Holland, Amsterdam, pp. 43-785, 1981.

57. Curatolo L, Colucci M, Cambini AL, Poggi A, Morasca L, Donati MB, Semararo N: Evidence that cells from experimental tumors can activate coagulation factor X. Br. J. Cancer 40:228-233, 1979.

58. Hilgard P, Whur P: Factor X-activating activity from Lewis lung carcinoma. Br. J. Cancer 41:642-643, 1980.

59. Honn KV, Cavanaugh PG, Evens C, Taylor JD, Sloane BF: Tumor cell-platelet aggregation: Induced by cathepsin B-like proteinase and inhibited by prostacyclin. Science 217:540-542, 1982.

60. Cavanaugh PG, Sloane BF, Bajkowski AS, Gasic GJ, Gasic TB, Honn KV: Involvement of a cathepsin B-like cysteine proteinase in platelet aggregation induced by tumor cells and their shed membrane vesicles. Clin. Exp. Metastasis 1:297-307, 1983.

61. Jamieson GA: (ed.) Interaction of Platelets and Tumor cells. Alan R. Liss, Inc., New York, 1982.

62. Ryan RE, Crissman JE, Honn KV, Sloane BF: Cathepsin B-like activity in viable tumor cells isolated from rodent tumors. Cancer Res. (In press).

63. Menter DG, Onoda JM, Taylor JD, Honn KV: Effects of prostacyclin on tumor cell induced platelet aggregation. Cancer Res. 44:450-456, 1984.

64. Menter D, Neagos G, Dunn J, Palazzo R, Tchen TT, Taylor JD, Honn KV: Tumor cell induced platelet aggregation: Inhibition by prostacyclin, thromboxane A_2 and phosphodiesterase inhibitors. In: Prostaglandins and Cancer (Powles TJ, Bockman RS, Honn KV and Ramwell PW, eds.) Alan R. Liss, New York, 809-814, 1982.

65. Grignani G, Pacchiarini L, Almasio P, Pagliasino M, Gamba G: Activation of platelet prostaglandin biosynthesis pathway during neoplastic cell induced platelet aggregation. Thromb. Res. 34:147-157, 1984.

66. Lerner WA, Pearlstein E, Ambrogio C, Karpatkin S: A mechanism for tumor-induced platelet aggregation. Comparison with mechanisms shared by other tumors with possible pharmacologic strategy toward prevention of metastases. Int. J. Cancer 31:463-469, 1983.

67. Bastida E, Ordinas A, Giardina SL, Jamieson GA: Differentiation of platelet-aggregating effects of human tumor cell lines based on inhibition studies with apyrase, hirudin and phospholipase. Cancer Res. 42:4348-4352, 1982.

68. Pearlstein E, Ambrogio C, Gasic G, Karpatkin S: Inhibition of the platelet-aggregating activity of two human adenocarcinomas of the colon and an anaplastic murine tumor with a specific thrombin inhibitor, Dansylarginine N-(3-ethyl-1,5-pentanediyl)amide. Cancer Res. 41:4535-4539, 1981.

69. Honn KV, Menter D, Moilanen D, Cavanaugh PG, Taylor JD, Sloane BF: Role of prostacyclin and thromboxanes in tumor cell platelet-vessel wall interactions. In: Protective Agents in Cancer. (McBrien DCH and Slater TF, eds.) Academic Press, New York, pp. 57-79, 1983.

70. Sindelar WF, Tralka TS, Ketcham AS: Electron microscopic observations on formation of pulmonary metastases. J. Surg. Res. 18:137-161, 1975.

71. Jones DS, Wallace AC, Fraser EF: Sequence of events in experimental metastases of Walker 256 tumor: Light, immuno-fluorescent and electron microscopic observations. J. Natl. Cancer Inst. 46:493-503, 1971.

72. Chew EC, Josephson RL, Wallace AC: Morphologic aspects of the arrest of circulating cancer cells. In: Fundamental Aspects of Metastasis. (Weiss L, ed.) North Holland Publishing Co., Amsterdam, p. 121-131, 1976.

73. Kinjo M: Lodgement and extravasation of tumor cells in blood borne metastasis: An electron microscopic study. Br. J. Cancer 38:293-303, 1978.

74. Warren BA: Origin and fate of blood-borne tumor emboli. Cancer Biol. Rev. 2:95-105, 1981.

75. Wood S, Jr: Pathogenesis of metastasis formation observed in vivo in the rabbit ear chamber. Arch. Pathol. 66:550-560, 1958.

76. Crissman JD, Hatfield J, Schaldenbrand M, Sloane BF, Honn KV: Arrest and extravasation of B16 amelanotic melanoma in murine lungs. A light and electron microscopic study. Lab. Invest. (In press).

77. Honn KV, Cicone B, Skoff A: Prostacyclin: A potent anti-metastatic agent. Science 212:1270-1272, 1981.

78. Honn KV: Inhibition of tumor cell metastasis by modulation of the vascular prostacyclin/thromboxane A_2 system. Clin. Exp. Metastasis 1:103-114, 1983.

79. Honn KV, Busse WD, Sloane BF: Prostacyclin and thromboxanes. Implications for their role in tumor cell metastasis. Biochem. Pharmacol. 32:1-11, 1983.

80. Stringfellow DA, Fitzpatrick FA: Prostaglandin D_2 controls pulmonary metastasis of malignant melanoma cells. Nature (London) 282:76-79, 1979.

81. Marcum JM, McGill M, Bastida E, Ordinas E, Jamieson GA: The interaction of platelets, tumor cells and vascular endothelium. J. Lab. Clin. Med. 96:1048-1053, 1980.

82. Gorelik E, Bere WW, Herberman RB: Role of NK cells in the antimetastatic effect of anticoagulant drugs. Int. J. Cancer 33:87-94, 1984.

83. Gasic TB, Gasic GJ, McEntee C, Viner ED, Gorelik: Role of immune cells in lung tumor colony (LTC) inhibition by leech salivary gland extracts (SGE) and anticoagulants. Proc. Am. Assoc. Cancer Res. 26:51, 1985.

84. Honn KV, Meyer J, Neagos G, Henderson T, Westley C, Ratanatharathorn V: Control of tumor growth and metastasis with prostacyclin and thromboxane synthase inhibitors: Evidence for a new antitumor and antimetastatic agent (Bay g 6575). In: Interaction of Platelets and Tumor Cells. (Jamieson GA, ed.) Alan R. Liss, Inc., New York, pp. 295-331, 1982.

85. Drago JR, Al-Mondhiry HAB: The effect of prostaglandin modulators on prostate tumor growth and metastasis. Anticancer Res. 4:391-394, 1984.

86. Agarwal KC, Parks RE: Forskolin: A potential antimetastatic agent. Int. J. Cancer 32:801-804, 1983.

87. Maniglia CA, Tudor G, Gomez J, Sartorelli AC: The effect of 2,6-Bis (diethanolamino)-4-piperidinopyrimido [5,4-d]-pyrimidine (RA233) on growth, metastasis and lung colony formation of B16 melanoma. Cancer Lett. 16:253-260, 1982.

88. Honn KV, Onoda JM, Pampalona K, Battaglia M, Neagos G, Taylor JD, Diglio CA, Sloane BF: Inhibition by dihydropyridine class calcium channel blockers of tumor cell-platelet-endothelial cell interactions in vitro and metastasis in vivo. Biochem. Pharmacol. 34:235-241, 1985.

CHAPTER 10. MECHANISMS OF INHIBITION OF CANCER DISSEMINATION BY WARFARIN

LEO R. ZACHARSKI

I. INTRODUCTION

Interest in the use of antithrombotic drugs for cancer therapy stems from studies in experimental animal tumor systems in which it has been shown that drugs of this class limit tumor dissemination (1,2). However, variability in responsiveness of various tumor types to individual agents suggests that the mechanisms of drug action may be complex. The pattern of responsiveness of human tumor types to antithrombotic drugs remains undefined, nevertheless, preliminary evidence suggests that the variability observed in experimental malignancy may exist for human tumors as well (3,4).

It is crucial that information on the possible mechanisms by which antithrombotic drugs might influence the course of cancer be carefully examined so that the results of current studies can be properly interpreted and future innovative studies can be designed. The purpose of this chapter is to examine several possible mechanisms of action of the anticoagulant, warfarin. Warfarin was chosen for this analysis because its coagulation-inhibitory properties can be measured in the laboratory (e.g., by the prothrombin time) and because warfarin is clearly of value in the treatment of thromboembolic diseases. Considerable information is available on the mechanism by which warfarin inhibits coagulation (5) and this may serve as a starting point for studies of warfarin's mechanism of action in malignancy. It is perhaps the most consistently effective single antithrombotic drug in experimental animal tumor systems (6). Efficacy for human malignancy has been claimed, based on uncontrolled trials, for several tumors such as breast cancer and lymphomas (7,8); and efficacy has been demonstrated in controlled trials for small cell carcinoma of the lung (3,4,9). For these reasons, and because it is feasible to achieve sustained, long-term anticoagulation on an outpatient basis, warfarin is applicable to further clinical investigation.

Available evidence suggests at least three possible mechanisms by which warfarin may influence neoplastic growth. These include a direct toxic effect on the tumor cells, enhancement of host defenses through augmentation of immune mechanisms, and inhibition of blood coagulation reactions. Each of these hypotheses will be considered along with strategies by which they can be tested.

146

II. WARFARIN CYTOTOXICITY

The hypothesis that warfarin ameliorates the course of cancer through a toxic mechanism presupposes the existence of metabolic pathways within neoplastic cells that are affected by this drug. A direct effect of warfarin on cells is viewed as an effect that is not mediated by the anticoagulant properties of this drug although it may be mediated by warfarin's ability to antagonize vitamin K. Alternatively, warfarin may have an adverse effect on cancer cells by an indirect mechanism, i.e., by enhancing the toxicity of other chemotherapeutic agents administered simultaneously. Evidence for the latter was presented by Kirsch and associates (10) who found that administration of warfarin results in slower clearing of 5-fluorouracil (5-FU) from plasma and in higher tissue levels of 5-FU in tumor-bearing mice. In several human subjects studied, plasma clearance of 5-FU is similarly delayed with warfarin treatment. In contrast, Chlebowski and associates (11) found that therapeutic anticoagulation with warfarin fails to alter the metabolic fate of 5-FU in humans or rabbits. Van Buskirk and Kirsch (12) observed that warfarin treatment of hepatoma-bearing mice results in a reduction of tumor cell RNA but observed no comparable warfarin effect on normal liver cells. Chang and Hill (13) reported a reduction in both DNA and RNA synthesis in tumor cells cultured in the presence of warfarin. Warfarin inhibits replication and motility of certain tumor cell lines maintained in continuous culture (10) and glioma cells cultured in the presence of warfarin exhibit cell cycle synchronization (14). Wood (15) also described reduced in vivo tumor cell motility in rabbits treated with warfarin.

The possibility of a direct effect of warfarin on tumor cells may be inferred from the structural resemblance of warfarin to quinone antibiotics which have a variety of effects on tumor cells which are of apparent therapeutic value (16). This quinone structure is a feature of both vitamin K and warfarin, and of the parent compound of warfarin, coumarin. Chlebowski et al. (17) observed a potentiating effect of vitamin K on tumor cell growth inhibition by warfarin in vitro. Both vitamin K_1 and K_3 inhibit the purine salvage pathway for DNA synthesis and this effect is synergized by warfarin. In the soft agar colony forming assay, vitamin K_3 is cytotoxic and both K_3 and warfarin potentiate the cytotoxicity of 5-FU for a variety of human tumor cell lines. Chlebowski et al. (18) also observed that in clinically achievable doses vitamin K_1 and warfarin enhance the cytotoxic effects of methotrexate and 5-FU on cultured L1210 cells. Finnegan and associates (19) found that certain coumarin derivatives are directly cytotoxic to sarcoma 180 cells in culture. The effect of warfarin on the potentiation of cytotoxic chemotherapy is apparently specific as warfarin does not potentiate the cytotoxic effects of radiation (20,21).

Warfarin may have potentially beneficial toxic effects on neoplastic cells apart from its ability to inhibit replication. Egilsson (22) showed that dicoumarol can induce differentiation in neuroblastoma cells. This effect is attributed to the ability of dicoumarol to release mitochondrial calcium. Complex theories linking disturbed vitamin K metabolism with chemical carcinogenesis have also been proposed (23,24). Israels and associates (25) found that adding warfarin or vitamin K$_3$, or creating vitamin K deficiency, inhibits benzo(a)pyrene-induced carcinogenesis resulting in delayed tumor appearance and a decreased death rate due to tumors in mice. Both Wattenberg and associates (26) and Feuer and associates (27) found inhibition of chemical carcinogenesis by coumarin. It was shown that the carcinogenicity of dimethylbenzanthracene (DMBA) is related to its metabolism by a hepatic hydroxylase. Depression of this enzyme system by coumarin is associated with a dramatic reduction in carcinogenicity (28). Hilgard (29,30) proposed that manipulation of vitamin K may alter the surface properties of neoplastic cells, which is suggested by the fact that warfarin treatment inhibits the locomotory behavior of V2 carcinoma cells in the rabbit (15,31).

The possibility that warfarin has a direct toxic effect on neoplastic cells served as the motivation for its therapeutic use in patients with malignancies (14,32). Should warfarin affect tumors by a cytotoxic mechanism, it is conceivable that cytopathic effects might be evident histologically and that warfarin may exaggerate the reduction in leukocyte and platelet counts that result from chemotherapeutic agents. One might predict that greater therapeutic benefit would be achieved by increasing the warfarin dose. Unfortunately, the dose of warfarin that can be safely administered is limited by the hypo-coagulable state induced by this drug. Accordingly, it would be logical to design therapeutic trials to capitalize on the possible potentiation of warfarin's effect upon simultaneous administration of vitamin K or anti-tumor quinone antibiotics. Compounds similar to warfarin may be discovered that possess anti-tumor but not anti-coagulant properties. These would be candidates for comparative trials.

III. WARFARIN IMMUNOPOTENTIATION

The hypothesis that warfarin ameliorates the course of cancer by enhancing host immune defenses presupposes the existence on neoplastic cells of features that are recognizable by immune mechanisms. Such cellular or humoral defenses are viewed as insufficient to destroy the tumor cells but are rendered more effective by warfarin. This mechanism for the effect of warfarin on malignancy has been supported by Thornes et al. (33) who advocate the use of coumarin rather than warfarin for this purpose in order to avoid the complications of anticoagulation. This hypothesis served as the basis for administration of both warfarin (7,8) and coumarin (33,34) to patients with malignancy.

Evidence supporting immune potentiation by warfarin or coumarin has emphasized their effects on cellular rather than humoral immunity. Thornes and colleagues (31) found that warfarin administration to rabbits bearing the V2 carcinoma results in increased tumor infiltration by granulocytes and macrophages. This group also claimed that coumarin therapy increases the number of helper T cells, decreases the number of suppressor T cells, and restores delayed hypersensitivity skin tests in anergic patients (31,33-35). Berkarda and associates (36) found that both warfarin and coumarin lead to increased lymphocyte responsiveness to phytohemagglutinin in normal subjects and cancer patients. This effect is more pronounced for coumarin than for warfarin. Hardt and Ritschel (37) observed that coumarin stimulates phagocytosis of latex particles by macrophages. Hilgard (38) claimed that vitamin K deficiency increases the phagocytic index of macrophages after nonspecific immunostimulation. Piller (39) presented evidence that coumarin treatment of rats results in increased macrophage adherence to subcutaneously implanted coverslips. These manifest increased pseudopod formation and an increased number of phagocytic vacuoles. Maat (40) showed that the beneficial effect of warfarin on experimental tumors is negated by carrageenan and silica. Since the latter two compounds depress macrophage function, he concluded that the beneficial effects of warfarin are mediated by macrophage activation. Gorelik and associates (41) observed that the antimetastatic effect of heparin and prostacyclin in the B16 melanoma in mice is abrogated by inhibition of natural killer (NK) cell activity (see also Chapter 15). Augmentation of NK activity by poly I:C potentiates the heparin effect. These authors proposed that a coating of fibrin on circulating tumor cells might protect the cells from destruction by NK cells and that anticoagulants may render circulating tumor cells more vulnerable to NK cells. It is conceivable that warfarin may work by a similar mechanism.

Should warfarin influence tumors by potentiating cellular immune mechanisms of the host, it is conceivable that infiltration of the tumor by inflammatory cells may be evident histologically and that a correlation may exist between increased immune function and tumor response to warfarin therapy. One might predict that greater therapeutic benefit would be achieved by administering warfarin together with some other immune adjuvant. Compounds similar to warfarin, such as coumarin, may be identified which have even greater immune-enhancing activity but lack anticoagulant properties. The antineoplastic properties of such compounds could be assessed by comparing their effects to warfarin in controlled clinical trials. Coumarin itself may be susceptible to such a study since recent evidence indicates that earlier fears of coumarin carcinogenicity may be unfounded (42). Considering the multiplicity of coumarin derivatives together with the importance and diversity of their physiologic effects (43,44), this could be a fruitful field for future clinical investigation.

IV. WARFARIN ANTICOAGULATION

The hypothesis that warfarin ameliorates the course of cancer by virtue of its anticoagulant action presupposes the existence on neoplastic cells of clot-inducing properties that are capable of activating the normally quiescent coagulation mechanism of the host (45). Such activation is viewed as favoring neoplastic dissemination (1,2,45).

Warfarin is probably the most consistently effective anti-thrombotic drug in limiting tumor dissemination in experimental animal tumors (6). An extensive literature has developed that supports the conclusion that warfarin's effects on malignancy are mediated by inhibition of coagulation. Hoover and associates (46) observed that the ability of warfarin to inhibit metastasis from 20 methylcholanthrene-induced sarcomas is directly related to the degree to which the prothrombin time is prolonged. However, a mechanism for the warfarin effect that is mediated by the coagulation mechanism is, perhaps, best illustrated by studies performed in the Lewis lung carcinoma (3LL) in mice. This literature has recently been reviewed (47,48). In the 3LL tumor model, warfarin has no effect when incubated with the tumor cells prior to inoculation. Rather, the host animal must be treated with warfarin. The benefits of warfarin therapy can be achieved even though warfarin is started several days after metastatic seeding has begun. However, in order for the effect to be maintained, warfarin must be given continuously. Interruption of treatment allows metastatic growth to commence. The most dramatic effect of warfarin is inhibition of metastasis, yet an effect on the primary tumor has also been observed. Metastasis following intravenous infusion of tumor cells or metastasis from a pre-existing subcutaneous tumor implant is inhibited by this drug.

In the experiments referred to, the beneficial effects of warfarin appear to be related to the ability of this drug to antagonize vitamin K-dependent reactions (for review see 47 and 48). Thus, warfarin's action is mimicked by dietary vitamin K deficiency but reversed by simultaneous administration of vitamin K. The effect on malignancy is observed with the vitamin K-antagonistic S-isomer of warfarin but not the inactive R-isomer. Infusion of vitamin K-dependent clotting factors present in the plasma does not diminish the beneficial effects of warfarin. However, warfarin therapy results in a reduction of the activity of a tumor cell-associated coagulant which is capable of directly activating factor X.

Warfarin treatment prevents the acute reduction in fibrinogen and platelets observed following intravenous infusion of 3LL tumor cells. Warfarin does not prevent the chronic changes in blood coagulation observed when a subcutaneous tumor mass is present even though metastatic seeding is inhibited (47,48).

Brown and Parker (49) found that warfarin reduces lung metastasis from both the immunogenic EMTG tumor and the non-immunogenic KHT sarcoma. In other studies, Brown (50) demonstrated that this effect is unrelated to a direct cytotoxic effect on the tumor cells. He also found that the beneficial effect on KHT metastasis, in both the spontaneous metastasis and tail vein injection models, is reversed by simultaneous administration of vitamin K. Similar numbers of isotopically tagged tumor cells are initially trapped in the lungs of warfarin treated and control animals. However, at one to twelve days following injection, retention of tumor cells in the lungs is significantly reduced in warfarin-treated animals. He attributed this

150

failure of retention, and hence the reduction in metastasis, to inhibition of thrombus formation about tumor cells lodged within pulmonary vessels.

The theory that warfarin exerts a beneficial effect on malignancy by virtue of its anticoagulant properties served as the basis for certain clinical trials of this drug (1,3,4,51). Evidence emerged from controlled trials that human small cell carcinoma of the lung (SCCL) may be responsive to warfarin therapy (3,4,9). SCCL is associated with systemic hypercoagulability evidenced by localized thromboembolic disease (52)as well as the coagulation changes of disseminated intravascular coagulation (53,54). Tissue factor (thromboplastin) antigen has been observed on SCCL cells in sections of fresh frozen tumor tissue and dense deposits of fibrin exist surrounding tumor nodules (55). These results indicate that induction of coagulation occurs in association with viable tumor cells in SCCL and suggest that the warfarin effect may be mediated by local inhibition of coagulation.

Should the salutary effects of warfarin on tumors be due to the anticoagulant properties of this drug, further benefit may be derived by combining warfarin with one or more agents that also have antithrombotic properties.

V. DISCUSSION

It is evident from the foregoing that the familiar anticoagulant, warfarin, has been administered for several decades to animals with experimental tumors and also to patients with malignancies but for different reasons and with variable results. The benefits for certain tumor types are strikingly favorable (3,4,6,9,46,48-50,56-61) although no effect is observed for other tumor types (3,62). Thus, the warfarin effect appears to be tumor-specific, but, to achieve its effect, warfarin must also be administered to the host over time. It is apparent that complex mechanisms are involved. If warfarin, in the usually effective doses, is acting by a toxic mechanism, one might expect this to be reflected by a reduction in peripheral blood leukocyte or platelet counts especially when given together with other cytotoxic agents. Despite evidence (reviewed above) supporting a toxic mechanism, such an effect has, in fact, never been described. It seems more likely that the warfarin effect is mediated either by blocking host-tumor interactions that are required for growth and spread of certain tumor types or by enhancement of ineffective host defenses.

Evidence favoring warfarin enhancement of host defenses has been presented above. Limited information is available on this subject and there is a need for expansion and clarification of existing data. For example, it may be premature to conclude that negation of the warfarin effect on experimental animal tumors by carrageenan means that warfarin exerts its influence through macrophage activation (40). The latter conclusion was based upon evidence that carrageenan is a macrophage inhibitor. However, carrageenan has multiple effects on the coagulation mechanism such as induction of disseminated intravascular coagulation (63), activation of platelets (64,65) and elevation of alpha-2 antiplasmin levels (66) that could also explain its ability to counteract warfarin. Coumarin, to which immune-potentiating properties have been attributed but which is said to lack anticoagulant properties (33), has been incriminated in the development of a hemorrhagic disorder associated with reduced vitamin K-dependent clotting factor activity (67). Thus, the possible benefits of coumarin may, after all, be in some way mediated by an effect on tumor cell coagulants or the the clotting mechanism of the host.

Goerner (68) was apparently the first to recognize the possibility of a cause-and-effect relationship between blood coagulation and neoplastic growth. A persuasive body of evidence suggests that the warfarin effect is in some way related to its anticoagulant properties. Thus, the host must be treated for the result to be achieved and antagonism of vitamin K is clearly involved. In addition, there are a number of reasons for postulating that activation of coagulation enhances tumor growth and spread. Evidence obtained from the 3LL tumor in mice suggests that it is the vitamin K-dependent, warfarin-inhibitable procoagulant properties of tumor cells themselves that may initiate the coagulation sequence of the host to promote tumor dissemination (47,48). The initial effect could be the generation of thrombin in the tumor cell periphery. The initial effect could be the generation of thrombin in the tumor cell periphery. Evidence indicates that increased thrombin generation, that is warfarin-inhibitable (69), is a feature of human malignancy. This thrombin is formed primarily in extravascular sites and is most likely tumor-derived. Local thrombin formation could promote the well-being of the tumor. For example, thrombin stimulates division of certain untransformed (70) and transformed (71) cell types, synergizes epidermal growth factor-induced cell growth (72,73), and is capable of inducing gaps between endothelial cells grown in confluent culture (74). Should thrombin be formed at the tumor cell periphery _in vivo_, a positive feedback mechanism for cell proliferation may be established and a mechanism would be afforded by which the tumor cell might more easily gain access to the subendothelial space. Certain tumor cells are capable of inducing platelet aggregation that is mediated by local thrombin formation (75). The creation of a platelet-tumor cell embolus might be conducive to tumor dissemination since endothelial attachment may be facilitated and tumor cell growth enhanced through local provision of platelet growth factor. Finally, local thrombin generation could be responsible for the investment of circulating tumor cells (50) as well as extravascular tumor deposits (55,76-78) with a fibrin coat. Such a coat on circulating tumor cells could, as suggested by Brown (50), be responsible for their persistence within the pulmonary vasculature, a prelude to metastasis. The formation of a fibrin investment around extravascular tumor masses might also provide conditions conducive to tumor well-being (55,77).

This seemingly tidy picture is subject to interpretation. Accepted at face value, existing evidence would lead to the conclusion that dissemination of methylcholanthrene-induced tumors is inhibited by warfarin (46,59) but not by phenprocoumon (79). Since both of these drugs are anticoagulants, differences in responsiveness may be attributable to subtle differences in molecular configuration that impart different chemical or physical properties to these compounds rather than to vitamin K antagonism as such. Granted that the effects for certain tumors are mediated by vitamin K antagonism, the end result of such antagonism, so far as the well-being of the tumor cell is concerned, need not be limitation of fibrin formation or even thrombin generation. For example, it is conceivable that vitamin K-dependent reactions are important to the economy of the tumor cell but are either unrelated or only indirectly related to blood coagulation. Perhaps, as has been suggested (15,31), these reactions contribute to tumor cell motility. Unfortunately, information on the occurrence of vitamin K-dependent enzyme systems within tumor cells is incomplete.

If warfarin exerts its effect by limiting thrombin formation, why then is heparin ineffective (or possibly even detrimental) in certain experimental (80) and clinical (81,82) settings? An explanation for this seeming paradox might be as follows. Antithrombin III, a plasma inhibitor of active coagulant enzymes, may leak out of damaged vessels in the vicinity of tumors along with intermediates in the coagulation sequence. The local effect of the antithrombin III would be to moderate the activity of such intermediates that are activated locally. Since heparin binds antithrombin III but also does not gain access to the extravascular space, it could limit the amount of antithrombin III that reaches the tumor site and thereby contribute to heightened local coagulation. Such an explanation would be consistent with the possible detrimental effects of heparin in disseminated SCCL (81,82) and also the possible beneficial effects of heparin in minimal disease colorectal cancer (83) in which tumor cells are more likely to reside within the vasculature.

Limitation of local fibrin formation is yet another level at which warfarin may exert its beneficial effect. In rats Shaeffer (84) found that tumor masses of the Murphy-Sturn lymphosarcoma avidly sequester labeled fibrinogen. Administration of warfarin in doses sufficient to produce therapeutic anticoagulation dramatically reduces fibrinogen incorporation into tumors. The reduced incorporation is attributed to reduced local coagulability rather than to accelerated local fibrinolysis (85). Unfortunately, the effects of warfarin on progression of this particular tumor were not determined. Paradoxically, the 3LL tumor, the classic example of a warfarin-responsive experimental tumor, lacks local fibrin associated with extravascular tumor deposits (86). In fact, fibrinolytic agents accelerate and antifibrinolytic agents inhibit progression of the 3LL tumor (47,48).

Granted that certain experimental tumors are associated with local fibrin deposition (76), it is possible that such fibrin may protect the tumor from invading host cells, serve as a substrate for new blood vessel formation, or serve as a scaffold that facilitates cell proliferation (45,76). However, Roszkowski and colleagues (87) showed that administration of low molecular weight fibrinogen degradation products along with injected L-1 (JW) sarcoma cells enhances primary tumor growth, increases metastasis formation and decreases survival in mice. Thus, local fibrin formation may be of importance primarily because of the consequences of local fibrinolysis.

Many, but not all, human tumor types sequester isotopically-labeled fibrinogen in vivo (for review see 1) but only a few human tumor types have been well characterized morphologically in terms of their fibrin content (55,77,78). Unfortunately, it is not known whether warfarin reduces fibrinogen incorporation into human tumors much less how such an effect might relate to therapeutic efficacy. Although evidence indicates that warfarin treatment reduces the increased thrombin generation that is associated with malignancy (69), this drug has no effect on the accelerated platelet consumption that occurs in cancer patients (88).

VI. CONCLUSIONS

Warfarin, the commonly used antithrombotic drug, has been reported to ameliorate the course of experimental animal and human malignancy. A multiplicity of possible mechanisms has been invoked but it is not possible to state with certainty whether the anticoagulant properties or some other chemical or physical characteristic accounts for the warfarin effect. The various mechanisms reviewed for this chapter are not mutually exclusive. Perhaps different mechanisms are relevant to different tumors or the drug may interfere with tumor progression at multiple points. Nevertheless, consideration of possible mechanisms suggests several therapeutic hypotheses that are testable by means of carefully controlled clinical trials. Insights from studies in experimental animals as well as positive results obtained in therapeutic trials in human malignancy point the way toward imaginative new approaches to cancer treatment (for a review of current clinical trials see 89).

REFERENCES

1. Zacharski LR, Henderson WG, Rickles FR, Forman WB, Cornell CJ, Jr., Forcier RJ, Harrower HW, Johnson RO: Rationale and experimental design for the VA Cooperative Study of Anticoagulation (warfarin) in the treatment of cancer. Cancer 44:732-741, 1979.
2. Zacharski LR, Henderson WG, Rickles FR, Forman WB, Van Eeckhout JP, Cornell CJ, Jr., Forcier RJ, Martin JF: Platelets and malignancy: Rationale and experimental design for the VA Cooperative Study of RA-233 in the treatment of cancer. Am. J. Clin. Oncol. 5:593-609, 1982.
3. Zacharski LR, Henderson WG, Rickles FR, Forman WB, Cornell CJ, Jr., Forcier RJ, Edwards RL, Headley E, Kim S-H, O'Donnell JF, O'Dell R, Tornyos K, Kwaan HC: Effect of warfarin anticoagulation on survival in carcinoma of the lung, colon, head and neck and prostate: Final report of VA Cooperative Study #75. Cancer 53:2046-2052, 1984.

4. Zacharski LR, Henderson WG, Rickles FR, Forman WB, Cornell CJ, Jr., Forcier RJ, Headley E, Kim S-H, O'Donnell JF, O'Dell R, Tornyos K, Kwaan HC: Effect of sodium warfarin on survival in small cell carcinoma of the lung. J. Am. Med. Assoc. 145:831-835, 1981.

5. Fasco MJ, Hildebrandt EF, Suttie JW: Evidence that warfarin anticoagulant action involves two distinct reductase activities. J. Biol. Chem. 257:11210-11212, 1982.

6. Maat B, Hilgard P: Critical analysis of experimental models for the antimetastatic effects of anticoagulants. In: Hellmann K, Hilgard P and Eccles S (eds.) Metastasis: Clinical and Experimental Aspects. Martinus Nijhoff, Boston, pp. 109-115, 1980.

7. Thornes RD: Oral anticoagulant therapy of human cancer. J. Med. 5:83-91, 1974.

8. Thornes RD: Adjuvant therapy of cancer via the cellular immune mechanism or fibrin by induced fibrinolysis and oral anticoagulants. Cancer 35:91-97, 1975.

9. Chahinian AP, Ware JH, Zimmer B, Comis RL, Perry MC, Hirsh V, Skarin AT, Raich PC, Weiss RB, Carey RW: Evaluation of anticoagulation with warfarin and of alternating chemotherapy in extensive small cell cancer of the lung (SCCL). Proc. Am. Soc. Clin. Oncol. 3:225, 1984.

10. Kirsch WM, Schulz D, Van Buskirk JJ, Young EE: Effects of sodium warfarin and other carcinostatic agents on malignant cells: A study of drug synergy. J. Med. 5:69-82, 1974.

11. Chlebowski RT, Gota CH, Chan KK, Weiner JM, Block JB, Bateman JR: Clinical and pharmacokinetic effects of combined warfarin and 5-fluorouracil in advanced colon cancer. Cancer Res. 42:4827-4830, 1982.

12. Van Buskirk JJ, Kirsch WM: Loss of hepatoma ribosomal RNA during warfarin therapy. Biochem. Biophys. Res. Commun. 52:562, 1973.

13. Chang JD, Hill TC: In vitro effect of sodium warfarin on DNA and RNA synthesis in mouse L1210 leukemia cells and Walker tumor cells. Oncology 28:232, 1973.

14. Kirsch WM, Van Buskirk JJ, Schulz DW, Tabuchi K: The biologic basis of malignant brain tumor therapy. In: Thompson RA and Green JR (eds.) Advances in Neurology. Raven Press, New York, pp. 301-313, 1976.

15. Wood S, Jr.: Mechanism of establishment of tumor metastases. In: Ioachim HI (ed.) Pathobiol. Ann., p. 281, 1971.

16. Lown JW: The mechanism of action of quinone antibiotics. Mol. Cell. Biochem. 55:17-40, 1983.

17. Chlebowski RT, Block JB, Dietrich M, Octay E, Barth N, Yanagihara R, Gota C, Ali I: Inhibition of human tumor growth and DNA biosynthetic activity by vitamin K and warfarin: In vitro and clinical results. Proc. Am. Assoc. Cancer Res. 24:165, 1983.

18. Chlebowski R, Block J, Dietrich M: Warfarin (W) and vitamin K_1 (K) enhance methotrexate (MTX) and 5-fluorouracil (FU) effects in L1210 cells. Clin. Res. 29:63, 1981.

19. Finnegan RA, Merkel KE, Back N: Constituents of Mammea americana L VIII: Novel structural variations on the mammein theme and antitumor activity of mammein and related coumarin and phloroglucinol derivatives. J. Pharmaceut. Sci. 161:1599-1603, 1972.

20. Baker D, Elkon D, Lim M-L, Constable W, Rinehart L, Wanebo H: The influence of warfarin or levamisol on the incidence of metastases following local irradiation of a solid tumor. Cancer 49:427-433, 1982.

21. Rottinger EM, Sedlacek R, Skuit HD: Ineffectiveness of anticoagulation in experimental radiation therapy. Eur. J. Cancer 11:743-749, 1975.

22. Egilsson V: Differentiation of malignant neuroblastoma cells: Evidence for a mitochondrial role. Cell. Biol. Int. Rep. 1:435-438, 1977.

23. Hadler HI, Cao TM: Vitamin K and chemical carcinogenesis. Lancet 1:397, 1978.

24. Egilsson V. Cancer and vitamin K. Lancet 2:254-255, 1977.

25. Israels LG, Walls GA, Ollmann DJ, Friesen E, Israels ED: Vitamin K as a regulator of benzo(a)pyrene metabolism, mutagenesis, and carcinogenesis. J. Clin. Invest. 71:1130-1140, 1983.

26. Wattenberg IW, Lam LKT, Fladmoe AV: Inhibition of chemical carcinogen-induced neoplasia by coumarins and α-angelica-lactone. Cancer Res. 38:1651-1654, 1979.

27. Feuer G, Kellen JA, Kovacs K: Suppression of 7,12-dimethylbenz (α) anthracene-induced breast carcinoma by coumarin in the rat. Oncology 33:35-39, 1976.

28. Feuer G, Kellen JA: Inhibition and enhancement of mammary tumorigenesis by 7,12-dimethylbenz (a) anthracene in the female Sprague-Dawley rat. Int. J. Clin. Pharmacol. 9:62-69, 1974.

29. Hilgard P: Cancer and vitamin K. Lancet 2:403, 1977.

30. Hilgard P: Experimental vitamin K deficiency and spontaneous metastases. Br. J. Cancer 35:891-892, 1977.

31. Thornes RD, Edlow DW, Wood S, Jr.: Inhibition of locomotion of cancer cells in vivo by anticoagulant therapy. Johns Hopkins Med. J. 123:305-316, 1968.

32. Bertolone SJ, Kirsch W: Chemotherapy with 5-FU + warfarin for cerebral metastasis. Proc. Am. Soc. Clin. Oncol. 17:287, 1976.

33. Thornes RD, Lynch G, Edwards GE, Coolican JE, Beesley W, Prenderville JB, O'Riain S, Sheehan MV: Coumarins and melanoma. Ir. J. Med. Sci. 152:252-253, 1983.

34. Thornes RD, Lynch G, Sheehan MV: Cimetadine and coumarin therapy for melanoma. Lancet 2:328, 1982.

35. Thornes RD: The anergy of chronic human brucellosis. Ir. Med. J. 70:480-483, 1977.

36. Berkarda B, Bouffard-Eyuboglu H, Derman U: The effect of coumarin derivative on the immunological system of man. Agents Action 13:50-52, 1983.

37. Hardt TJ, Ritschel WA: The effect of coumarin and 7-hydroxycoumarin on in vitro macrophage phagocytosis of latex particles. Meth. Find. Exp. Clin. Pharmacol. 5:39-43, 1983.

38. Hilgard P. Coumarin anticoagulation and experimental metastases. Thromb. Haemostasis 42:353, 1979.

39. Piller NB: A morphological assessment of the stimulatory effect of coumarin on macrophages. Br. J. Exp. Pathol. 59:93-96, 1978.

40. Maat B: Selective macrophage inhibition abolishes warfarin-induced reduction of metastasis. Br. J. Cancer 41:313-316, 1980.

41. Gorelik E, Bere WW, Herberman RB: Role of NK cells in the antimetastatic effect of anticoagulant drugs. Int. J. Cancer 33:87-94, 1984.

42. Shilling WH, Crampton RF, Longland RC: Metabolism of coumarin in man. Nature (London) 221:664-665, 1969.

43. Feuer G: The metabolism and biological actions of coumarin. Prog. Med. Chem. 10:85-144, 1974.

44. Mabry TJ, Ulubelen A: Chemistry and utilization of phenyl-propanoids including flavonoids, coumarins, and ligans. J. Ag. Food Chem. 28:188-196, 1980.

45. Zacharski LR: The biologic basis for anticoagulant treatment of cancer. In: Jamieson G (ed.) Interaction of Platelets and Tumor Cells. Alan R. Liss, New York, pp. 113-129, 1982.

46. Hoover HC, Jones D, Ketcham AS: The optimal level of anti-coagulation for decreasing experimental metastases. Surgery 79:625-630, 1976.

47. Zacharski LR: Basis for selection of anticoagulant drugs for therapeutic trials in human malignancy. Haemostasis (In press).

48. Donati MB, Semeraro N, Gordon SG: Relationship between pro-coagulant activity and metastatic capacity of tumor cells. In: Honn KV and Sloane BF (eds.) Hemostatic Mechanisms and Metastasis. Martinus Nijhoff, The Hague, pp. 84-95, 1984.

49. Brown JM, Parker ET: Host treatments affecting artificial pulmonary metastases: Interpretation of loss of radioactively labelled cells from lungs. Br. J. Cancer 40:677-688, 1979.

50. Brown JM: A study of the mechanism by which anticoagulation with warfarin inhibits blood borne metastases. Cancer Res. 33:1217-1224, 1973.

51. Zacharski LR: Anticoagulation in the treatment of cancer in man. In: Donati MB, Davidson JF and Garattini S (eds.) Malignancy and the Hemostatic System. Raven Press, New York, pp. 113-129, 1981.

52. Byrd RB, Divertie MB, Spittell JA, Jr.: Bronchogenic carcinoma and thromboembolic disease. J. Am. Med. Assoc. 202:1019-1022, 1967.

53. Brugarolas A, Elias EG, Takita H, Mink IB, Mittelman A, Ambrus JL: Blood coagulation and fibrinolysis in patients with carcinoma of the lung. J. Med. 4:96-105, 1973.

54. Hagedorn AB, Bowie EJW, Elvebach LR, Owen CA, Jr.: Coagulation abnormalities in patients with inoperable lung cancer. Mayo Clin. Proc. 49:647-653, 1974.

55. Zacharski LR, Schned AR, Sorenson GD: Occurrence of fibrin and tissue factor antigen in human small cell carcinoma of the lung. Cancer Res. 43:3963-3968, 1983.

56. Berkarda FB, D'Sousa JP, Bakemeier RF: The effect of anti-coagulants on tumor growth and spread in mice. Proc. Am. Assoc. Cancer Res. 15:99, 1974.
57. Kolenich JJ, Mansour EG, Flynn A: Haematological effects of aspirin. Lancet 2:714, 1972.
58. Mooney B, Serlin M, Taylor I: The effect of warfarin on spontaneously metastasizing colorectal cancer in the rat. Clin. Oncol. 8:55-59, 1982.
59. Ryan JJ, Ketcham AS, Wexler H: Warfarin treatment of mice bearing autochthonous tumors: Effect on spontaneous metastases. Science 162:1493, 1968.
60. Tseng MH, Mittelman A, Holyoke ED: The limitation of combined coumadin or aspirin with chemotherapy in experimental metastasis. Clin. Res. 28:653, 1980.
61. Williamson RCN, Lyndon PT, Tudway AJC: Effects of anticoagulation and ileal resection on the development and spread of experimental intestinal carcinomas. Br. J. Cancer 42:85-94, 1980.
62. Higashi H, Heidelberger C: Lack of effect of warfarin (NSC-59813) alone or in combination with 5-fluorouracil (NSC-19893) on primary and metastatic L1210 leukemia and adenocarcinoma 755. Cancer Chemother. Rep. 55:29-33, 1971.
63. Davidson RJL, Simpson JG, Whiting PH, Milton JI, Thomson AW: Haematological changes following systemic injection of purified carrageenans (kappa, lambda and iota). Br. J. Exp. Pathol. 62:529, 1981.
64. Vargaftig BB, Fouque F, Chignard M, Dumarey C: Carrageenan-induced activation of human platelets is independent of phospholipase A_2 and of formation of thromboxanes. J. Pharm. Pharmacol. 32:740-745, 1980.
65. McMillan RM, MacIntyre DE, Gordon JL: Stimulation of human platelets by carrageenans. J. Pharm. Pharmacol. 31:148-512, 1979.
66. Kosugi T, Kinjo K, Takagi I, Matsuo O, Mihara H, Mishikaze O: Antiplasmin activity in carrageenan-induced inflammation of rats. Int. J. Tiss. React. 3:173-176, 1981.
67. Hogan RP, III: Hemorrhagic diathesis caused by drinking an herbal tea. J. Am. Med. Assoc. 249:2679-2680, 1983.
68. Goerner A: The influence of anticlotting agents on transplantation and growth of tumor tissue. J. Lab. Clin. Med. 16:369-372, 1930.
69. Rickles FR, Edwards RL, Barb C, Cronlund M: Abnormalities of blood coagulation in patients with cancer. Fibrinopeptide A generation and tumor growth. Cancer 51:301-307, 1983.
70. Glenn KC, Cunningham DD: thrombin-stimulated cell division involves proteolysis of its cell surface receptor. Nature (London) 278:711-714, 1979.
71. Bruhn HD, Zurborn KH: Influences of clotting factors (thrombin, factor XIII) and of fibronectin on the growth of tumor cells and leukemic cells in vitro. Blut 46:85-88, 1983.
72. Baker JB, Simmer RL, Glenn KC, Cunningham DD: Thrombin and epidermal growth factor become linked to cell surface receptors during mitogenic stimulation. Nature (London) 278:743-746, 1979.

158

73. Cherington PV, Pardee AB: Synergistic effects of epidermal growth factor and thrombin on the growth stimulation of diploid hamster fibroblasts. J. Cell. Physiol. 105:25-32, 1980.

74. Laposata M, Dovnarsky DK, Shin HS: Thrombin-induced gap formation in confluent endothelial cell monolayers in vitro. Blood 62:549-556, 1983.

75. Jamieson GA, Bastida E, Ordinas A: Mechanisms of platelet aggregation by human tumor cell lines. In: Jamieson GA (ed.) Interaction of Platelets and Tumor Cells. Alan R. Liss, New York, pp. 405-413, 1982.

76. Dvorak HF, Orenstein NS, Dvorak AM: Tumor-secreted mediators and the tumor microenvironment: Relationship to immunologic surveillance. Lymphokines 2:203-233, 1981.

77. Dvorak HF, Dickersin GR, Dvorak AM, Manseau EJ, Pyne K: Human breast carcinoma: Fibrin deposits and desmoplasia. Inflammatory cell type and distribution. Microvasculature and infarction. J. Natl. Cancer Inst. 67:335-345, 1981.

78. Harris NL, Dvorak AM, Smith J, Dvorak HF: Fibrin deposits in Hodgkin's disease. Am. J. Pathol. 108:119-129, 1982.

79. Hagmar B: Effect of heparin, coumarin and E-aminocaproic acid (EACA) on spontaneous metastasis formation. Pathol. Eur. 4:283-292, 1969.

80. Hagmar B: Cell surface change and metastasis formation. Acta Pathol. Microbiol. Scand. 80:357-366, 1972.

81. Stanford CF: Anticoagulants in the treatment of small cell carcinoma of the bronchus. Thorax 34:113-116, 1979.

82. Jamieson GG, Angove RC: Heparinized chemotherapy in the treatment of disseminated lung cancer. Aust. NZ. J. Med. 9:381-384, 1979.

83. Kohanna FH, Sweeney J, Hussey S, Zacharski LR, Salzman EW: Effect of perioperative low-dose heparin administration on the course of colon cancer. Surgery 93:433-438, 1983.

84. Shaeffer JR: Interference in localization of I^{131} fibrinogen in rat tumors by anticoagulants. Am. J. Physiol. 206:573-579, 1964.

85. Shaeffer JR: Lack of enhanced lysis of fibrinogen-I^{131} by anticoagulants in tumor-bearing rats. Am. J. Physiol. 206:1251-1254, 1964.

86. Tanaka N, Ogawa H, Kinjo M, Kohga S, Tanaka K: Ultrastructural study of the effects of tranexamic acid and urokinase on metastasis of Lewis lung carcinoma. Br. J. Cancer 46:428-435, 1982.

87. Roszkowski W, Stachurska J, Gerdin B, Saldeen T, Kopec M : Peptides cleaved from fibrinogen by plasmin enhance the progression of L-1 sarcoma in BALB/c mice. Eur. J. Cancer Clin. Oncol. 17:889-892, 1981.

88. Slichter SJ, Weiden PL, O'Donnell MR, Storb R: Interruption of tumor-associated platelet consumption with platelet enzyme inhibitors. Blood 59:1252-1258, 1982.

89. Temple WJ, Ketcham AS: Current clinical trials with anticoagulant therapy in the management of patients. In: Honn KV and Sloane BF (eds.) Hemostatic Mechanisms and Metastasis. Martinus Nijhoff, The Hague, pp. 409-425, 1984.

CHAPTER 11.   CANCER CELL PROCOAGULANTS AND THEIR POSSIBLE ROLE IN METASTASIS

STUART G. GORDON

I.   INTRODUCTION

    For more than two decades, investigators have sought to understand the possible role of the coagulation system and fibrin in the metastatic process. The first suggestion of a tumor cell thrombus dates back to 1936 when Warren and Gates (1) observed a "hyaline thrombus" associated with blood-borne Walker 256 cells. However, the early observations by Sumner Wood (2-5) showing that fibrin was associated with blood-borne malignant cells in the ear chamber of rabbits provided the first convincing evidence that the coagulation system may be involved in the metastatic process. This has been confirmed more recently by several investigators (6-11). Data supporting the deposition of fibrin on arrested tumor cells include histologic data using selective immunofluorescent staining and electron microscopic data showing that malignant cells in the lung or other organs of an experimental animal have fibrin strands attached to them. In addition, several investigators have demonstrated that anticoagulant therapy of animals with heparin (2,12,13), warfarin (2,12,14-18), proteinase inhibitors (19) and defibrination (20,21) as well as fibrinolytic therapy (2,22-24) decreases metastasis. On the other hand, agents that promote coagulation increase metastasis (25). At face value, these lines of evidence indicate that activation of the coagulation system enhances metastasis, but there is not universal agreement on this hypothesis (26).

    In an oversimplified view, the metastatic process is composed of three general phases: intravasation, transport and extravasation. Briefly, as a primary solid tumor grows and becomes vascularized, it will invade through the basement membrane of vessels and surrounding tissue; at some point during this process it invades through the wall of the lymphatic or vascular system and tumor cells are shed into either the lymph or bloodstream, a process that is call intravasation. The blood-borne malignant cells are transported in the blood to organs that are susceptible for metastasis. The malignant cells will arrest in small capillaries of these organs and they will invade through the capillary endothelium, a process known as extravasation, where they multiply to form a metastatic tumor. Since the metastatic process is described in detail in other chapters in this volume, it is not appropriate to reiterate such detail here. Instead, I would like to focus on those aspects of the metastatic process that involve the blood coagulation system and fibrin deposition.

II. ACTIVATION OF COAGULATION AND FIBRIN DEPOSITION

Fibrin is deposited within and at the advancing margin of solid tumors (27-32).   This fibrin network or "cocoon" may provide a supporting mesh for the growth of new tumor cells.   In addition, this fibrin network may limit access of the host immune cells to the tumor site and thus diminish the capacity of the host's immune system to destroy the neoplastic cells.   During intravasation, as the tumor cells are shedding into the lymph or blood the fibrin network in the primary tumor may decrease the releasse of tumor cells.   Thus, some investigators hypothesize that cancer cell procoagulant activity and fibrin deposition may decrease metastasis whereas anticoagulants and fibrinolytic activity may increase metastasis by reducing fibrin (32).

Most of the tumor cells shed into the circulation do not survive (33-35).   The current belief is that fibrin deposition on blood-borne malignant cells may protect them from the host immune system by masking antigenic sites on the tumor cell with the host's fibrin so that the tumor cells are not recognized by the monocytes (28,32). Alternatively, fibrin may physically protect the tumor cells from contact with cytotoxic blood cells (36).   Recently, Gorelik et al. (36) have shown that anticoagulant therapy with either heparin or warfarin decreases metastasis of B16 melanoma cells.   Inhibition of NK cell activity with asialo GM_1 blocks this antimetastatic effect whereas augmentation of NK cell activity with poly I:C enhances the effect. These data suggest that anticoagulation makes malignant cells more vulnerable to the cytotoxic effects of NK cells.

A critical step in the metastatic process is the arrest of the blood-borne tumor cell within a capillary of an organ susceptible for a metastatic tumor (2-11).   Several studies have shown that tumor cell-blood cell aggregates lodge within small capillaries.   Injection of clumps of malignant cells into the circulation of experimental animals results in significantly more metastases than injection of the same number of cells as single cell suspensions (37-39).   In addition, far fewer clumps of cells are observed in animals that are anticoagulated than in control animals.   Fibrin deposition on the tumor cells is thought to facilitate clumping of tumor cells with other cells whereas inhibition of fibrin deposition with either anticoagulants or fibrinolytic agents is thought to decrease clumping and metastasis.

Thus, activation of the coagulation system and fibrin deposition is thought to participate in each of the three phases of the metastatic process.   In the first, activation of coagulation is thought to diminish metastasis but in the other two phases, it is thought to enhance metastasis.

III. PROCOAGULANTS

These lines of evidence have led several investigators to look for procoagulant activity associated with malignant cells. Currently, there are at least two procoagulants that are believed to participate in this process (Figure 1): tissue factor and cancer procoagulant. Other procoagulant factors have been postulated (28,40-42) but their existence awaits confirmation.

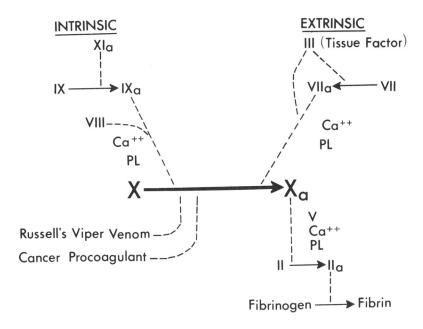

Blood Coagulation Pathway

FIGURE 1. Schematic Diagram of the Coagulation System. Note the distinction between tissue factor that requires factor VII (VIIa) for activity and cancer procoagulant that directly activates factor X. Russell's viper venom is a common control procoagulant for studies of factor X activation.

Tissue factor is a well known lipoprotein cofactor on the surface of normal cells that is exposed during an insult to the cell (43-47). Exposure of this lipoprotein facilitates the conversion of factor VII to its activated form, factor VIIa, such that the tissue factor-factor VIIa complex in the extrinsic coagulation pathway catalyzes the conversion of X to Xa very efficiently. Monocytes and macrophages from tumor bearing animals have been found to be activated and to express tissue factor activity (48-51). However, in chronic lymphocytic leukemia, monocyte tissue factor is diminished and is refractory to endotoxic stimulation (52). Prior to the mid 1970s, the procoagulant activity of cells was assumed to be tissue thromboplastin and was not characterized further (53,54). Since the factor X activator (cancer procoagulant) has been identified (40,55), it is now necessary for investigators to confirm either the enzymatic (usually factor VII dependence) or immunologic characteristics of a procoagulant associated with malignant cells in order to determine whether it is tissue factor or cancer procoagulant. Tissue factor is the procoagulant associated with some malignant cells from both leukemias (56,57) and solid tumors (58,59). Promyelocytic leukemia is associated with a high frequency of disseminated intravascular coagulation and other thrombotic abnormalities. Promyelocytes have high levels of procoagulant activity that cross reacts immunologically with an antibody to tissue factor (60,61). In addition, tissue factor and tissue-factor-like activity have been found in many experimental tumors and malignant cells (62-64).

Cancer procoagulant is a cysteine proteinase that has been purified from rabbit V2 carcinoma (65,66), amnion-chorion tissue from human placenta (67) and murine B16 melanoma cells (68,69). Cancer procoagulant is a 68,000 molecular weight protein that is rich in serine and glycine and does not contain carbohydrate (66,70). It has an isoelectric point of 4.8. Cancer procoagulant initiates coagulation by directly activating factor X in the coagulation cascade (55,66,70). Its activity has also been identified in a variety of other malignant cells listed in Table 1 (69,71-75). Cancer procoagulant does not appear to be associated with normal cells and tissues (69,71,72).

What are the relative roles of tissue factor and cancer procoagulant in the activation of the coagulation system in malignant disease? This is a very difficult question to answer; it is impossible to "take a snapshot" of a cancer cell at some point in time in the malignant or metastatic process and then dissect out the relative contribution of these two procoagulant activities as they may affect the malignant cell's extracellular environment. The tissue factor-factor VIIa complex probably has much greater specific activity for the conversion of factor X to Xa than does cancer procoagulant (68). However, the specific nature of the "insult" to the malignant cell that would facilitate exposure of tissue factor or activation of the extrinsic pathway is not clear. Furthermore, other factors in the microenvironment around the cancer cell may influence the relative contribution of the extrinsic pathway and/or cancer procoagulant in the activation of the coagulation system. The expression of cancer procoagulant activity by the malignant cell might be influenced by cell density, cell cycle characteristics and other parameters of the growth properties of the tumor cell (76). Such factors may affect tissue factor activity also.

Table 1. Identification of Cancer Procoagulant or Cancer Procoagulant-Like Activity in Malignant Samples.

Source of Procoagulant		Species	Reference
Adenocarcinoma - colon, kidney	(n = 9)	Human	72
Carcinoma - breast, liver, kidney, lung	(n = 8)	"	72
Neuroblastoma - liver		"	72
Sarcoma - abdomen		"	72
Liposarcoma - abdomen, leg	(n = 2)	"	72
Osteogenic sarcoma	(n = 5)	"	68
HT-29 carcinoma		"	72
LVP hepatoma		"	72
V2 carcinoma		Rabbit	55,65,66
SV-40 transformed fibroblasts	(n = 5)	Hamster	71
Chemically transformed fibroblasts	(n = 2)	"	71
Parietal yolk sac carcinoma		Mouse	72
B16 melanoma	(n = 2)	"	69,76
Lewis lung carcinoma		"	73,74,75,79
JW sarcoma		"	82
Ehrlich carcinoma		"	86
Ca 755		"	73
DMBA induced		"	73
HT3		"	73
BP8		"	73
Glioma 261		"	73
C1498		"	73
EAKR		"	73

A list of tissues and cell lines in which a factor X activator (cancer procoagulant-like) or cancer procoagulant activity has been identified. This procoagulant activity has been distinguished from tissue factor by either factor VII independent activity or inhibition by DFP or other substances that do not inhibit tissue factor, or both. The presence of cancer procoagulant has been confirmed in some samples immunologically (unpublished observation).

There is substantial heterogeneity among malignant cells within a primary tumor as well as within selected clones of cells with similar phenotypic properties (e.g., B16-Fl and B16-F10) as described in other chapters of this volume (see Chapters 4 and 5). From the perspective of procoagulant activity, does this mean that some cells in a population will express tissue factor and others will express cancer procoagulant? If so, it may be virtually impossible to define the relative contribution of each procoagulant in activation of the coagulation system in the malignant and metastatic process. Many investigators are looking for better tools such as specific inhibitors and antibodies to dissect out these factors within well characterized experimental animal model systems in an effort to futher delineate the importance of each factor in the malignant and metastatic process.

Before one is able to fully evaluate results of experiments with animal models and malignant (metastatic) cells, it is appropriate to mention a few words about two animal model systems, a spontaneous metastasis model and a hematologic phase metastasis model. These models are discussed in more detail in other chapters of this volume and elsewhere (77,78). There are advantages and disadvantages to both. In one spontaneous metastasis model, a primary tumor is grown on a limb for a designated period of time thereby allowing cells from the primary tumor to shed into the circulation. The limb is then amputated to terminate intravasation. Several days later the cells that have shed from the primary tumor into the circulation and successfully metastasized to secondary tumor sites (frequently the lung) are counted. This model is clearly the most authentic. In the hematologic phase model, a suspension of malignant cells is injected directly into the bloodstream of the experimental host animal, and 2 to 3 wk later the number of metastatic tumors is scored in the secondary organ. This is an artificial model of the metastatic process because most of the malignant cells are removed from the blood in the first capillary bed they pass through (often the lung). However, this model has the important advantage that the cells that are actually entering the bloodstream can be characterized biochemically and morphologically. Thus the investigator can effectively correlate particular properties of the malignant cells with the metastatic capacity of those cells. In the spontaneous metastasis models, the cells released into the circulation that develop metastatic foci cannot be characterized. It is widely accepted by investigators in the field that a population of cells either directly injected into the vein of an animal host or shed spontaneously from a primary tumor are composed of a heterogeneous population of cells, i.e., some of these cells are highly metastatic while other cells have very low metastatic capacity. Again, this heterogeneity and variability of malignant cell populations makes it very difficult to clearly establish the characteristics that participate in the metastatic process.

Taking into consideration the limitations imposed on research by the models, let us review the available information on studies of the relationship between procoagulant activity and the metastatic capacity of malignant cells. One very active group of investigators in this area of coagulation and metastasis research is at the Mario Negri

Institute in Milan, Italy (16,17,21,32,53,64,75,79-88). They have examined the Lewis lung carcinoma (16,79-81,84,87), the JW sarcoma (64,75,82,83), the colon 26 carcinoma (88), the Ehrlich carcinoma ascites (75,88), the B16 melanoma (88), and the MN/MCA1 and mFS6 fibrosarcoma (85,88). These investigators have used the spontaneous model described above to examine the effect of either dietarily or pharmacologically induced vitamin K deficiency on the metastatic capacity of Lewis lung carcinoma cells (3LL; 16,80,88). There is a significant reduction in the number and mass of lung metastases in mice that are treated continuously with warfarin starting 7 da before tumor implantation until death and in mice fed a vitamin K deficient diet for the same period of time. There is a reduction in cell procoagulant activity that parallels the reduction in weight and number of metastastic tumors. Repletion of vitamin K to vitamin K depleted animals(both pharmacologically and dietarily induced) restores the metastatic capacity and procoagulant activity of the tumor cells. When mice are treated with heparin or are defibrinated (by treatment with Batroxobin snake venom) there is a minimal effect on the metastatic behavior or procoagulant activity of the cells. These investigators demonstrated that the cellular procoagulant activity in the 3LL cells is active in the absence of factor VII and presumably might be classified as cancer procoagulant. The cancer procoagulant from the 3LL cells is vitamin K dependent and may contain gamma-carboxyglutamic acid for the binding of calcium (81). Two other murine malignant cell lines, JW sarcoma (64,75,82,83), and the mFS6 benzopyrene-induced fibrosarcoma (85,88), have been examined in the same type of metastasis model. The JW sarcoma has activity that is similar to that of the 3LL and which has been tentatively identified as cancer procoagulant, because it initiates coagulation in factor VII-deficient plasma. Both of these cell lines also exhibit parallel decreases in cellular procoagulant activity and in metastatic capacity. The JW cell line contrasts with the mFS6 cell line; mFS6 cells contain a procoagulant that is inactive in factor VII-deficient plasma and that is probably tissue factor. Neither cellular procoagulant activity nor metastatic capacity are affected by vitamin K depletion. Thus, these studies suggest that the 3LL, JW sarcoma and B16 melanoma produce cancer procoagulant and are sensitive to vitamin K depletion.

The factor or factors that are responsible for metastasis are difficult to dissect out due to all the events that take place between tumor implantation and formation of metastatic lung tumors. However, studies with the B16 melanoma in the hematologic phase metastasis model, although artificial, may provide some additional data on the relationship between cellular procoagulant activity and metastatic capacity of B16 melanoma cells. B16 mouse melanoma cells produce a cysteine proteinase procoagulant with the same enzymatic and immunologic properties as cancer procoagulant. Two metastatic variants of the B16 mouse melanoma were studied: B16-F1, with a low incidence of lung colonization and B16-F10, with a high incidence of lung colonization. To study the relationship between cellular procoagulant activity and metastatic capacity, a cell suspension of cultured B16 cells was obtained, and an aliquot of 50,000 cells was analyzed for cellular procoagulant activity. Other aliquots of 50,000 cells from the same cell suspension were injected into the tail vein of mice; 17 da later the number of melanotic lung tumors was counted and correlated with the procoagulant activity. Figure 2 shows the strong positive correlation (r = 0.9) between these two parameters. These data suggest that cellular procoagulant activity may have a direct positive effect on the metastatic capacity of a blood-borne tumor cell by promoting fibrin formation. These results are consistent with those described previously with the spontaneous metastasis model and would suggest that the role of fibrin formation in the B16 melanoma, the 3LL carcinoma and the JW sarcoma is to either protect the blood-borne malignant cell from destruction by the host immune system or to promote aggregation and arrest of the blood-borne malignant cell within the lung capillaries. The data suggest that the procoagulant activity is not participating in the diminished capacity of the malignant cell to enter the bloodstream from the primary tumor.

There are some important therapeutic implications in the information presented here. Activation of the coagulation system and fibrin deposition are associated with the metastatic process and inhibition of coagulation or decreased fibrin deposition diminishes tumor growth and metastasis. Selective inhibition of cancer cell procoagulant activity with specific inhibitors or antibodies may break the chain of events involved in the metastatic process and provide a mechanism for diminishing or preventing metastatic dissemination of malignancies.

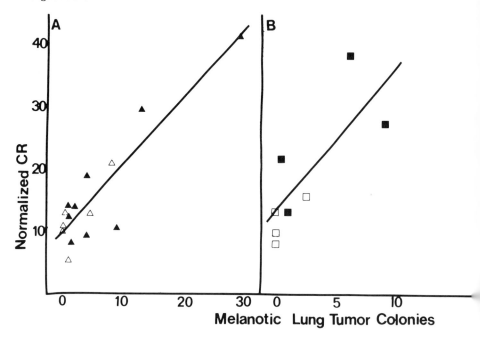

FIGURE 2. Regression Analysis of Procoagulant Activity (Normalized CR) versus the Number of Melanotic Lung Tumor Colonies for the B16-F1 (open symbols) and B16-F10 (closed symbols) Cell Lines. Each point represents the average of 2 to 4 values for procoagulant activity and the median of 4 to 5 values for metastatic capacity for the same cell suspension sample. The correlation coefficient is 0.90 for Expt. 1 (triangles) and 0.79 for Expt. 2 (squares). [From Gilbert and Gordon (76) with permission].

REFERENCES

1. Warren S, Gates O: The fate of intravenously injected tumor cells. Am. J. Cancer 27:485-492, 1936.
2. Wood S, Jr.: Experimental studies on the spread of cancer, with special reference to fibrinolytic agents and anticoagulants. J. Med. 5:7-22, 1974.
3. Wood S, Jr., Strauli P: Tumor invasion and metastasis. IN: Gregory JE (ed.) The Pathogenesis of Cancer. Fremont Foundation, Pasadena, pp. 140-151, 1955.
4. Wood S, Jr., Baker RR, Marzocchi B: In vivo studies of tumor behavior: Locomotion of and interrelationships between normal cells and cancer cells. IN: The Proliferation and Spread of Neoplastic Cells, collection of papers presented at 21st Annual Symposium on Fundamental Cancer Research. William & Wilkins Co., Baltimore, pp. 495-507, 1968.
5. Wood S, Jr.: Mechanisms of establishment of tumor metastases. IN: Ioachim HL (ed.) Pathobiology Annual 1971. Appleton Century-Crofts, New York, pp. 281-308, 1971.
6. Jones DS, Wallace AC, Fraser EE: Sequence of events in experimental metastasis of Walker 256 tumor: Light, immuno-fluorescent, and electron microscopic observations. J. Natl. Cancer Inst. 46:493-504, 1971.
7. Chew EC, Josephson RL, Wallace AC: Morphologic aspects of the arrest of circulating cells. IN: Weiss L (ed.) Fundamental Aspects of Metastasis. North-Holland Pub. Co., Amsterdam, pp. 121-150, 1976.
8. Hagmar B: Tumour growth and spontaneous metastasis spread in two syngeneic systems. Acta Pathol. Microbiol. Scand. Section A 78:131-142, 1970.
9. Kinjo M: Lodgement and extravasation of tumour cells in blood-borne metastasis: An electron microscope study. Br. J. Cancer 38:293-300, 1978.
10. Warren BA: Environment of the blood-borne tumor embolus adherent to vessel wall. J. Med. 4:150-177, 1973.
11. Roos E, Dingemans KP: Mechanisms of metastasis. Biochim. Biophys. Acta 560:135-166, 1979.
12. Millar RC, Ketcham AS: The effect of heparin and warfarin on primary and metastatic tumors. J. Med. 5:23-31, 1974.
13. Skolnik G, Alpsten M, Ivarsson L: Studies on mechanisms involved in metastasis formation from circulating tumor cells. J. Cancer Res. Clin. Oncol. 97:249-256, 1980.

168

14. Hilgard P, Thornes RD: Anticoagulants in the treatment of cancer. Eur. J. Cancer 12:755-762, 1976.

15. Brown JM: A study of the mechanism by which anticoagulation with warfarin inhibits blood-borne metastases. Cancer Res. 33:1217-1224, 1973.

16. Poggi A, Colucci M, Delaini F, Semeraro N, Donati MB: Reduced procoagulant activity of Lewis lung carcinoma cells from mice treated with warfarin. Eur. J. Cancer 16:1641-1642, 1980.

17. Colucci M, Delaini F, Vitti G, Vita G, Locati D, Poggi A, Semeraro N, Donati MB: Cancer cell procoagulant activity, warfarin and experimental metastases. IN: Hellmann K, Hilgard P and Eccles S (eds.) Metastasis: Clinical and Experimental Aspects. Martinus Nijhoff, The Hague, pp. 90-94, 1980.

18. Zacharski LR, Henderson WG, Rickles FR, Forman WB, Cornell CJ, Jr., Forcier RJ, Edwards R, Headley E, Kim S-H, O'Donnell JF, O'Dell R, Tornyos K, Kwaan HC: J. Am. Med. Assoc. 245:831-835, 1981.

19. Saito D, Sawamura M, Umezawa K, Yoshiyuki K, Furihata C, Matsushima T, Sugimura T: Inhibition of experimental blood-borne lung metastasis by protease inhibitors. Cancer Res. 40:2539-2542, 1980.

20. Wood S, Jr., Hilgard PH: Arvin-induced hypofibrinogenemia and metastasis formation from blood-borne cancer cells. Johns Hopkins Med. J. 133:207-213, 1973.

21. Donati MB, Poggi A, Mussoni L, de Gaetano G, Garattini S: Hemostasis and experimental cancer dissemination. IN: Day SB (ed.) Cancer Invasion and Metastasis: Biologic Mechanisms and Therapy. Raven Press, New York, pp. 151-160, 1977.

22. Kodama Y, Tanaka K: Effect of urokinase on growth and metastases of rabbit V2 carcinoma. GANN 69:9-18, 1978.

23. Ambrus JL, Ambrus CM, Pickern J, Slodes S, Bross I: Hematologic changes and thromboembolic complications in neoplastic disease and their relationship to metastasis J. Med. 6:433-458, 1975.

24. Brown JM: A study of the mechanism by which anticoagulation with warfarin inhibits blood-borne metastases. Cancer Res. 33:1217-1224, 1973.

25. Cliffton EE, Agostino D, Minde K: Effect of hyperlipemia on pulmonary metastases of the Walker 256 carcinoma in the rat. Cancer Res. 21:1062-1067, 1961.

26. Glaves D, Weiss L: Initial tumor cell arrest in animals of defined coagulative status. Int. J. Cancer 21:741-746, 1978.

27. Ogura T, Tsubura E, Yamamura Y: Localization of radioiodinated fibrinogen in invaded and metastasized tumor tissue of Walker carcinosarcoma. GANN 61:443-449, 1970.

28. Dvorak HF, Dvorak AM, Manseau EJ, Wilberg L, Churchill WH: Fibrin gel investment associated with Line 1 and Line 10 solid tumor growth, angiogenesis, and fibroplasia in guinea pigs. Role of cellular immunity, myofibroblasts, microvascular damage and infarction in Line 1 tumor regression. J. Natl. Cancer Inst. 62:1459-1472, 1979.

29. O'Meara RAQ, Jackson RD: Cytological observations on carcinoma. Ir. J. Med. Sci. 391:327-328, 1958.

30. Day ED, Planinsek JA, Pressman D: Localization in vivo of radioiodinated anti-rat-fibrin antibodies and radioiodinated rat fibrinogen in the Murphy rat lymphosarcoma and in other transplantable rat tumors. J. Natl. Cancer Inst. 22:413-416, 1959.

31. Goodall CM, Saunders AG, Shubik P: Studies of vascular patterns in living tumors with a transparent chamber inserted in hamster cheek pouch. J. Natl. Cancer Inst. 35:495-521, 1965.

32. Donati MB, Poggi A, Semeraro N: Coagulation and malignancy. IN: Poller L (ed.) Recent Advances in Blood Coagulation. Churchill-Livingston, Edinburgh, pp. 227-259, 1981.

33. Hart IR, Fidler IJ: Role of organ selectivity in the metastatic patterns of B16 melanoma. Cancer Res. 40:2281-2287, 1980.

34. Raz A, Bucana C, McLellan W, Fidler IJ: Distribution of membrane anionic sites on B16 melanoma variants with differing lung colonising potential. Nature (London) 284:363-364, 1980.

35. Weiss L, Mayhew E, Glaves-Rapp D, Holmes JC: Metastatic inefficiency in mice bearing B16 melanomas. Br. J. Cancer 45:44-53, 1982.

36. Gorelik E, Bere WW, Herberman RB: Role of NK cells in the antimetastatic effect of anticoagulant drugs. Int. J. Cancer 33:87-94, 1984.

37. Liotta LA, Kleinerman J, Saidel GM: The significance of hematogenous tumor cell clumps in the metastatic process. Cancer Res. 36:889-894, 1976.

38. Fidler IJ: The relationship of embolic homogeneity, number, size and viability to the incidence of experimental metastasis. Eur. J. Cancer 9:223-227, 1973.

39. Watanabe S: Metastasizability of tumor cells. Cancer 7:215-223, 1954.

40. Pineo GF, Rogoeczi E, Hatton MWC, Brian MC: The activation of coagulation by extracts of mucus: A possible pathway of intravascular coagulation accompanying adenocarcinomas. J. Lab. Clin. Med. 82:255-266, 1973.

41. Boggust WA, O'Brien DJ, O'Meara RAW, Thornes RD: The coagulative factors of normal human and human cancer tissue. Ir. J. Med. Sci. 447:131-144, 1963.

42. Dvorak HF, Quay SC, Orenstein NS, Dvorak AM, Hahn P, Bitzer AM: Tumor shedding and coagulation. Science 212:923-924, 1981.

43. Nemerson Y, Bach R: Tissue factor revisited. IN: Spaet TH (ed.) Progress in Hemostasis and Thrombosis. Grune & Stratton, New York, Vol. 6, pp. 237-261, 1982.

44. Nemerson Y, Pitlick FA: The tissue factor pathway of blood coagulation. IN: Spaet TH (ed.) Progress in Hemostasis and Thrombosis. Grune & Stratton, New York, Vol. 1, pp. 1-37, 1972.

45. Bach R, Nemerson Y, Konigsberg W: Purification and characterization of bovine tissue factors. J. Biol. Chem. 256:8324-8331, 1981.

46. Maynard JR, Fintel DJ, Pitlick FA, Nemerson Y: Tissue factor in cultured cells. Lab. Invest. 35:550-556, 1976.

47. Zeldis SM, Nemerson Y, Pitlick FA: Tissue factor (thromboplastin): localization to plasma membranes by peroxidase-conjugated antibodies. Science 175:766-767, 1972.

48. Ewan VA, Edwards RL, Rickles FR: Expression of procoagulant activity in a human monocyte-like cell line. J. Lab. Clin. Med. 101:401-410, 1983.

49. Schwartz BS, Levy GA, Edgington TS: Immune complex-induced human monocyte procoagulant activity. II. Cellular kinetics and metabolic requirements. J. Immunol. 128:1037-1042, 1982.

50. Edwards RL, Rickles FR, Cronlund M: Abnormalities of blood coagulation in patients with cancer: Mononuclear cell tissue factor generation. J. Lab. Clin. Med. 98:917-928, 1981.

51. Prydz H, Allison AC: Tissue thromboplastin activity of isolated human monocytes. Thromb. Haemostasis 39:582-591, 1978.

52. Scortellazzo PV, Barbui T, Colucci M, Semeraro N: Impaired production of mononuclear cell procoagulant activity in chronic lymphocytic leukaemia. J. Clin. Pathol. 36:37-40, 1983.

53. Frank LA, Holyoke ED: Tumor fluid thromboplastin activity. Int. J. Cancer 3:677-682, 1968.

54. Holyoke ED, Ichihashi H: The c3H/St/Ha mammary tumor. I. Thromboplastin content. J. Natl. Cancer Inst. 36:1049-1056, 1966.

55. Gordon SG, Franks JJ, Lewis B: Cancer procoagulant A: A factor X activating procoagulant from malignant tissue. Thromb. Res. 6:127-137, 1975.

56. Sakuragawa N, Takahashi K, Hoshiyama M, Jimbo C, Matsuoka M, Onishi Y: Pathologic cells as procoagulant substance of disseminated intravascular coagulation syndrome in acute promyelocytic leukemia. Thromb. Res. 8:263-273, 1976.

57. Garg SK, Niemetz J: Tissue factor activity of normal and leukemic cells. Blood 42:729-735, 1973.

58. Kohga S: Thromboplastic and fibrinolytic activities of ascites tumor cells of rats, with reference to their role in metastasis formation. GANN 69:461-470, 1978.

59. Sakuragawa N, Takahashi K, Hoshiyama M, Jimbo C, Ashizawa K, Matsuoka M, Ohnishi Y: The extract from the tissue of gastric cancer as procoagulant in disseminated intravascular coagulation syndrome. Thromb. Res. 10:457-463, 1977.

60. Ishikawa K: Tissue fibrinolyte activity in malignant skin tumors: Correlation with blood fibrinolytic and coagulative factors. Iwate Igaki Zasshi 32:825-835, 1980.

61. Goualt-Heilman M, Chardon E, Sultan E, Josse F: The procoagulant factor of leukaemic promyelocytes: Demonstration of immunologic cross-reactivity with human brain tissue factor. Br. J. Haematol. 30:151-158, 1975.

62. Pearlstein EP, Ambrogio C, Gasic GJ, Karpatkin S: Inhibition of platelet-aggregating activity of two human adenocarcinomas of the colon and an anaplastic murine tumor with a specific thrombin inhibitor, dansyl arginine N-(3-ethyl-1, 5-pentanediyl)amide. Cancer Res. 41:4533-4539, 1981.

63. Svanberg L: Thromboplastic activity of human ovarian tumours. Thromb. Res. 6:307-313, 1975.

64. Colucci M, Giavazzi R, Alessandri G, Semeraro N, Mantovani A, Donati MB: Procoagulant activity of sarcoma sublines with different metastatic potential. Blood 57:733-735, 1981.

65. Gordon SG, Cross BA: A factor X activating cysteine protease from malignant tissue. J. Clin. Invest. 67:1665-1671, 1981.
66. Falanga A, Gordon SG: Isolation and characterization of cancer procoagulant: A cysteine proteinase from malignant tissue. (Submitted).
67. Gordon SG, Hasiba U, Poole MA, Falanga A: A cysteine proteinase procoagulant from amnion-chorion. (Submitted).
68. Unpublished observation.
69. Gordon SG, Gilbert LC, Lewis BJ: Analysis of procoagulant activity of intact cells from tissue culture. Thromb. Res. 26:379-387, 1982.
70. Gordon SG: A proteolytic procoagulant associated with malignant transformation. J. Histochem. Cytochem. 29:457-463, 1981.
71. Gordon SG, Lewis B: Comparison of procoagulant from normal and transformed fibroblasts. Cancer Res. 38:2467-2472, 1978.
72. Gordon SG, Franks JJ, Lewis BJ: Comparison of procoagulants in extracts of normal and malignant human tissue. J. Natl. Cancer Inst. 62:773-776, 1979.
73. Cattan A, Bresson ML: Murine tumor cell activity on in vitro hemostasis. Biomedicine 25:252-254, 1976.
74. Hilgard P, Whur P: Factor X-activating activity from Lewis lung carcinoma. Br. J. Cancer 41:642-643, 1980.
75. Curatola L, Colucci M, Cambini AL, Poggi A, Morasca L, Donati MB, Semeraro N: Evidence that cells from experimental tumours can activate coagulation factor X. Br. J. Cancer 40:228-233, 1979.
76. Gilbert LC, Gordon SG: Relationship between cellular procoagulant activity and metastatic capacity of B16 mouse melanoma variants. Cancer Res. 43:536-540, 1983.
77. Donati MB, Semeraro N, Gordon SG: Relationship between procoagulant activity and metastatic capacity of tumor cells. IN: Honn KV and Sloane BF (eds.) Hemostatic Mechanisms and Metastasis. Martinus Nijhoff, The Hague, pp. 84-92, 1984.
78. Markus G: The role of hemostasis and fibrinolysis in the metastatic spread of cancer. Semin. Thromb. Hemostasis 10:61-70, 1984.
79. Donati MB, Mussoni L, Poggi A, De Gaetano G, Garattini S: Growth and metastasis of the Lewis lung carcinoma in mice defibrinated with Batroxobin. Eur. J. Cancer 14:343-347, 1978.
80. Colucci M, Delaini F, De Bellis Vitti G, Locati D, Poggi A, Semeraro N, Donati MB: Warfarin inhibits both procoagulant activity and metastatic capacity of Lewis lung carcinoma cells. Biochem. Pharmacol. 32:2689-2691, 1983.
81. Delaini F, Colucci M, De Bellis Vitti G, Locati D, Poggi A, Semeraro N, Donati MB: Cancer cell procoagulant: A novel vitamin K-dependent activity. Thromb. Res. 24:263-266, 1981.
82. Chmielewska J, Poggi A, Mussoni L, Donati MB, Garattini S: Blood coagulation changes in JW sarcoma, a new metastasizing tumour in mice. Eur. J. Cancer 16:1399-1407, 1980.
83. Chmielewska J, Poggi A, Janik P, Latallo ZS, Donati MB: Effect of defibrination with Batroxobin on growth and metastasis of JW sarcoma in mice. Eur. J. Cancer 16:919-923, 1980.

172

84. Poggi A, Polentarutti N, Donati MB, De Gaetano G, Garattini S: Blood coagulation changes in mice bearing Lewis lung carcinoma, a metastasizing tumor. Cancer Res. 37:272-277, 1977.
85. Delaini F, Giavazzi R, De Bellis Vitti G, Alessandri G, Mantovani A, Donati MB: Tumour sublines with different metastatic capacity induce similar blood coagulation changes in the host. Br. J. Cancer 43:100-104, 1983.
86. Colucci M, Curatolo L, Donati MB, Semeraro N: Cancer cell procoagulant activity: Evaluation by an amidolytic assay. Thromb. Res. 18:589-595, 1980.
87. Poggi A, Donati MB, Polentarutti N, De Gaetano G, Garattini S: On thrombocytopenia developing in mice bearing a spontaneously metastasizing tumor. Z. Krebsforsch. 86:303-306, 1976.
88. Giavazzi R, Alessandri G, Spreafico F, Garattini S, Mantovani A: Metastasizing capacity of tumour cells from spontaneous metastases of transplanted murine tumours. Br. J. Cancer 42:462-469, 1980.
89. Poggi A, Mussoni L, Kornblihtt L, Ballabio E, Gaetano G, Donati BM: Warfarin enantiomers, anticoagulation, and experimental tumour metastasis. Lancet I:163-164, 1978.

CHAPTER 12. ROLE OF GROWTH STIMULATORY FACTORS IN DETERMINING THE SITES OF METASTASIS

PETER ALEXANDER, PAUL V. SENIOR, PAUL MURPHY AND RICHARD CLARKE

I. INTRODUCTION

Two theories have been put forth to explain why cancer emboli show a degree of selectivity for the organs in which they give rise to metastases. There is Ewings opinion that "the mechanism of the circulation will doubtlessly explain most of these peculiarities" and there is the concept of Paget who likened tumor emboli to seeds which need to fall into a suitable soil if they are to grow. In this Chapter we describe experiments designed to elucidate the role of host factors in causing site selectivity of blood borne metastasis in three chemically induced rat tumors, a carcinoma, a sarcoma and a hepatoma. To perform such studies it is essential to eliminate the hemodynamic factors which dictate the first organ encountered by the embolus as these can obscure other mechanisms.

The tumors used in our studies were induced in our syngeneic hooded Lister rats and transplanted within rats of this colony. The sarcoma had been produced by a subcutaneous implant of methyl-cholanthrene and the breast carcinoma by an implant of estrogen. The breast carcinoma remains estrogen dependent and all rats injected with this tumor require an implant of a pellet containing estrogen. The hepatoma had been induced by feeding dimethylazobenzene. All tumors had been transplanted a number of times. To avoid biological drift we restricted ourselves to five subcutaneous passages before returning to frozen stock. Tumor cells were prepared by enzymatic disaggregation with neutral bacterial protease DNAse.

A. Initial Arrest of Cancer Cells

Depending on the site of the primary cancer, cancer cells will be discharged into the portal vein, where the first capillary bed in which trapping can occur will be the liver, or into the vena caval system where the organ of first encounter is the lung. Only with cancers in the lung do tumor cells gain immediate access to the systemic arterial circulation. Detailed autopsy investigations (1-3) show conclusively that metastases occur most frequently in the liver for cancers such as those of the colon which drain to the liver and in the lung for cancers arising above the abdomen which drain to the lung. Hemodynamic considerations also explain why with tumors that drain into the portal system, the second most common site for metastasis, after the liver, is the lung. The lung is the second capillary bed which will be encountered by tumor cells which have passed through, or derive from, the liver. Dissemination beyond the lung must stem from cells that have gained access to the systemic arterial circulation via the pulmonary vein and the left ventricle. Tumor cells may also be carried directly from the vena cava to bone through venous plexuses to the vertebrae (4). But this caveat apart, blood borne dissemination must be divided into A) organ of the first encounter and B) systemic via the arterial system; the latter can also of course result in lung and liver metastases coming from cancer cells which have gained access through the bronchial or hepatic artery.

A question having potential clinical relevance is whether cells reach the arterial circulation as a result of having traversed the capillary bed of the lung with their reproductive integrity unimpaired, or whether blood borne cancer cells are initially contained within lung or liver because they are either wholly trapped or irreversibly damaged while passing through the lung or liver. If the latter situation pertains then systemic dissemination would stem from cells released by metastases growing in these organs of first encounter (metastasis from metastases; see Chapter 23). For the three experimental rat tumors with which this report is concerned, there is strong experimental evidence (5) that the cells are completely trapped in lung and liver following intravenous or intraportal inoculation. A variety of procedures failed to detect transpulmonary passage of intact cells. The sensitivity of the methods was such as to have detected passage through lung or liver of 1% of the cancer cells. In general these studies are in accord with a large body of data by others using experimental carcinomas and sarcomas; following intravenous injection such tumors were either seen only in the lung or if they occurred in other organs did so at a time when they could have occurred as a metastasis which stemmed from a lung lesion. Transpulmonary passage of fully viable cells of lymphoid and myeloid origin is to be anticipated and has been reported. Zeidman and Buss (6) found evidence for the presence in systemic arterial blood of rabbit tumor cells that had been injected intravenously, but the manner in which these experiments were performed did not permit quantitation.

The data in experimental animals seem to mirror those seen in man. On the basis of detailed post-mortem studies, Willis has questioned whether carcinoma and sarcoma cells traverse the lung (1).

B. Role of Host Factors

There is compelling evidence, both experimental and clinical, that the incidence of metastases beyond the lung is dictated by the environment and not by blood flow. Although the whole of the venous blood traverses the lung and the whole of the portal blood traverses the liver, only a fraction of the arterial blood traverses any one organ or tissue. If mechanical factors of the circulation are the sole determinant of the distribution of metastases, then the incidence of metastases deriving from the arterial circulation should be proportional to the fraction of the cardiac output received by the different organs. The facts are the opposite. Blood borne metastases are rare in muscle and gut which between them take more than half of the cardiac output yet occur predominantly in organs such as liver and adrenal which receive a very small fraction of the cardiac output. The high frequency of liver metastases from primary cancers with initial drainage into the vena caval system was considered by Willis (1) to provide a striking illustration of the discordance between cardiac output and incidence of metastases, since in this situation the cancer emboli reach the liver via the hepatic artery which only received a few percent of the arterial blood. The remarkable site selectivity of metastases stemming from cells in the arterial circulation can be investigated experimentally by inoculating tumor cells directly into the left side of the heart. The few studies (7,8) that have been performed show that the relative incidence of metastases in different organs bears no relationship to cardiac output.

Host factors which determine whether a cancer embolus develops into a metastasis fall into one of two classes: A) negative effects which result in the intravascular death of the cancer cells, i.e., before it has extravasated and B) stimulatory effects such as might stem from growth factors provided by the host tissue. Our initial working hypothesis (9) was that the probability of an embolus developing to a metastasis depended critically on the rate at which the cancer cells are killed after arrest in a capillary bed, as this decided whether the cancer cell succeeds in extravasating. Our initial concept was that once the cell has extravasated it has a high probability of developing into a metastasis. Accordingly we investigated the various mechanisms that can cause the death of circulating cancer cells. The studies summarized below indicate that the rate of cell destruction is a key factor in determining the overall metastatic incidence, but that the organ selectivity beyond the lung (i.e., after entry of cancer cells into the arterial circulation) cannot be explained by differences in cell death in the various capillary beds. The site preference - after the organ of first encounter - is more likely to be determined by the supply of host-derived growth factors.

II. MECHANISMS OF INTRAVASCULAR CELL DEATH

Evidence that the vast majority of cancer cells shed from tumors into the venous circulation fail to develop into metastases is overwhelming. This phenomenon which Leonard Weiss has very aptly referred to as metastatic inefficiency has been reviewed several times (9 and Chapter 3). Mechanisms which contribute to the destruction or sterilization of cancer emboli are listed in Table 1.

A. Specific Immunity

That specific T-cell dependent immunity to antigenic tumors contributes to an important degree to the destruction of tumor emboli from some, but by no means all cancers, has been demonstrated in experimental systems in which immunosuppression has been found to facilitate metastasis (for review see 9). There are many sarcomas and some lymphomas where from 80-100% of the animals can be "cured" by surgery, yet if the animals are immunosuppressed almost all will die of distant metastases. Moreover, sarcomas and lymphomas which do not

Table 1.

A. ESCAPE OF TUMOR EMBOLI FROM MICROVASCULATURE DETERMINED BY:

    1. Rate of cell death while <u>intravascular</u>:

       Specific immunity

       Non-specific destruction by leukocytes

       Mechanical trauma

       Oxygen toxicity

       Thrombus formation

    2. Rate of extravasation:

       Accessibility of basement membrane

       Attachment to basement membrane

       Penetration

B. FATE OF TUMOR CELLS AFTER EXTRAVASATION DETERMINED BY:

       Growth factors produced by tumor cells

       Growth factors produced by host tissue

       Dormancy

       Differentiation

metastasize in normal syngeneic mice do so in genetically athymic "nude" mice. However, there are experimental tumors, particularly carcinomas, in which immunosuppression does not facilitate metastatic spread (9). Furthermore, immunity can play no part in the rapid destruction within the lung of cancer cells inoculated intravenously into normal (i.e., non-tumor bearing) animals, as this occurs much more rapidly than the induction of immunity (10).

B. Destruction by Leukocytes

Granulocytes, monocytes, mitogen-stimulated lymphocytes and NK cells from normal animals that have not been exposed to tumors will all kill cells in vitro. The susceptibility of different cancer cells to different classes of leukocytes varies and the order of in vitro sensitivity of a range of tumor cells depends on the type of leukocyte tested (Table 2 and 11). There is some evidence (12) that killing by granulocytes and monocytes contributes to the intravascular lysis of cancer cells, however, claims that NK cells play a role have not been supported (13). [An opposing viewpoint is discussed in Chapter 15.] At best, however, non-specific destruction by leukocytes can only be a minor component in the rapid autolysis of tumor cells after arrest in the lung (10) as this occurs to nearly the same extent and rate in mice that are grossly leukopenic following total body irradiation.

C. Damage in Passing through Capillaries

Sato and Suzuki (14) have shown that rat ascites cells sustain irreversible mechanical damage from shearing forces experienced in passing through narrow capillaries. Our experiments (5) in which we compared the cell dose needed to induce lesions in the lung by intravenous as compared to arterial injection indicate that intravascular mechanical trauma irreversibly damages sarcoma, hepatoma and carcinoma tumor cells. Experiments with radiolabeled cancer cells show that these cells do not pass morphologically intact through lung or liver but approximately one third can traverse the major capillary beds (e.g., skin, muscle and gut) supplied by arterial blood following left ventricle injection. Following intravenous or intraportal injection essentially all of the radioactivity associated with morphologically intact cancer cells is found in the lung or liver immediately after inoculation. Eighty-nine percent of the radioactivity found in the lung immediately after injection is lost from this organ within 16 hr. This disappearance is not associated with recirculation of viable tumor cells to other organs, but is a consequence of cell damage. The activity builds up initially in the liver and then as a result of autolysis appears as free iodide. If the cells have been slowly released over 24 hr into the systemic circulation, they will be distributed as observed after left ventricular inoculation (see Table 3), but this is not the case in detailed studies of sarcoma cells.

Table 2. Susceptibility in Vitro of Tumors to Immunologically Non-Specific Leukocyte Effectors.

	Tumor Cells Used	NK Cells	MAF Activated Macrophages	% Lysis By: Stimulated Granulocytes	"Lymphotoxin" Diluted to: 1:64	1:256
Sarcoma (C57/BL)	FS6	15	21	9	100	95
Sarcoma (CBA)	FS29	27	26	13	65	47
Melanoma (C57/BL)	B16	20	12	11	8	4
Lymphoma (DBA/2)	L5178Y	19	50	28	6	0
Lymphoma (C57/BL)	TLX9	4	62	18	0	0

Evidence that a proportion of blood borne cancer cells can pass through the capillaries comes from experiments in which the distribution of radioactive plastic microspheres of 15 μm diameter is compared with that following inoculation of ^{125}IUdr-labeled sarcoma cells. The microspheres are completely trapped in the capillaries and the fraction of radioactivity counted in an organ represents the proportion of cardiac output received by this organ.

The data in Table 3 demonstrate that the distribution of radioactivity in different organs immediately after injection of labeled sarcoma cells differed in two respects from the cardiac output received by these organs as measured by the microsphere method. First, a much higher proportion of the cell associated radioactivity appeared in lung (and also liver - data not shown) than corresponded to the cardiac output. In all of the other organs the radioactivity from cells ran parallel to that from microspheres and was approximately 35% less than the microspheres. These differences between cardiac output and distribution of radiolabeled tumor cells suggest that a fraction of the cancer cells were capable of traversing the capillary beds of muscle, kidney, skin, gut, etc. to be trapped via venous circulation in the lung or liver.

Table 3. Relationship between Fraction of Cardiac Output Received by Different Organs in Male Rats and Fraction of Radiolabeled Sarcoma Cells Trapped following Left Ventricular Injection.

	Cardiac Output (%) Distribution as Determined by Microsphere Injection	Sarcoma Cells (%) Trapped at 5 min
Muscle/Bone	37.0 ± 7.0	26.7 ± 4.1
Kidney	14.8 ± 4.7	9.3 ± 3.3
Skin	12.5 ± 2.4	5.73 ± 2.6
Heart	8.3 ± 3.4	5.1 ± 1.6
Brown Fat	5.1 ± 2.1	5.5 ± 3.2
Brain	3.3 ± 0.7	1.4 ± 0.7
Adrenals	0.4 ± 0.2	0.2 ± 0.1
Lung	1.16 ± 0.29	20.6 ± 2.8

However, cancer cells which had gained access to the lung or liver following intracardiac injection were much less tumorigenic than cells that had reached these organs directly. Thus, the number of sarcoma cells needed to produce a lung tumor following intravenous injection was of the order of 10^4 cells and 5 of 8 rats developed a lung tumor. Via the portal vein 5×10^3 cells caused liver lesions in 4 of 4 rats. In contrast, following an arterially administered dose (left ventricle) of 2×10^6 sarcoma cells neither lung or liver tumors were observed. From the results of injecting radiolabeled cells we can conclude that the lung received 20% of the injected dose of cells (i.e., 4×10^5 cells) and the liver 10% (i.e., 2×10^5 cells). Therefore, 10^4 sarcoma cells deposited directly via the venous circulation produced tumors in lung or liver whereas $2-5 \times 10^5$ cells reaching these organs following transcapillary passage were not tumorigenic.

III. OXYGEN TOXICITY

Normal cells, with the exception of those lining blood vessels, as well as the majority of cancer cells replicate in a milieu provided by extracellular fluid in which the concentration of dissolved oxygen is approximately one quarter that in arterial blood (i.e., that attained by equilibration with air). Cancer emboli arrested in a capillary bed will be exposed, prior to extravasation, to concentrations of oxygen that are much higher than those found extravascularly. The precise oxygen concentration encountered will depend on their position within the microvasculature. Thus, in the lung the oxygen concentration will be at its lowest on the arterial side of the capillary and at its highest at the venous end. In other organs (except those provided with a portal blood supply) the oxygen concentration will be higher for cells stopped in small arteries or precapillary sphincters than in the actual capillaries. A large embolus consisting of either an aggregate of several cancer cells or a cancer cell around which a clot has formed is likely to be arrested at the arterial side and a single cancer cell is likely to penetrate into the capillaries. Accordingly, in the lung a large embolus will be retained in an environment which has a lower oxygen concentration than that of an isolated blood-borne cancer cell whereas in other organs - particularly those with a high rate of oxygen consumption - the reverse will be the case.

We have been testing the hypothesis that oxygen at a concentration approaching that of blood in equilibrium with air is harmful to blood borne cancer cells and that oxygen toxicity may contribute to the death of cancer cells trapped in capillary beds. This suggestion is not at variance with general tissue culture experience. There can be no doubt that long established cell lines which can proliferate _in vitro_ from low cell numbers (or indeed as single cells) are not inhibited by oxygen at normal concentrations. However, this does not necessarily apply to the growth _in vitro_ of recently explanted cells, i.e., cells not adapted to standard _in vitro_ conditions. Successful growth of such cells usually requires large cell inocula. When the cell concentration is high (greater than 10^4 cells/ml) the actual oxygen concentration to which the cells are exposed _in vitro_ can be very much lower than atmospheric. Consumption of oxygen by the cultures is not compensated for by the slow diffusion in the tissue culture vessels. The magnitude of this effect depends on the seeding density and the metabolic rate of the cells (16). Therefore, to determine the effect of oxygen tension on growth, cells need to be seeded at low densities to minimize depletion of oxygen. Indeed, at high cell densities in vitro, the oxygen concentration may be below that needed for optimum growth even when the culture is exposed to the atmosphere. There have been several reports (17,18) that cells isolated directly from animals will grow (at low seeding densities) better in cultures exposed to atmospheres containing 5% oxygen than to air.

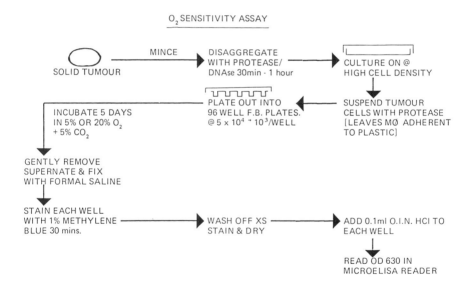

Figure 1.

We have investigated the effect of oxygen concentration on the rate of proliferation of sarcoma and carcinoma cells taken from mice and rats with tumors using the procedure outlined in Figure 1 (9). Most, but not all, of the cancers so far studied grow at low cell numbers only in atmospheres with low oxygen concentrations. The toxic effect of atmospheres rich in oxygen is lost as the initial seeding density is increased (see Figure 2). Indeed, at the highest seeding densities, cells do not grow in atmospheres of low oxygen concentrations. The depletion by metabolism of oxygen in the medium is then so great that the oxygen concentration with which the cells are in contact, measured with an oxygen microelectrode, is now insufficient for optimal growth. The general pattern for many cancer cells prior to adaptation to tissue culture is that they proliferate optimally at oxygen concentrations equivalent to atmospheres of 2% to 5% (as found in extracellular fluid) and die at concentrations greater than 10%. We have noted that cancer cells rapidly adapt to oxygen when grown in vitro. Sometimes after as few as two passages in vitro and usually after five passages, the cells grow equally well when exposed to 18% as to 5% oxygen. This is true even at low cell densities when measurements with oxygen microelectrodes show that high oxygen concentrations are achieved at the point of contact between the culture medium and the cells.

A. Mechanism of Toxicity of Oxygen at Atmospheric Concentrations

There have been many investigations into the cytotoxicity of oxygen. Two mechanisms can be considered (see Table 4). The experiments summarized in Table 5 have failed to provide any direct evidence for the involvement of H_2O_2 or O_2^- (i.e., no protection by catalase or superoxide dismutase, respectively). Mannitol, a scavenger for OH radical, only protects the cultures against 20% O_2 at very high concentrations and then only to a marginal degree. The effect of changing the glutathione content of the cancer cells by culturing in medium containing an inhibitor of glutathione synthetase, buthionine sulphoximine (BSO), is complex in that one of the oxygen resistant cancers becomes sensitive to 20% oxygen. On the other hand, cells that have "adapted" to growing in air after prolonged in vitro culture do not become sensitive to oxygen when grown in medium with BSO. An alternative mechanism is that the oxygen sensitive cells rely for intermediate metabolism on enzymes which are poisoned by oxygen (19,20). Table 4 lists examples.

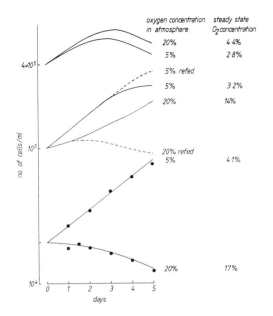

FIGURE 2. Freshly Explanted Murine Sarcoma Cells (FS19) Cultured in Atmospheres of Either 5% O_2, 5% CO_2, 90% N_2 or 20% O_2, 5% CO_2, 75% N_2. Starting inocula were 2 x 10^4, 10^5 and 4 x 10^5 cells/ml. The actual concentration of oxygen in the culture medium of the microwell was measured with a microelectrode. Replenishing the medium every day renders cells more sensitive to 20% O_2.

Table 4. Mechanisms for Cytotoxicity to Cancer Cells of Oxygen at Atmospheric Concentrations.

A. Peroxy Compounds:

    1. H_2O_2 (protection by catalase)

    2. Peroxy radicals (protection by superoxide dismutase)

    3. OH radicals (protected by scavengers like mannitol)

    4. Sensitivity of cells depends on glutathione content of cells. If this is lowered, cells become more sensitive.

B. Oxygen Sensitive Enzymes Essential for Intermediate Metabolism:

    1. Lactic dehydrogenase isoenzyme present in cancer cells, and inhibited by O_2 > corresponding to 5% in gas (19).

    2. Pyruvate oxidase in spirochetes inhibited by O_2 > 7% in gas; reason for failure of organisms to grow aerobically (20).

Table 5. Effects on Inhibition by Oxygen of Growth in Vitro of Freshly
Explanted Murine Sarcoma Cells.

Protective Agent[*] Added	Number of Cells/ml[†]	
	in 5% O_2[‡]	in 20% O_2
None	8.4 (± .7) x 10^4	1.7 (± 0.2) x 10^4
0.1% Catalase	8.6	1.3
0.1% Superoxide Dismutase	8.2	1.6
5 mg/ml Mannitol	8.3 (± 0.2)	2.4 (± 0.3)
1 mg/ml Mannitol	8.8 (± 0.3)	2.4 (± 0.2)
0.25 mg/ml Mannitol	9.0 (± 0.3)	2.1 (± 0.5)
0.05 mg/ml Mannitol	9.3 (± 0.4)	1.7 (± 0.4)

[*]Agents which interfere with cytotoxicity of peroxy compounds.

[†]Determined after 3 da of culture; 4 x 10^4 cells/ml:inoculum.

[‡]Atmospheric concentration of O_2.

B. Effect of Changing Oxygen Content of Gas Breathed on Behavior
    of Pulmonary Metastases

In the pulmonary microcirculation, cancer cells will be exposed to
high (i.e., approaching atmospheric) concentrations of oxygen if
trapped at the tips of the capillaries where the blood becomes
reoxygenated. If they are arrested in small arteries, they will be in
an oxygen-depleted environment. Accordingly, if oxygen at atmospheric
concentrations is toxic to cancer emboli, lung metastases would be
expected to occur more commonly from large emboli that have arrested in
arterioles, than from small emboli arrested in the capillaries. Support
for this hypothesis came from the finding (21) that emboli containing a
cluster of cancer cells give rise to lung metastases more frequently
than single cancer cells.   This would also explain why admixture of
small microspheres of synthetic polymers with cancer cells increases by
a factor of between 10 and 100 the numbers of lung colonies produced by
intravenously administered cancer cells (22).

We have attempted to study more directly whether changing the oxygen concentration breathed by mice and rats following i.v. injection of cancer cells changes the number of lung tumors produced or the rate of autolysis of the trapped cancer cells. In initial experiments exposure of mice to hyperbaric (2.5 atmospheres) oxygen reduced the incidence of lung tumors, but in repeated experiments the results were extremely variable. Therefore, we were unable to reach any conclusions. Others (23) had similar experiences in that hyperbaric oxygen is only effective in reducing the capacity of cancer cells to grow in the lung on some occasion. One reason for this could be that the physiological response to hyperbaric oxygen is complex and the actual change in blood oxygen concentration difficult to evaluate.

We have, therefore, decided to approach the question of the role of oxygen concentration on tumor growth in vivo from an opposite point of view. Namely we will study the role of oxygen in mice and rats breathing a low concentration of oxygen. We find that 8% is the lowest oxygen concentration in which mice and rats can survive for six hours. There is a dramatic increase in the number of lung tumors produced by syngeneic sarcomas in both mice and rats if they are kept for six hours in an atmosphere containing only 8% oxygen compared with air. The trapping in the lung of sarcoma cells injected intravenously is essentially complete (i.e., greater than 95%) under both conditions. Their rate of autolysis two to six hours after inoculation is markedly slowed for rodents breathing 8% oxygen. These experiments suggest that the toxicity of oxygen observed in vitro may have a counterpart in vivo.

IV. ORGAN SELECTIVITY OF METASTASES FOLLOWING INTRAARTERIAL INJECTION OF CANCER CELLS

Like others (7,8), we (5) have found that the distribution of tumors in the different organs of rats following left ventricular injection of sarcoma, hepatoma or carcinoma cells does not parallel the proportion of cardiac output received. In these experiments a cannula is inserted via the right carotid artery into the left side of the heart. The cannulae are kept patent using saline only and are removed 6 to 24 hr after injection; injections are done in conscious rats held in a restraining cage. As already mentioned (see Table 3), the proportion of cardiac output reaching different organs is determined by intra-cardiac injection of 15 μm diameter plastic microspheres and by measuring the proportion of radioactivity in each organ. Table 3 also shows that radiolabeled tumor cells are trapped in the different organs in the same proportion as the microspheres, i.e., the arrest of cancer cells follows cardiac output. This is true with the exception of the fraction of cancer cells that have succeeded in traversing the systemic arterial beds to be finally stopped in the lung or liver.

The incidence of tumors following left ventricular injection is shown in Table 6; by comparison with Table 3 it is clear that the development of metastases is not related to cardiac output. The adrenal was the most common site for tumor growth, occurring in almost every rat that developed tumor colonies. Bony growths were also common (probably more frequent than recorded due to problems of visualizing them). Lung colonies were uncommon except for the breast carcinoma. Liver, pancreas, kidney, heart, mesentery, muscle, skin and eye colonies are rare. Gut, brain, spleen, thymic and thyroid colonies were not seen. Brown fat growths were almost entirely confined to the rats injected with sarcoma cells and grew in thoracic, abdominal and interscapular brown fat. Lesions were multiple in adrenals, brown fat and bone, but usually single in less favorable sites. With the sarcoma a range of cell doses (10^3 - 2 x 10^6) was used. The organ selectivity did not vary detectably in the range of 10^4 to 2 x 10^6 cells. With 10^3 sarcoma cells three of four rats developed tumor colonies; these were restricted to bone and brown fat without the development of adrenal lesions.

Autoradiography indicated that intraarterially injected cancer cells are deposited as isolated cells within the different organs. The susceptibility of different organs to developing metastases can therefore be quantitatively expressed as "the probability of a single cancer cell trapped in the organ giving rise to a tumor colony." The number of cancer cells trapped in an organ can be calculated from the distribution of radioactivity immediately following the injection of radiolabeled tumor cells as shown in Table 3. The number of tumor foci can be counted microscopicallly by killing rats between 15 and 22 da after intracardiac injection of living tumor cells. The latter is imprecise, but the differences in the probabilities are so great that the reality of the phenomenon of site selectivity cannot be in doubt.

With the sarcoma a cell arrested in an adrenal has a greater than 1 in 20 probability of causing a tumor, whereas in the kidney the probability is less than 1 in 10^5. Brown fat is a "good soil" for the sarcoma, but when expressed as a probability for a single cell it is less favorable than the adrenal. The lowest intracardiac dose required to produce metastases in brown fat and in the adrenal respectively is 10^3 and 10^4 sarcoma cells, yet the proportion of cells arrested in brown fat is 50 times greater than those arrested in the adrenal.

Table 6. Sites of Tumor Growth following Left Ventricular Injection of
Tumor Cells.[*]

	Sarcoma (N=52) $(10^4 - 2 \times 10^6)$ cells	Hepatoma (N=11) $(3 \times 10^5 - 10^6)$ cells	Breast Carcinoma (N=18) $(10^6$ cells)
Adrenals	96%	100%	100%
Bone	54%	27%	33%
Lung	12%	9%	61%
Brown Fat	85%	0%	6%
Kidney	0%	9%	0%
Heart	2%	0%	6%
Liver	2%	0%	0%
Ovaries	81%	100%	94%

[*]84 male and female rats were injected with 10^4 tumor cells; only 3 of
these failed to develop tumors. In this group, 38 of 81 rats were
female.

A. Organ Preference Is Not Related to Rate of Intravascular Cell Death

We set out to test the hypothesis that the rate at which trapped
cancer cells are killed within the vasculature is a determining factor
in the organ preference for metastasis after intraarterial injection.
The rate of cell death was measured by following the rate of
disappearance in different organs of radioactivity associated with
sarcoma cells, the DNA of which had been labeled with ^{125}IUDr. The
cell associated radioactivity was determined one, three, five and
sixteen hours after intraarterial inoculation. No significant loss of
label was observed until three hours after injection; at sixteen hours
between 5 and 35% of the radioactivity was retained in an ethanol
insoluble form in the different organs. There was no correlation
between organ susceptibility to metastasis and retention of radioactivity. For example, the rate of lysis within the kidney (which is
very refractory) was the same within experimental error as that in the
adrenal, the organ in which a sarcoma cell is most likely to grow into
a metastasis. Sixteen hours after injection, 21% of the initial

188

radioactivity was retained in the kidney and 19% in the adrenal. Although the destruction of the majority of cancer emboli intravascularly by one or more of the mechanisms discussed is no doubt responsible for the overall inefficiency of the metastatic process, it does not appear that the preferential growth of metastases following intracardiac injection is due to differences in the rate of cell death of cancer emboli in the different capillary beds.

B. Rate of Extravasation

Organ selectivity could in theory arise from differences in the rate of extravasation. If this is rapid a higher proportion of trapped cells would escape destruction in the hostile environment of the blood. To some extent the fate of a blood borne cancer cell is the outcome of two competing and opposed processes, extravasation and intravascular death. To extravasate the cells in the cancer emboli need to bind to the basement membrane; specific receptors for intercellular macromolecules may bring about such an attachment (see Chapter 19). Cancer cells do not seem to interact directly with the endothelial cells but instead with exposed basement membrane. This may explain why metastasis is facilitated in organs damaged by radiation or cytotoxic drugs which cause retraction of the endothelium and exposure of basement membrane. It is, however, unlikely that organ preference stems from differences in the proportion of basement membrane that is accessible to trapped cells.

C. Dormant State of Some Extravasated Cancer Cells

Growth of a cancer cell that has successfully extravasated is not guaranteed. A clinical metastasis may not develop from a cancer cell after extravasation because the cancer cell remains dormant while retaining the capacity to divide. Outgrowth of dormant cells seems to be determined by the environment. In experimental animals manipulation of the host has caused dormant cancer cells to grow into macroscopic metastases after long periods of quiescence (24).

D. Need for Growth Factors

Failure of a cancer cell to grow after successful extravasation may result from the requirement by cancer cells for growth factors. The evidence is now overwhelming that division of normal cells requires specific growth factors which bind to receptors on the plasma membrane (25). DNA synthesis is an adaptive response to extracellular signals and in their absence the cell is "out of cycle." Growth control is not brought about by inhibitors of division but is the consequence of controlled mitogenic stimuli. One of the processes that ensures the physiological control of division of normal cells within an organism is that one type of cell produces the growth factors to which another type of cell responds. The difference between cancer and normal cells is apparently not that the cancer cells do not require such growth factors. Cancer cells seem to derive their autonomy by producing growth factors for which they have membrane receptors and this results in autocrine stimulation - a hypothesis first put forward by Sporn and Todaro (26). These autocrine factors appear to be released from cancer cells into the surrounding medium whence they bind to the cells that produce them; this self stimulation is an essential component of the uncontrolled growth of cancer cells. An attractive but as yet unproved possibility (24) is that after extravasation cancer cells can remain quiescent and perhaps eventually die because the local concentration of a diffusible growth factor released by any one isolated cell is too low to initiate mitosis. This could explain why transplantation by direct injection into tissue of all but the most bizarre tumors requires an inoculum of many cells, the cells cooperating to establish a local concentration of autologous growth factor sufficient to initiate mitosis. When cells are delivered via the arterial blood they are dispersed throughout the organ as single cells and the distance between them is too great for interaction to give an adequate concentration of growth factors. If this is so the blood borne cancer cell that has succeeded in passing through the blood vessel into an extravascular space will not initially grow autonomously, but must rely for its mitogenic stimulus on factors released by the cells in the tissues in which it finds itself. Once the isolated cancer cell has started to divide it will create its own environment in which tumor derived growth factors are adequate for growth independent of the host.

The concept that the favorable "soil" is the product of growth stimuli released by the organ in which the cancer cell finds itself was suggested 50 years ago by Alexander Haddow to explain the high incidence in man of liver metastases of cancers that drain into the vena caval system. He stressed that the incidence is much higher than would be expected from the proportion of blood flowing through the hepatic artery.

Evidence is accumulating 1) that different organs produce different growth factors (or co-factors which act synergistically) and 2) that growth factors from normal cells can interact with the growth factors produced by tumor cells themselves so as to facilitate the autocrine stimulation of cancer cells. This hypothesis predicts that different types of cancer will show different organ preferences for metastasis. It also explains why there is no organ preference if the cancer cells are inoculated directly as opposed to being delivered by the blood stream since such transplantation requires the injection of many cancer cells which cooperate with one another.

V. SUMMARY

The site of growth following injection into the blood by three routes has been determined for three syngeneic rat tumors: a carcinoma, a sarcoma and a hepatoma. If given intravenously all of the tumors grow only in the lung; after intraportal injection growth is confined to the liver. No evidence could be found that following intravenous injection any of the cancer cells tested passed intact through the lung into the systemic circulation. Spread beyond the lung must, therefore, stem from cells released from a lung metastasis into the pulmonary vein and thence into the arterial circulation. If the cancer cells are injected through the left ventricle, metastases occur preferentially in certain organs, notably the adrenal, despite the fact that the cancer cells are arrested in the microvasculature of all of the organs in proportion to the cardiac output received by the organs. The organ selectivity of metastasis development from cancer cells in arterial blood is not related to the rate at which cancer cells died after arrest in a capillary bed as a consequence of such cytotoxic processes as mechanical trauma or poisoning by oxygen. The data are compatible with the hypothesis that after blood borne dissemination cancer cells are deposited in the tissues singly. As isolated cells they do not establish a local concentration of autocrine (i.e., self-produced) growth factors at a concentration which is mitogenic. We postulate that such isolated cells will grow if the host tissue produces growth stimuli which are able, perhaps in conjunction with factors released by the cancer cell, to initiate mitosis of the cancer cell. The distribution of metastases beyond the organ first encountered seems to be dictated by local growth factors and not by hemodynamic considerations.

ACKNOWLEDGMENTS

This investigation was supported by a grant from the Cancer Research Campaign.

REFERENCES

1. Willis RA: Pathology of Tumours. 4th Edition, Butterworths, London, p. 174, 1964.
2. Bross DJ, Blumenson LE: In: Weiss L (ed.) Fundamental Aspects of Metastasis. North Holland Publishing Co., Amsterdam, pp. 359-375, 1976.
3. Weiss L, Haydock K, Pickren JW, Lane W: Organ vascularity and metastatic frequency. Am. J. Pathol. 101:101-113, 1980.
4. Coman DR, Delong RP: The role of the vertebral venous sytem in the metastases of cancer to the spinal column. Cancer 4:610-618, 1951.
5. Murphy P, Taylor I, Alexander P: The efficiency of trapping blood borne cancer in the organ of first encounter using experimental rat tumours. Br. J. Surgery (In press).
6. Zeidman I, Buss JM: Transpulmonary passage of tumour cell emboli. Cancer Res. 12:731-733, 1952.
7. Weiss L: Cancer cell traffic from the lungs to the liver: An example of metastatic inefficiency. Int. J. Cancer 25:385-392, 1980.
8. Sugarbaker ED: The organ selectivity of experimentally induced metastases in the rat. Cancer 5:606-612, 1952.

9. Alexander P, Eccles SA: Host mediated mechanisms in the elimination of circulating cancer cells. In: Nicolson GL and Milas L (eds.) Cancer Invasion and Metastasis: Biologic and Therapeutic Aspects. Raven Press, New York, pp. 293-308, 1984.

10. Fidler IJ: Metastasis: Quantitative analysis of distribution and fate of tumour emboli labelled with ^{125}I-5-iodo-2-deoxyridine. J. Natl. Cancer Inst. 45:773-782, 1970.

11. Parr IB, Jackson LE, Alexander P: Role of "lymphotoxin" in the local anti-tumour action associated with inflammation. Br. J. Cancer 48:395-403, 1983.

12. Glaves D: Role of neutrophils in the destruction of tumour cells trapped in the lung. Invasion Metastasis 3:160-161, 1983.

13. Bishop CJ, Whiting VA: The role of the natural killer cells in the intravascular death of intravenously injected murine tumours cells. Br. J. Cancer 48:441-449, 1983.

14. Sato H, Suzuki M: Deformability and viability of tumour cells by transcapillary passage with reference to organ affinity of metastasis in cancer. In: Weiss L (ed.) Fundamental Aspects of Metastasis. North Holland, Amsterdam, pp. 311-317, 1976.

15. Tsulhiya M, Ferrone RA, Walsh GM, Frohlich EO: Regional blood flows measured in conscious rats by combine fick and microsphere methods. Am. J. Physiol. 235:H357-H449, 1978.

16. Werrlein RJ, Glinos AD: Oxygen microenvironment D and respiratory oscillations in cultured mammilian cells. Nature (London) 251:317-319, 1974.

17. Richter A, Sanford KK, Evans VJ: Influence of oxygen and culture media on plating efficiency of some mammalian tissue cells. J. Natl. Cancer Inst. 49:1705-1712, 1972.

18. Packer L, Fuehr K: Low oxygen concentration extends the lifespan of cultured human diploid cells. Nature (London) 267:423-425, 1977.

19. Anderson GR, Farkas BK: Asp56/LDH$_K$ in the Kirsten and Harvey sarcoma system. Transplantation Proc. 16:449-451, 1984.

20. Barbieri JT, Cox CD: Influence of oxygen on respiration and glucose catabolism by Treponema pallidum. Infection Immunity 31:992-997, 1981.

21. Liotta AL, Kleinerman J, Saidel GM: The significance of hematogenous tumor cell clumps in the metastatic process. Cancer Res. 36:889-894, 1976.

22. Steel GG, Adams K: Stem cell survival and tumor control in the Lewis lung carcinoma. Cancer Res. 35:1530, 1975.

23. Kluft O, Boereme I: Hyperbaric oxygen in experimental cancer in mice. In: Clinical Application of Hyperbaric Oxygen. Proceedings of the 1st International Congress. Elsevier, Amsterdam, pp. 126-136, 1964.

24. Alexander P: Dormant metastases - Studies in experimental animals. J. Pathol. 141:379-383, 1983.

25. Alexander P, Currie G: Concomitant synthesis of growth factors and their receptors - an aspect of malignant transformation. Biochem. Pharmacol. 33:941-943, 1984.

26. Sporn MB, Todaro GJ: Autocrine secretion and malignant transformation of cells. N. Engl. J. Med. 303:878-880, 1980.

CHAPTER 13. INTERLEUKINS, LYMPHOKINES AND LYMPHOID NEOPLASIA

RICHARD J. FORD, FRANCES DAVIS, NICOLA KOUTTAB AND SHASHI MEHTA

I. INTRODUCTION

As this volume clearly indicates, human cancer biology has recently focused to a large extent on the area of metastatic spread of tumor cells throughout the body. The delineation of biological consequences of such invasion to the host is for the first time beginning to be understood on more than a phenomenologic basis. Recent studies with a wide variety of experimental tumor systems, as reported here and in the literature, have begun to elucidate many of the biological mechanisms involved in the pathophysiology of neoplasia and have greatly improved our current understanding of the consequences of the spread of tumor cells. Another related area of emphasis has focused on the host's immune system and its role in preventing the development of neoplasia through various putative immunosurveillance mechanisms available, or in suppressing the progression of the neoplastic process once the surveillance mechanism(s) are either interdicted or circumvented (1,2). This latter area is generally referred to as tumor immunology, dealing with the contest between the host's immune system and the incipient or established tumor (usually of epithelial or mesenchymal origin). In this Chapter, we would like to discuss a related but somewhat more insidious condition, wherein the tumor is actually present within the host's immune system. In such conditions of lymphoreticular neoplasia, one does not usually observe metastasis in the conventional sense. However, these neoplasms do "spread" or progress, but usually within the confines of the immune or lymphatic system itself in a manner similar to normal lymphocyte homing mechanisms (3,4). The consequence of this progressive spread of the neoplastic process within the immune system, like metastatic processes in other organ systems, is the eventual loss of normal physiologic functions. In the lymphoid system this usually leads to immuno-deficiency and often the eventual demise of the host from infection. We will now consider the general organization of the human immune system, several functional aspects of soluble factors or immunoregulatory molecules controlling lymphocyte proliferation, and their relationship to neoplastic disease processes involving the immune system.

II. THE HUMAN IMMUNE SYSTEM

The human immune system is composed of complex networks of interacting lymphoid and mononuclear accessory cells, working in concert to provide protection against the hostile environment to which the body is constantly exposed. These lymphoid cell interactions occur through genetically programmed cell surface recognition molecules of both the histocompatability (5) and non-histocompatibility types (6), and also through secreted soluble factors referred to as lymphokines (7,8). This latter group of biologically active molecules, of which the Interleukin growth factors are an important component, comprise the principal repertoire of regulatory molecules through which the human immune system appears to be controlled (9). The Interleukin growth factors IL-2 (TCGF; 10) and B cell growth factor (BCGF, BSF; 11) are basically non-specific biological amplification factors that expand various subsets of lymphoid cells that have been specifically activated by the immunological recognition of antigen [i.e., by interaction with either the T cell receptor for antigen or cell surface immunoglobulin (SIg) on B lymphocytes]. The monocyte/macrophage series which includes the various types of dendritic or interdigitating reticulum cells (12) is an important accessory cell component of the immune system, functioning to present antigen to T lymphocytes probably in the presence of HLA-DR antigens (13). Cells of this lineage also secrete the monokine Interleukin 1 (IL-1, LAF; 14) which is important in triggering the concatenation of cellular events believed necessary for human T and B cell activation (15), by stimulating T cells to make their respective growth factors (i.e., TCGF and BCGF). In addition, IL-1 has many other biological activities, acting on a variety of different cell types with various functional effects (16). Together, cells of the many subsets of the T, B, and monocyte/macrophage lineages interact functionally and give rise to biologically active molecules. These molecules include antibodies, lymphokines and other immunological mediators that are the effector molecules active in the various types of immune responses that the organism can muster. These mechanisms provide immunologic protection against the constant antigenic challenge provided by the environment.

III. HUMAN LYMPHOID NEOPLASIA

The cells of the immune system: lymphocytes, monocytes, plasma cells, etc., like those of any other organ system, are potentially susceptible to neoplastic transformation giving rise to tumors of the immune system referred to as lymphomas and leukemias (17). In the non-Hodgkin's lymphomas (NHL), apparently normal T or B lymphoid cells of various phenotypes, maturation states, and functional capabilities are transformed into monoclonally expanded lymphoid tumor cell populations (18); the protector becomes the incipient attacker. At the very least, transformed lymphoid cells become immunologically effete and slowly appear to supplant or "crowd out" the normal lymphoid cell constituents of the immune system. This process usually gives rise to progressive immune deficiency states within the patient. This immuno-logically deteriorating condition often leaves the patient at risk to environmental pathogen exposure, which when combined with the immuno-suppressive effects of chemotherapy or radiotherapy can lead to the eventual demise of the patient. Death due to infection in patients with lymphoid tumors is sometimes due to usually innocuous microbes that in the immunocompromised host give rise to opportunistic infections (19). Human lymphoid tumors, due to their common occurrence and to their intrinsic involvement with the immune system itself, are among the most studied human cancers. Pathologists have written endlessly about their varied morphologic appearances (20) and devised numerous controversial schemes for classification. Unfortunately, however, little scientific information about these common human tumors exists beyond hypothetical speculations and extrapolations to the putative normal human lymphoid cell counterparts of these tumors.

IV. EXPERIMENTAL SYSTEMS

One of the major problems in studying human lymphoid tumors is the lack of appropriate experimental systems. The main difficulty in establishing such systems relates to the inability to identify the tumor cell populations with certainty and the subsequent inability to grow the tumor cells in vitro. A number of T and B neoplastic cell lines have been established but these have been transformed with either the human T cell leukemia virus (HTLB; 21) or the Epstein-Barr virus (EBF; 22), respectively. Some of the permanent tumor cell lines, due to the apparent viral transformation event involved in their establishment, are of questionable relevance to the study of the tumor biology of the lymphoma in question as, apparently, non-virally transformed tumor populations do not spontaneously proliferate in vitro. The recent identification of viral and cellular oncogenes and their expression in lymphoid tumor cells (23) may provide some answers to this dilemma. Clearly something is missing in the in vitro conditions that is involved in the lymphoreticular disease process in vivo, where lymphoid tumor cell growth can be followed by various clinical parameters.

A. Non-Hodgkin's Lymphomas (NHL)

One of the relatively recent advances in the study of human lymphoma has been the ability to immunologically phenotype the putative tumor cells, first through conventional cell membrane immunological markers (24) and more recently through the use of monoclonal antibodies (MCA) to cell surface antigens (25). These cell marking techniques have allowed the apparent cell lineage in most of the T and B cell NHL to be established and have provided at least some information on the apparent stage of normal lymphocyte differentiation represented by the tumor cell clone. We have recently combined MCA phenotyping of the NHL with the use of the human malignancy associated nucleolar antigen (HMNA), which can discriminate neoplastic human lymphoid cells from their putative normal lymphocyte counterparts (26). Table 1 shows representative NHL of T and B cell type that have been assayed for the expression of HMNA, along with suitable controls. HMNA is found to be

Table 1.   Phenotypic Analysis of Non-Hodgkin's Lymphomas with Monoclonal Antibodies and HMNA Antisera.

Lymphoma Type[*]	SIg[†]	Monoclonal Antibodies[‡]	HMNA[◊]
Small Cell			
N-PDL-B cell	μκ	Leul, Bl, DR	+
N-PDL-B cell	μδκ	Leul, Bl, B2, DR	+
D-WDL-B cell	μδκ	Leul, Bl, DR	+
D-PDL-B cell		T3, T4	+
HCL-B cell	μκ	Bl, DR	+
Large Cell			
D-LCL-B cell	μκ	Leul, Bl, DR	+
N-LCL-B cell	μδκ	Bl, DR	+
D-LCL-T cell		T3, T4, T10	+
D-LCL-B cell	μκ	Bl, B2	+
Controls			
Normal LN	polyclonal	Multiple T and B	+
Reactive LN	polyclonal	Multiple T and B	+
Normal LN	polyclonal	Multiple T and B	+

[*]Modified Rappaport histopathologic classification, diagnosis made from paraffin H & E sections.

[†]Surface immunoglobulin determined by immunofluorescence.

[‡]Monoclonal antibody phenotype was determined by direct or indirect immunofluorescence on fixed frozen sections. Leul (Becton Dickinson), Bl (Dr. Lee Nadler), OKTs (Ortho).

[◊]HMNA was determined by immunofluorescence as described in (26).

present in the morphologic and phenotypical neoplastic cell populations, whereas normal or reactive lymphoid cell populations do not express the antigen(s).   When the HMNA is combined with MCA cell surface phenotyping on the same lymphoid cell population, one can thus establish simultaneously the neoplastic nature of the cell as well as its lineage and/or stage of differentiation by various immuno-fluorescent or immunoenzyme staining techniques. Closer analysis of the cell populations identified with HMNA reveals them to be monoclonal by cell surface immunoglobulin light chain typing and to show cytogenetic abnormalities characteristic of human lymphoid neoplasms (26).

The capability of precisely identifying the neoplastic cell population in lymphomatous lesions, which often do not show striking cytologic abnormalities, allows one to subject purified tumor cells to experimental studies with some confidence that the results are reflective of lymphomatous T or B cells rather than the ubiquitous normal or reactive lymphoid cells that are constantly present in the lesions of human lymphoid neoplasms (27). Since virtually all studies have shown that NHL tumor cells retain the cell surface phenotype of their putative normal T or B cell counterparts, it is of interest to determine if this phenotypic concordance also corresponds to functional similarities. A fundamentally important question here relates to the control of cell proliferation in these tumors. In the past few years it has become clear that normal T and B cell proliferation is dependent on the appropriate Interleukin growth factor, a hormone-like low molecular weight protein that drives activated lymphoid cells into cell division (28). Do lymphoid tumor cells require or are they sensitive to normal Interleukin growth factors for cell division or alternatively is cell proliferation autonomous in the neoplastic cell? A third possibility might be that the tumor cell makes its own growth factor and that the tumor proliferates through autocrine stimulation.

We therefore assayed a variety of purified, well-characterized NHL cell populations to determine if autonomous cell growth occurred or if normal purified growth factors for the putative lineage of the tumor cells would stimulate their proliferation. Table 2 shows that only background levels of thymidine were incorporated by nonstimulated tumor cells but that the corresponding lineage specific Interleukin growth factor could stimulate a significant increase in cell proliferation in the small cell T and B cell NHL. Interestingly, the large cell T and B cell NHL appeared to be refractory to growth factor stimulation but showed little spontaneous proliferative capacity as well. Thymidine incorporation in NHL cells, when observed, was however considerably less than that seen in separated T and B cell populations obtained from normal or reactive (hyperplastic) control lymph nodes.

What does this data signify with regard to the biology of the tumor? The observation that the tumor cell populations after removal from the host are not proliferating to any significant extent and that the cells simply die in vitro indicates that the tumor microenvironment must be an important factor. It could also be inferred that in vitro conditions, regardless how nutrient rich the media or the serum supplements added, may not provide an adequate artificial environment to support lymphoid tumor cell growth. Exactly what is missing in vitro remains obscure, but our data suggests that at least some proliferative stimuli can be provided for NHL by normal Interleukin growth factors. The magnitude of stimulation in the sensitive NHL cells suggests that only a small percentage of the tumor cells are dividing and preliminary studies utilizing cytofluorometry suggest that

Table 2. Growth Factor Mediated Proliferation in Non-Hodgkin's Lymphoma.

Lymphoma Type*	BCGF[†]	α-μ[‡]	α-μ + BCGF
SC-WDL (B cell)[◊]	11935[ƒ]	1692	13620
SC-NPDL (B cell)	6758	1290	11840
SC-WDL (B cell)	8159	5166	30574
LC (B cell)	256	320	220
LC (B cell)	347	116	690
Control lymph nodes			
Normal LN	5856	2620	16640
Normal LN	2483	1297	11940

*Modified Rappaport histopathologic classification abbrev. SC - small cell, WDL - well differentiated lymphocytic lymphoma, N-DPL - nodular poorly differentiated lymphocytic lymphoma, LC - large cell.

[†]BCGF preparations were obtained from PHA stimulated lymphocyte conditioned media after DEAE and P-30 gel filtration (42) and used at 10% v/v in culture wells containing 0.2×10^6 cells/well.

[‡]Anti-mu (α-μ) conjugated agarose beads (Biorad) were added at a final concentration of 15 μg/ml.

[◊]Tumor cell populations were En-rosetted and adherent cell depleted prior to phenotyping using MCA and anti-HMNA.

[ƒ]CPM of experimental minus control of triplicate cultures.

not more than 10% of the tumor cell population is proliferating after exposure to the growth factor. In fact our studies have shown that most NHL cells present in a given lymphoma tumor cell population cannot be stimulated in vitro by mitogens, phorbol esters, and even non-specific mitogenic substances such as calcium ionophores (29). These findings suggest that the majority of the lymphoma cells present in the lymphoma lesion may be functionally inert and that only a small percentage of the tumor cell population represents the actual proliferating pool of the neoplasm. It is possible that in the small cell NHL, the cells of the proliferating pool (tumor "stem" cells, etc.) may be sensitive to, if not dependent upon, normal immuno-regulatory factors such as Interleukin growth factors. It is also interesting that the large cell NHL appear to be refractory to growth factor stimulation. These tumors often appear more aggressive clinically than the small cell variety and one might speculate that they may have lost the capacity to be immunoregulated either in a positive or negative sense. Further studies on the biology and immunoregulatory aspects of human lymphoid tumors should add a great deal to the developing of new therapeutic modalities, possibly through biological response modifiers.

B. Hodgkin's Disease (HD)

More than 150 years ago, an English physician by the name of Thomas Hodgkin described a curious disease of the lymphatic system or the "absorbant glands," as lymph nodes were then called, which now bears his name. HD has been controversial since its original description, and only in recent years has its neoplastic nature been generally accepted (30). HD is primarily a pleomorphic lymphoreticular neoplasm of adolescents and young adults, but the disease does occur in older adults as well as in children. In young adults, HD is one of the most common forms of cancer. Fortunately, HD is also one of the most successfully treated human tumors since the advent of high voltage radiotherapy several decades ago and, more recently, the addition of combination chemotherapy. The therapeutic success story of HD can be contrasted with our lack of understanding of the disease process involved. Unfortunately, we know very little about the biological nature of the disease. In fact, we do not even know for certain the nature of the putative neoplastic cell, the Reed-Sternberg cell (RSC) and its mononuclear variants, often referred to as Hodgkin's cells (HC).

These cells have been attributed to virtually every cell lineage in the reticuloendothelial system (31) but convincing evidence to substantiate these claims has been largely lacking. Our in vitro studies on HC over the past several years have suggested that their origin lies somewhere in the monocyte/macrophage (MØ) lineage (32). Most experiments have shown that the large mononuclear cells from HD lesions that can be maintained in culture have some if not all the characteristics of MØ's. When one studies the phenotypes of the cell populations derived from HD lesions, the predominant cell initially is the T lymphocyte, but the cells with the morphologic appearance of HC usually have some antigenic and/or enzymatic properties consistent with the MØ lineage (Table 3). It has recently been suggested that the Interdigitating reticulum cell, which has some but not all of the characteristics of the macrophage, may be the actual precursor cell of the RSC and the HC (33). Unfortunately, little experimental information is available about these rather obscure cells and in vitro techniques for their study are just beginning to be developed. A number of permanent cell lines from heavily treated HD patients have been developed by Diehl and his colleagues (34). These cell lines appear to have some characteristics of HC but their origin, as determined by standard lineage-specific MCA remains obscure. In addition, MCA made against these cell lines, which react with most HC in tissue sections, also stain a variety of other lymphoid and myeloid cell types present in HD lesions and in control lymphoid tissue. One thing that emerges clearly from all of these studies is that the experimental systems for studying HD, at the present time, are inadequate to answer the most cogent questions regarding the nature of the disease. These questions involve the possible viral etiology of the disease, the presence of defined or possibly undefined oncogenes in HC, and the role of the HD tumor cells in characteristic immuno-deficiency of HD.

Table 3.   Cellular Phenotype in Hodgkin's Disease Cell Cultures.

Pt#[*]	DX[†]	T_4/T_8[‡]	B[◊]	MO[ƒ]	NK[Ψ]	HMNA[ψ]
1	NSHD	72/6	2	14	2	10
2	NSHD	64/10	5	12	4	11
3	NSHD	69/6	3	20	2	14
4	NSHD	59/14	2	21	1	18
5	NSHD	68/6	5	18	2	ND
6	NSHD	66/8	0	22	3	17

[*]Frozen sections were cut from lymph node biopsies from untreated patients. The sections were fixed in cold absolute methanol for 10 min and stored at -70°C until assayed.

[†]Diagnosis of nodular sclerosing Hodgkin's disease was made from paraffin sections from the same lymph node as the frozen sections above.

[‡]Direct or indirect immunofluorescence assays utilized OKT4 and OKT8 monoclonal antibodies (Ortho). The numbers indicate the percentage of viable cells staining with the antibody.

[◊]B1 monoclonal antibody (provided by Dr. Lee Nadler).

[ƒ]LeuM1 monoclonal antibody (Becton Dickinson).

[Ψ]NKP15 (Leu 11; provided by Dr. George Babcock).

[ψ]Human malignancy associated Nucleolar antigens heteroantibody (26).

Studies done in our laboratory have indicated that short term cultures of HC, with most of the characteristic of MØ's, secrete the monokine Interleukin 1 (IL-1; 32). Due to the pleomorphic histopathologic nature of the HD lesion, where an admixture of chronic and acute inflammatory cells are seen interspersed with the RSC and HC, we have hypothesized that the secretion of IL-1 by the putative neoplastic cells could account for the unique appearance of the nodular sclerosing HD lesion. The multiple biologic activities of IL-1 (16) could easily account for the presence of proliferating helper T cells and fibroblasts, as well as for various chemotactic activities which in turn account for the presence of eosinophils and other granulocytes usually observed in the lesions. At least one of Diehl's cell lines, incidently, has also been reported to secrete IL-1 (35). These studies suggest that HD may in fact be a disease of neoplastically transformed but functionally active cells of the monocyte/macrophage lineage, and perhaps of one of the more specialized interdigitating or dendritic reticulum cell subtypes (33).

Another major question in HD is the cause of the characteristic immunodeficiency observed in virtually all patients at the time of presentation. Now that HD is very effectively treated with radiation and chemotherapy, patients are often at risk for infectious complications, due to not only their intrinsic immune defect(s) but also from the iatrogenic component as a result of the therapy. The immunologic defect in HD patients has been extensively studied by many groups (36,37) and is most readily demonstrated as decreased responsiveness to skin test delayed hypersensitivity reactions and hyporesponsiveness to T cell mitogens such as phytohemagglutin (PHA). A variety of mechanisms have been invoked to explain the cause of the immune defect including suppressor T cells (38), and monocytic suppression mediated through the excessive secretion of prostaglandins (39). Recently, we have studied this defect in relation to our current understanding of how the human T lymphocyte system is regulated (see Section II). We were interested to ascertain if we could identify a site in the cascade of events leading to T cell activation where an abnormality or defect is present. To evaluate this system, we studied 1) the patient's peripheral blood monocytes for IL-1 production, 2) the patient's peripheral blood mononuclear cells (PBMC) for Interleukin 2 (IL-2) production, and 3) the proliferative response of the patient's activated T lymphocytes to exogenously provided IL-2 in vitro (40). We found that the HD patient's IL-1 response to bacterial lipopolysaccharide was normal, as was their T cell proliferative response to exogenous partially purified IL-2. The HD patient's IL-2 production, however, was only 50% of the age-matched controls (Table 4). The degree of impairment seen in the patient's IL-2 response roughly correlated with the decrement observed in the patients PHA responses and skin test reactivities. This finding raises the question of whether the IL-2 production deficiency is the actual cause or possibly only a contributory component to the T cell deficiency. Assuming that IL-2 deficiency is in fact involved in the phenomenon, what could be the cause? Two immediate possibilities include a regulatory abnormality such as excessive immunosuppression and/or an intrinsic cellular defect in IL-2 production. The former explanation may be consistent with the previous findings of PGE_2-mediated immuno-suppression in HD, as PGE_2 has been shown to inhibit IL-2 production (41). Therefore, HC, due to their apparent MØ lineage, may be responsible for T cell immunodeficiency by a PGE_2-mediated mechanism.

V. CONCLUSIONS

We have discussed a number of the approaches that we have used to study human lymphoid tumors experimentally. These studies have focused on the group of lymphoid growth factors referred to collectively as the Interleukins. These studies have begun to elucidate the role of immunoregulatory factors in some human lymphoid malignancies as well as in one type of concomitant immunodeficiency associated with these diseases. We feel that this type of approach can contribute a great deal to our understanding of the biology of these common neoplastic diseases. Similar studies may eventually suggest strategies for therapy, perhaps through the use of biologic response modifiers, that may augment if not replace conventional therapy.

Table 4. Summary of Growth Factor Responses of Hodgkin's Patients' PBMC as Compared to Age-Matched Controls.

Assay	Percent of Age/Sex Matched Controls[*]	p Value[†]
PHA responsiveness of PBMC	70.5 ± 11.6 (11)[‡]	p < 0.1
IL-1 generation by MØ	90.9 ± 11.1 (13)	p < 0.3
IL-2 generation by PBMC	49.6 ± 8.3 (14)	p < 0.02
Response of T blasts to exogenous IL-2	101 ± 24 (14)	p > 0.5

[*] $\dfrac{[^3H]Tdr \text{ in patient cells}}{[^3H]Tdr \text{ in age/sex matched control}}$ x 100 ± SEM

[†]Derived from paired t test

[‡]Number in parentheses represents the number of patients/controls studied.

ACKNOWLEDGMENTS

This investigation was supported by Grant Numbers CA36243 and CA314797 awarded by the National Cancer Institute, Department of Health and Human Services. We would also like to thank Tammy Hazelrigs and Linda Kimbrough for typing the manuscript.

REFERENCES

1. Burnet FM: The concept of immunological surveillance. Prog. Exp. Tumor Res. 13:1-27, 1970.
2. Old LJ, Stockert E, Boyse E, Kim JH: Antigenic modulation. Loss of TL antigen from cells exposed to TL antibody. J. Exp. Med. 127:523-539, 1968.
3. Warnke R, Levy R: Immunopathology of follicular lymphomas: A model of B lymphocyte homing. N. Engl. J. Med. 298:481-486, 1978.
4. Crowther D, Wagstaff J: Lymphocyte migration in malignant disease. Clin. Exp. Immunol. 5:413-420, 1983.
5. Thorsby E, Berle E, Nousiainen H: HLA-D region molecules restrict proliferative T cell response to antigen. Immunol. Rev. 66:39-56, 1982.
6. LoCascio NJ, Haughton G, Arnold LW, Corley RB: Role of cell surface immunoglobulin in B-lymphocyte activation. Proc. Natl. Acad. Sci. USA 81:2466-2469, 1984.
7. Maizel AL, Lachman L: Control of human lymphocyte proliferation by soluble factors. Lab. Invest. 50:369-377, 1981.
8. Cohen S, Pick E, Oppenheim JJ: Biology of the Lymphokines. Academic Press, New York, 1979.
9. Ruscetti FW, Gallo RC: Human T-lymphocyte growth factors; regulation of growth and function of T lymphocytes. Blood 57:379-394, 1981.
10. Morgan D, Ruscetti FW, Gallo RC: Selective growth of T-lymphocyte from normal human bone marrows. Science 193:1007-1009, 1976.
11. Ford RJ, Mehta SR, Franzini D, Montagna R, Lachman LB, Maizel AL: Soluble factor activation of human B lymphocytes. Nature (London) 294:261-263, 1981.
12. Steinman RM, Nussenzweig MC: Dendritic cells: Features and functions. Immunol. Rev. 53:127-147, 1980.
13. Thorsby E, Nousiainen H: In vitro sensitization of human T lymphocytes to Hapten (TNP)-conjugated and non-treated autologous cells is restricted by self HLA-D. Scand. J. Immunol. 9:183-189, 1979.
14. Lachman LB: Human Interleukin 1: Purification and properties. Fed. Proc. Fed. Am. Soc. Exp. Biol. 42:2639-2645, 1983.
15. Smith KA, Lachman LB, Oppenheim JJ, Favata MF: The functional relationship of the interleukins. J. Exp. Med. 151:1551-1555, 1980.
16. Oppenheim JJ, Stadler BM, Seraganian RP, Mage M, Mathieson B: Lymphokines: Their role in lymphocyte responses: Properties of interleukin 1. Fed. Proc. Fed. Am. Soc. Exp. Biol. 41:258-265, 1981.

17. Ford RJ, Maizel AL: Immunobiology of lymphoreticular neoplasms. IN: Twomey JJ (ed.) The Pathophysiology of Human Immunologic Disorders. Urban and Schwartzenberg, Baltimore, pp. 199-217, 1982.
18. Levy R, Warnke R, Dorfman RF, Hamovich J: The monoclonality of human B cell lymphomas. J. Exp. Med. 145:1014-1028, 1977.
19. Glicksman AS, Pajak TF: Early and late effects of lymphoma treatment in the expectation of cure. IN: Rosenberg SA and Kaplan HS (eds.) Malignant Lymphomas: Etiology, Immunology, Pathology, Treatment. Academic Press, New York, pp. 639-661, 1982.
20. Lukes RJ, Parker JW, Taylor CR: Immunologic approach to non-Hodgkin's lymphomas and related leukemias. Semin. Hematol. 15:322-338, 1978.
21. Gallo RC, Mann D, Broder S, Ruscetti FW, Maeda M, Reitz MS: Human T cell leukemia-lymphoma virus (HTLV) is in T but not B lymphocytes from a patient with cutaneous T-cell lymphoma. Proc. Natl. Acad. Sci. USA 79:3680-3683, 1982.
22. Nilsson K: The nature of lymphoid cell lines and their relationship to the virus. IN: Epstein MA and Achong BG (eds.) The Epstein-Barr Virus. Springer-Verlag, New York, pp. 225-266, 1979.
23. Marcu KB, Harris LJ, Stanton LW, Erikson J, Watt R, Croce CM: Transcriptionally active c-myc oncogene is contained within NIARD, a DNA sequence associated with chromosome translations in B cell neoplasia. Proc. Natl. Acad. Sci. USA 80:519-523, 1983.
24. Aisenberg AC, Wilkes BM, Long JC, Harris NL: Cell surface phenotype in lymphoproliferative disease. Am. J. Med. 68:206-213, 1980.
25. Warnke RA, Link MP: Identification and significance of cell markers in leukemia and lymphoma. Ann. Rev. Med. 34:117-131, 1983.
26. Ford RJ, Cramer M, Davis FM: Identification of human lymphoma cells by antisera to malignancy-associated nucleolar antigens. Blood 63:559-565, 1984.
27. Harris NL, Data RE: The distribution of neoplastic and normal B-lymphoid cells in nodular lymphomas. Hum. Pathol. 13:610-617, 1982.
28. Maizel AL, Mehta SR, Hauft S, Lachman LB, Ford RJ: Human lymphocyte/monocyte interaction in response to lectin: Kinetics of entry into the S-phase. J. Immunol. 127:1058-1064, 1981.
29. Ford RJ: Unpublished observations.
30. Kaplan HS: Hodgkin's disease: Biology, treatment, prognosis. Blood 57:813-822, 1981.
31. Kaplan HS: Hodgkin's disease: Unfolding concepts concerning its nature, management and prognosis. Cancer 45:2439-2474, 1980.
32. Ford RJ, Mehta SR, Davis F, Maizel AL: Growth factors in Hodgkin's disease. Cancer Treat. Rep. 66:633-638, 1982.
33. Kadin ME: Possible origin of the Reed-Sternberg cell from the Interdigitating reticulum cell. Cancer Treat. Rep. 66:601-608, 1982.

34. Diehl V, Kirchner H, Schaadt M, Stein H, Gerdes J, Boie C: Hodgkin's disease: Establishment of four in vitro cell lines. J. Cancer Res. Clin. Oncol. 101:111-124, 1981.

35. Diehl V, Burrichter H, Schaadt M, Hirchner H, Stein H, Gerdes J: Hodgkin's cell lines: Characteristics and possible pathogenic implications. Hematol. Oncol. 1:139-147, 1983.

36. Levy R, Kaplan HS: Impaired lymphocyte function in Hodgkin's disease. N. Engl. J. Med. 290:181-186, 1974.

37. Hersh EM, Oppenheim JJ: Impaired in vitro lymphocyte transformation in Hodgkin's disease. N. Engl. J. Med. 273:1006-1012, 1965.

38. Vanhaelen CP, Fisher RI: Increased sensitivity of lymphocytes with patients with Hodgkin's disease to concanavalin A induced suppressor cells. J. Immunol. 127:1216-1220, 1981.

39. Goodwin JS, Messner RP, Bankhurst AD, Peake GT, Saiki JH, Williams RC: Prostaglandin-producing suppressor cells in Hodgkin's disease. N. Engl. J.·Med. 297:963-968, 1977.

40. Ford RJ, Tsao J, Kouttab N, Sahasrabuddhe CG, Mehta SR: Association of an Interleukin abnormality with the T cell defect in Hodgkin's disease. Blood (In press).

41. Rappaport RS, Dodge GR: Prostaglandin G inhibits the production of human Interleukin 2. J. Exp. Med. 155:943-946, 1982.

42. Maizel A, Sahasrabuddhe C, Morgan J, Lachman L, Ford RJ: Biochemical separation of a human B cell mitogenic factor. Proc. Natl. Acad. Sci. USA 79:5998-6002, 1982.

CHAPTER 14. THE USE OF ACTIVATED MACROPHAGES FOR THE DESTRUCTION OF HETEROGENEOUS METASTASIS

ALAN J. SCHROIT AND ISAIAH J. FIDLER

I. INTRODUCTION

Metastasis, the spread of malignant cells from the primary tumor to distant sites, is the major cause of cancer mortality. Indeed, by the time many malignancies are diagnosed, metastases have already been established in a variety of sites distant from the primary tumor, making selective excision or destruction by irradiation or chemo-therapeutic agents extremely difficult. Exacerbating the problem of treating metastatic disease is the fact that cancer cells in different metastases originating from the same primary tumor, and in some instances even different zones within the same metastatic nodule, may respond completely differently to treatment. For example, although new and highly promising chemotherapeutic agents have been developed, their overall effectiveness is hindered by the common occurrence of drug resistance due to the rapid emergence of drug-resistant tumor cell variants, which then populate drug-resistant metastases (1,2; see also Chapters 5 and 6).

The potential for cellular heterogeneity of neoplastic tissue has been recognized for over a century since the initial pathological descriptions of "pleomorphism," describing heterogeneous morphology. However, only recently has it become clear that cells from malignancies of human and animal origin exhibit an apparently endless potential for biological diversity with regard to almost every measurable phenotypic characteristic, such as growth rates, antigenic and immunogenic properties, membrane receptors, the ability to invade and metastasize, sensitivity to cytotoxic drugs, etc. (1,2; see also Chapter 5). Although the biological basis for a tumor cell's incredible potential for phenotypic alteration is unclear, the demonstration of nonrandom proliferation of specialized subpopulations of cells within a primary tumor (3), the finding that metastasis can be clonal in origin, and the observation that different metastases can originate from different progenitor cells (4) does provide some explanation for the clinical observations of highly variable responses to cancer therapy. The corollary to these observations on the varied response of tumor cells to conventional treatment modalities is that the successful therapy of disseminated metastatic disease will have to circumvent the problems of cellular heterogeneity.

A good candidate for such a phenotype-insensitive therapeutic modality appears to be the patient's own mononuclear phagocytes. Indeed, there is now an overwhelming body of data demonstrating that cells of the reticuloendothleial system (RES), i.e., macrophages, appropriately activated to the tumoricidal state, can fulfill the demanding needs of cellular heterogeneity and phenotypic diversity (5).

In this chapter, we present some of the evidence that supports this observation. In addition, we review the salient points in the use of liposome-based delivery systems aimed at rendering macrophages tumoricidal in situ. We place particular emphasis on the chemical properties of the macrophage activator, the lipid composition and structure of the liposomes, and the potential for synergistic activation through the use of combined and multiple therapies.

II. THE INTERACTION OF MACROPHAGES WITH HETEROGENEOUS NEOPLASMS

Tumoricidal macrophages acquire the ability to recognize and destroy neoplastic cells both in vitro and in vivo, while leaving normal cells unharmed (6-10), by a nonimmunological mechanism that requires cell-to-cell contact (11-15). The ability of tumoricidal macrophages to discriminate between tumorigenic and normal cells has been demonstrated with syngeneic and allogeneic tumors of rodents (6-10) and allogeneic human tumors (16,17). Thus, although tumor cell populations can exhibit heterogeneity with respect to many phenotypes, they are all susceptible to lysis mediated by activated macrophages (5). For example, variant B16 melanoma lines that have low or high metastatic potentials and that are either susceptible or resistant to T-cell-mediated lysis are all lysed in vitro by macrophages activated by a lymphokine with macrophage-activating factor (MAF) activity (18). Similarly, several UV-2237 fibrosarcoma sublines that vary greatly in their invasive and metastatic potentials in vivo, in their immuno-genicity, and in their susceptibility to natural killer (NK) – cell mediated lysis are all susceptible to destruction in vitro by tumoricidal macrophages (19; see also Chapter 15).

A typical example of this phenomenon can be seen in Figure 1, where we have attempted to select in vitro for a tumor cell variant that exhibits a phenotypic resistance to macrophage-mediated lysis. In this experiment cells from either the B16 melanoma or the UV-2237 fibrosarcoma were incubated with the selective T-killer cells (cyto-toxic T cells), NK cells, or tumoricidal macrophages. The surviving target cells were then grown into monolayers and again incubated with the respective effector cells. After four or five sequential selections carried out in this manner, tumor cell variants resistant to cytolysis mediated by T cells (B16) or NK cells (UV-2237) were obtained. In contrast, variants resistant to macrophage-mediated lysis could not be obtained even though the selection pressure (90% killing) exceeded that of the T and NK cells. Moreover, as already stated, despite their resistance to T-cell-mediated lysis (B16-Fl^r) or NK-cell-mediated lysis (UV-2237-NK^r), both variants were still susceptible to destruction by the tumoricidal macrophages.

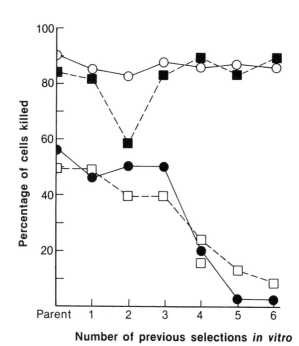

FIGURE 1. Variation in the Frequency of Selection of Tumor Cell Variants Resistant to Killing in Vitro by NK Cells (open squares = UV-2237), by Immune Cytotoxic T Lymphocytes (CTL) (closed circles = B16) and by Activated Macrophages (closed squares = UV-2237; open circles = B16). Monolayer cultures of B16 melanoma cells or UV-2237 fibrosarcoma cells were incubated in vitro with the indicated effector cells. This process was then repeated for a total of six times using the cultures of surviving tumor cells. This procedure results in the selection of tumor cell variants that are resistant to killing by CTL or NK cells. In contrast, no significant change in cellular susceptibility to destruction by activated macrophages was detected.

210

Additional evidence that appropriately activated macrophages are capable of tumor cell destruction without regard to the cell's phenotypic diversity has recently been obtained by Giavazzi et al. (20) using drug resistant tumor cell variants (21). They succeeded in selecting a variant line of the UV-2237 fibrosarcoma that is 100-fold more resistant to Adriamycin than are the parental cells (Figure 2). Not surprisingly, the Adriamycin-resistant cells have been shown to be as susceptible to activated macrophage-mediated destruction as the drug-sensitive parental tumor cells (Table 1).

Table 1. Tumoricidal Activity of Activated Macrophages Against Adriamycin-Resistant Tumor Cells.

	Tumor Targets			
	UV-2237 Parent		UV-2237	
Macrophage Treatment	cpm[*]	% cytolysis	cpm[*]	% cytolysis
No Macrophages	3041	--	4638	--
Control Macrophages	3147	0	4403	0
MAF-Activated Macrophages	1967	37	2609	40
MTP-PE-Activated Macrophages	1302	58	2150	51

[*]cpm remaining in viable tumor cells (^{125}I-UDR) three days after the addition of macrophages to the cultures [See (20) for detailed description of the experimental protocols employed.]

Taken together, our data and those from many other laboratories indicate that, at least in vitro, tumoricidal macrophages discriminate between neoplastic and non-neoplastic cells by a process that is independent of transplantation antigens, species-specific antigens, tumor-specific antigens, cell cycle time, or other various phenotypes associated with transformation. Although the exact mechanisms by which macrophages recognize and lyse tumor cells is unclear at this time, they are most probably determined by a yet-unidentified cell surface moiety associated with the tumorigenic phenotype.

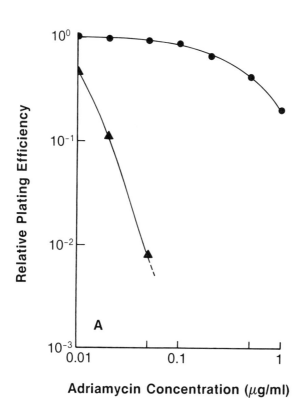

FIGURE 2. Plating Efficiency of UV-2237 Adriamycin-Resistant Cells in the Presence of Adriamycin. Plating efficiency was evaluated for the ability of the cells to form colonies in the presence of Adriamycin (see 41). UV-2237 parent, closed triangles ; tumor cells selected for Adriamycin resistance, closed circles.

212

III. ACTIVATION OF MACROPHAGES TO THE TUMORICIDAL STATE

Since macrophages in general, and macrophages from tumor-bearing animals in particular, can respond to activating stimuli and become tumoricidal, finding a nontoxic means to activate them in situ becomes desirable.

One of the major pathways for macrophage activation in vivo is believed to result from the action of MAF, a lymphokine released from mitogen or antigen sensitized lymphocytes. The therapeutic use of MAF has, however, been hindered by a lack of purified preparations. In addition, efforts to activate the tumoricidal properties of macrophages in vivo by parenteral injection of crude lymphokine preparations have proved to be unsuccessful for several reasons: 1) lymphokines injected intravenously have a short half-life, probably due to serum protein binding (22), 2) only a small fraction of the mononuclear phagocyte system may be capable of responding to free MAF, 3) macrophages can be activated by lymphokines only within a relatively short period of time following their extravasation from the peripheral circulation to the tissues (22), and 4) the tumoricidal properties of MAF activated macrophages are short lived (2-3 da) and macrophages become refractory to reactivation by free lymphokines (22). For further discussion of lymphokines see Chapter 13.

A second major pathway for the activation of macrophages in vivo involves their direct interaction with microorganisms or their products. For example, Mycobacteria, Corynebacteria and Nocardia cell walls interact directly with macrophages to activate them (23). However, the chemical constituents responsible for activation are poorly understood and their use in vivo is, with two notable exceptions, accompanied by significant toxicity. The exceptions are the synthetic moiety N-acetyl-muramyl-L-alanyl-D-isoglutamine (MDP; 24,25), which has been shown to be the minimal structural unit of Mycobacteria that has immune-potentiating activity (26), and the recently synthesized lipophilic MDP derivative, N-acetyl-muramyl-L-alanyl-D-isoglutamyl-L-alanyl-phosphatidylethanolamine (MTP-PE) shown in Figure 3 (27). Although MDP influences several macrophage functions in vitro (28), comparable effects have initially not been observed in vivo because it is cleared extremely rapidly after parenteral administration (25). Even when injected at very high doses, MDP fails to induce significant macrophage-mediated antitumor activity in vivo (29). Consequently, to be effective in vivo the agent must be capable of activating macrophages irrespective of the normal physiologic pathways of the drug.

Fortunately, many of the problems discussed above have been overcome with the introduction of liposome-based drug delivery systems which have provided a mechanism for activating macrophages in situ with soluble MAF, MDP or both.

IV. THE USE OF LIPOSOMES AS CARRIERS FOR AGENTS THAT ACTIVATE MACROPHAGES IN SITU

The use of liposomes for carriers of drugs and macromolecules has become widespread in recent years (30,31). Encapsulation of a variety of compounds within liposomes dramatically alters the in vivo behavior and localization of entrapped drugs and markedly enhances the therapeutic potential of drugs in certain situations. Indeed, it has been possible to appropriately engineer the biochemical and biophysical properties of the liposome membrane, which has made it possible to "target" these structures to particular cell types in vivo.

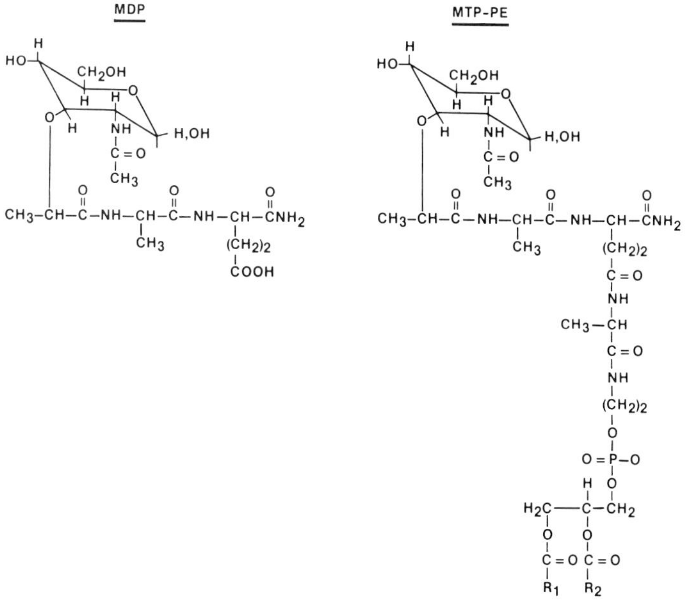

FIGURE 3.   Chemical Structures of MDP and MTP-PE (R = C16:0).

A. Activation of Macrophage Tumoricidal Properties in Vivo by Liposomes Containing Immunomodulators

Although liposomes provide a particularly convenient carrier vehicle for the delivery of biologically active agents to mononuclear phagocytes in vivo, several demanding criteria must be met for such systems to be ideal carriers for macrophage activators. They must: 1) readily bind to and be phagocytosed by reticuloendothelial cells, 2) retain the entrapped drug for reasonable periods of time, i.e., be nonleaky, 3) demonstrate preferential localization to tissues other than those rich in reticuloendothelial activity, i.e., to the lung parenchyma (since the lung is a major site of metastatic disease) following intravenous administration, and 4) have a relatively stable shelf life.

In order to better define these problems and in turn design efficient liposome carrier targeting systems, we have systematically evaluated the role of liposome lipid composition on macrophage-liposome interactions (32,33).

B. Binding and Phagocytosis of Liposomes by Macrophages

As discussed above, in order for liposomes to serve as vehicles for the delivery of compounds to cells of the RES, they must avidly bind to and become phagocytosed by the cells. Following extensive experimentation it became clear that macrophages might be able to recognize certain classes of phospholipids when we and other investigators observed that the inclusion of negatively charged lipids in liposomes greatly enhances their binding to, and subsequent phago-cytosis by, macrophages (32,34). Specifically, negatively charged liposomes containing phosphatidylserine (PS) are phagocytosed at rates 5- to 10-fold faster than are liposomes containing phosphatidylcholine (PC) alone. Neutral multilamellar vesicles (MLV) composed exclusively of PC are inefficiently bound to (Figure 4) and phagocytosed by (Figure 5) the macrophages. On the other hand, the inclusion of 30 mol % PS in these structures results in a dramatic increase in the binding (Figure 4) and phagocytosis of the liposomes by these cells (Figure 5).

It now appears that most cells of the RES recognize liposomes containing PS since enhancement of phagocytosis has been shown to occur in mouse peritoneal macrophages (34), Kupffer cells (35), alveolar macrophages (32) and human peripheral blood monocytes (17,36).

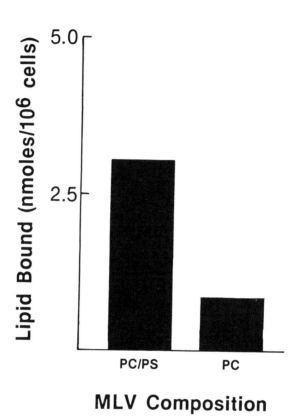

FIGURE 4. Binding of MLV to Macrophages. MLV containing trace amounts of iodinated lipid were incubated with macrophages for 1 hr at 37°C in the presence of 10^{-1} M NaN$_3$ [From (33) with permission.]

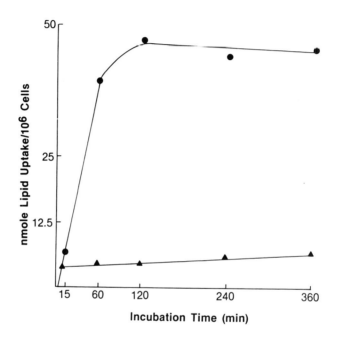

FIGURE 5. Phagocytosis of MLV by Macrophages. MLV containing trace amounts of iodinated lipid were incubated with macrophages at 37°C. At various times, the cells were washed and uptake quantified. Triangles, PC; circles, PC/PS (7:3) [From (33) with permission.]

C. Lung Localization of Liposomes Injected Intravenously

Since the lung is a major site of disseminated metastatic disease, we next identified those liposomes with increased efficiency for localization to the lung parenchyma. The retention of radiolabeled liposomes of differing structure and composition within the lungs of mice after i.v. injection is shown in Table 2. The data indicate that large multilamellar vesicles (MLV) or reverse evaporation (REV) liposomes are retained in the lungs more efficiently than small unilamellar liposomes (SUV) of identical lipid composition. In addition, the lipid composition of liposomes also significantly affects retention in the lungs. Liposomes of the same structural class are more efficiently retained in the lungs when they contain negatively charged lipids (PS) than when they contain neutral lipids (PC; 33).

Table 2. Pulmonary Retention of Liposomes of Differing Charge, Size and Lipid Composition after I.V. Injection into Mice[*]

Composition (mol ratio)	Structure[†]	% of Injected Dose Retained in Lungs
PC	MLV	2.2
PC	SUV	0.5
PC/PS (7/3)	SUV	0.9
PC/PS (7/3)	REV	7.2
PC/PS (9/1)	MLV	2.2
PC/PS (8/2)	MLV	2.3
PC/PS (7/3)	MLV	6.6

[*]Mice were injected with various liposome preparations containing iodinated lipids (2 μmol lipid in 0.2 ml) and the radiation was measured in the lungs four hours later.

[†]MLV, multilamellar vesicles; REV, reverse evaporation phase vesicles; SUV, small unilamellar vesicles.

The foregoing data demonstrate that MLV prepared from PC and PS (7/3 mol ratio) are more efficiently phagocytosed by macrophages and arrest more efficiently in the lungs than MLV composed exclusively of PC. However, these results do not show whether these liposomes are efficiently engulfed by alveolar macrophages, a prerequisite for them to become tumoricidal. The results of experiments based on the morphological examination of alveolar macrophages did, however, prove that at least some of the liposomes arrested in the lungs were recognized and subsequently phagocytosed by alveolar macrophages. Liposomes composed of PC/PS (7/3 mol %) containing 0.1% of the fluorescent lipid analog N-(7-nitro-2,1,3-benzoxadiazol-4-yl) phosphatidylethanolamine (NBD-PE) were injected into the tail veins of mice. Twenty-four hours later we assessed the total number of lung macrophages containing phagocytosed liposomes by analyzing all the cells from enzymatically dissociated tissue for Fc receptors (macrophages) and fluorescence (liposome positive). As can be seen in Table 3, about 12-15% of the total macrophage population (as identified by the formation of rosettes between opsonized erythrocytes and macrophages) were fluorescent, suggesting that MLV composed of PC and PS are the most efficient vehicles for the delivery of encapsulated compounds to lung macrophages (33,37).

Table 3. Lung Localization of Macrophages Containing MLV.

Treatment Group	% of Total Cells Containing Fluorescent MLV	% Fluorescent Macrophages[*]
No treatment	0	0
MLV	4.4	15.2

[*]Comparison of the number of fluorescent macrophages to total macrophages isolated from the samples.

D. Stability of Liposomes

The observations indicating that low molecular weight solutes entrapped in liposomes can leak from the liposome interior, and become rapidly diluted in the external media to concentrations at which they have no biological effect, are extremely disturbing, especially considering that serum proteins are potent inducers of liposome leakage (32). Conceivably this problem can be eliminated by converting potent water-soluble compounds to lipophilic pro-drugs. An example of such a lipophilic conversion is the covalent attachment of MDP to the primary functional amino group of phosphatidylethanolamine (PE), MTP-PE, shown in Figure 3.

As can be seen in Table 4, MLV formed from PC, PS and MTP-PE were indeed stable. In these experiments MLV were formed under sterile conditions 1, 4 and 8 wk before use and sealed in ampules under nitrogen to prevent oxidation. The data show that all of the MLV preparations produced similar levels of macrophage activation whether they were assessed by in vitro or in vivo techniques.

Another advantage of using lipophilic pro-drugs is shown in Table 5, where it can be seen that approximately 93% of the MTP-PE became incorporated in the PC/PS MLV. In contrast, only 3% of the water-soluble MDP became entrapped in the MLV. Moreover, it has also been shown that the MTP-PE was inserted directly into the liposome bilayer. We conclude this from the demonstration that MDP antibodies specifically precipitated more than 95% of the liposomes following their conversion into SUV by ultrasonication.

Table 4. Stability of Liposomes.

Cytotoxicity Assay	% Cytotoxicity after MLV Storage for:			
	Fresh	1 Week	4 Weeks	8 Weeks
in vitro[*]	55	54	54	28
in vivo[†]	42	44	49	43

[*]MLV containing MTP-PE were added to macrophages cultivated in vitro for 24 hr, washed and radiolabeled tumor cells were added.

[†]MLV were injected i.v. Twenty-four hours later alveolar macrophages were harvested and their cytotoxic activity was assessed in vitro.

Table 5. Incorporation of MDP and MTP-PE into MLV.

Liposome[*]	% MLV Recovered[†]	% Total Recovery[‡]
MLV Containing ^{3}H-MDP	78	3
MLV Containing ^{3}H-MTP-PE	82	93

[*]MLV were prepared by vortexing 10 μmol lipid (PC/PS = 7.3) containing 0.1% NBD-PE with ^{3}H-MTP-PE in 1.0 ml PBS.
[†]Percent recovery was calculated as the percentage of total NBD fluorescence present in MLV pellets after centrifugation at 15,000 x g for 30 min.
[‡]Values obtained are corrected for extent of MLV recovery.

V. TREATMENT OF SPONTANEOUS METASTASIS BY MULTIPLE INTRAVENOUS INJECTIONS OF LIPOSOMES CONTAINING IMMUNOMODULATORS

Previous studies have shown that immunomodulators such as MAF and MDP are most efficient in activating macrophages in vitro whether incorporated into liposomes alone or in combination (38). These data raised the possibility that macrophages could be activated to the tumoricidal state in situ by systemically administered immunomodulators encapsulated in liposomes, and that this could provide a therapeutic modality for enhancing host destruction of metastasis.

The results of our previous studies have indicated that multiple i.v. injections of liposomes containing MDP or MTP-PE, but not free drug or control preparations, eradicated spontaneous visceral metastasis in C57BL/6 mice from which a syngeneic melanoma growing intradermally had been surgically removed (29,39). In this experimental system, each mouse was given an intrafootpad injection of viable B16-BL6 melanoma cells. When the primary tumor reached a size of 0.8-1.0 cm in diameter (4 wk of growth), the tumor-bearing leg including the popliteal lymph node was amputated, and treatment begun three days later. As can be seen in Table 6, multiple administration of liposomes containing MDP or MTP-PE led to the eradication of established pulmonary and lymph node metastases. By da 90 of the experiment, 85-90% of the animals treated with the control had died. In contrast, 40% and 70% of the mice injected with MLV containing MDP or MTP-PE, respectively, survived at least 200 da after the last injection.

Table 6. Treatment of Spontaneous Lung and Lymph Node Melanoma Metastases by the Systemic Administration of Liposomes Containing MDP or MTP-PE.

Treatment	Percentage of mice surviving on day:						
	30	60	90	120	150	180	200
HBSS	100	69	14	10	10	10	10
MLV containing HBSS and suspended in 10 µg MDP	100	75	15	14	14	14	14
MLV containing 10 µg MDP	100	95	40	40	40	40	40
MLV containing 10 µg MTP-PE	100	83	66	66	66	66	66

It should be noted that studies using tumor cells isolated from the growing metastasis of the "treatment failures" have revealed that the tumor cells from these lesions are still susceptible to macrophage-mediated killing as assessed by in vitro techniques. Indeed, this result is consistent with the data discussed earlier, which suggest that tumor cell resistance to macrophage-mediated killing is not likely to be a limiting factor in the efficacy of this treatment modality. The more challenging and significant limitation to this treatment regimen is likely to be the extent of tumor burden at the time therapy is initiated. Thus, potential therapeutic protocols designed to stimulate host immunity must be used in combination with other treatment modalities in order to first reduce tumor burden.

In an effort to enhance the efficacy of macrophage-mediated destruction of metastases we have recently shown that the combination of MAF and MDP at suboptimal concentrations in the same liposome dramatically enhances the therapeutic potential (40).

A. Synergistic Activation of Mouse Alveolar Macrophages (AM) by MAF and MDP Encapsulated within the Same Liposomes

In experiments designed to evaluate the efficacy of this approach, mice were injected i.v. with MLV containing various dilutions of MAF, various dilutions of MDP, combinations of MAF and MDP, or control preparations. AM were harvested 24 hr after i.v. treatment and their tumoricidal properties were determined by an in vitro assay. As can be seen in Table 7, MLV containing 1:2 dilutions of MAF or MLV containing 6.25 μg MDP were highly effective in rendering AM cytolytic to B16 melanoma cells, whereas MLV containing either a 1:20 dilution of MAF or a 1:20 dilution of MDP (equivalent to 0.3 μg entrapped MDP) were not. On the other hand, when MLV containing a 1:20 dilution of MAF and a 1:20 dilution of MDP (0.3 μg) were injected, significant in situ activation of AM occurred (44%), one that was as effective as a 1:2 dilution of MAF and 6.25 μg MDP within the same MLV (42%).

In order to determine whether the regimen would be efficacious in the treatment of relatively large tumor burdens, the therapy experiments described above were carried out again, but this time i.v. administration of liposomes began 7 da after the surgical removal of the primary (subcutaneous) B16-BL6 melanoma. At that time, spontaneous pulmonary metastases were well established, with some lung metastases as large as 1 mm in diameter. Liposomes were injected twice weekly for 4 wk (eight injections). Practically all the mice receiving HBSS alone and MLV suspended in encapsulated MAF and MDP had died by da 90 of the experiment (Figure 6). On the other hand, multiple i.v. injections of liposomes containing either 6.25 μg MDP or a 1:2 dilution of MAF resulted in long-term survival (~ 250 da) of 27% of the animals (5/18). Neither MAF at a 1:20 dilution nor MDP at doses lower than 0.6 μg was therapeutically effective. In contrast, mice treated with MLV containing both agents at individual subthreshold concentrations had enhanced survival rates, with 50% (9/18) of the mice alive at da 250.

222

Table 7. Synergistic Activation of Mouse AM by MAF and MDP Encapsulated in the Same Liposomes.

Liposome Content for Intravenous Treatment of AM Donor	Percent AM-Mediated Cytolysis[*]
HBSS	2
MAF 1:2	45
MAF 1:20	8
MDP 6.25 μg	38
MDP 0.30 μg	9
MAF 1:2 + MDP 6.25 μg	49
MAF 1:20 + MDP 0.30 μg	38

[*]Percentage cytolysis was derived by comparison with control AM (alveolar macrophages).

VI. CONCLUSION

The optimal conditions for systemic therapy with liposome-encapsulated immunomodulators and the efficacy of this modality alone, or in combination, in treating large metastatic tumor burdens has not been completely defined. Although the experimental observations reported here have been encouraging, it is unlikely that this therapeutic approach could serve as the single treatment for advanced metastatic disease. As with many other antitumor therapies, optimal application of these modalities will probably require their use in combination with other antitumor agents. For example, if the ratio of macrophages to tumor cells required for optimal macrophage-mediated tumoricidal activity _in vivo_ is similar to that operating _in vitro_, then, even allowing for maximum recruitment of monocytes from the blood, there are insufficient macrophages in the lung to permit effective destruction of metastatic tumor burdens exceeding 10^8 tumor cells/lung. Since tumor burdens of this size are much too often observed both clinically and experimentally, potential therapeutic

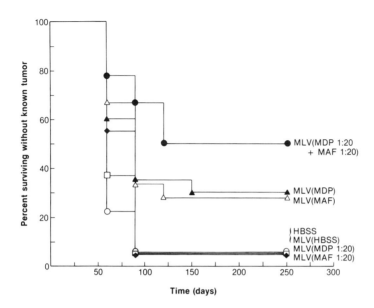

FIGURE 6. Effect of Treatment of Spontaneous Metastasis by the Systemic Administration of Liposomes Containing MDP, MAF or Combined MDP/MAF.

regimens designed to stimulate the antitumor properties of macrophages exclusively will meet with limited success. Therefore, the development of potential therapeutic protocols designed to stimulate host defenses must be used in combination with other treatment modalities which can first reduce the tumor burden to within acceptable limits. Activated macrophages could then be employed to destroy those few remaining tumor cells which are probably resistant to conventional therapies.

REFERENCES

1. Poste G, Fidler IJ: The pathogenesis of cancer metastasis. Nature 283:139-146, 1979.
2. Fidler IJ, Hart IR: Biological diversity in metastatic neoplasms: Origins and implications. Science 217:998-1003, 1982.
3. Fidler IJ, Kripke ML: Metastasis results from pre-existing variant cells within a malignant tumor. Science 197:893-895, 1977.

224

4. Talmadge JE, Wolman SR, Fidler IJ: Evidence for the clonal origin of spontaneous metastasis. Science 217:361-363, 1982.
5. Fidler IJ, Poste G: Macrophage mediated destruction of malignant tumor cells and new stratagies for the therapy of metastatic disease. Springer Semin. Immunopathol. 5:161-174, 1982.
6. Fidler IJ: Recognition and destruction of target cells by tumoricidal macrophages. Isr. J. Med. 14:177-191, 1978.
7. Hamilton TA, Fishman M: Characterization of the recognition of target cells sensitive or resistant to cytolysis by activated rat peritoneal macrophages. J. Immunol. 127:1702-1706, 1981.
8. Hibbs JB, Jr.: Discrimination between neoplastic and non-neoplastic cells in vitro by activated macrophages. J. Natl. Cancer Inst. 53:1487-1492, 1974.
9. Piessens WF, Churchill WH, Jr.: Macrophages activated in vitro with lymphocyte mediators kill neoplastic but not normal cells. J. Immunol. 114:293-299, 1975.
10. Tucker RW, Meltzer MS, Sanford KK: Susceptibility to killing by BCG-activated macrophages associated with "spontaneous" neoplastic transformation in culture. Int. J. Cancer 27:555-562, 1981.
11. Hibbs JB, Jr.: Heterocytolysis by macrophages activated by bacillus Calmette-Guerin: Lysosome exocytosis into tumor cells. Cancer Res. 184:468-471, 1974.
12. Bucana CD, Hoyer LL, Hobbs B, Breesman S, MacDaniel M, Hanna MG, Jr.: Morphological evidence for the translocation of lysosomal organelles from cytotoxic macrophages into the cytoplasm of tumor target cells. Cancer Res. 36:4444-4458, 1976.
13. Marino PA, Adams DO: Interaction of bacillus Calmette-Guerin-activated macrophages and neoplastic cells in vitro. I. Conditions for binding and selectivity. Cell. Immunol. 54:11-25, 1980.
14. Marino PA, Adams DO: Interaction of bacillus Calmette-Guerin-activated macrophages and neoplastic cells in vitro. II. The relationship of selective binding to cytolysis. Cell. Immunol. 54:26-35, 1980.
15. Bucana CD, Hoyer LL, Schroit AJ, Kleinerman E, Fidler IJ: Ultrastructural studies of the interaction between lipsosome-activated human blood monocytes and allogeneic tumor cells in vitro. Am. J. Pathol. 112:101-111, 1983.
16. Kleinerman ES, Erickson KL, Schroit AJ, Fidler IJ: Activation of tumoricidal properties in human blood monocytes by liposomes containing lipophilic muramyl tripeptide. Cancer Res. 43:2010-2014, 1983.
17. Kleinerman ES, Schroit AJ, Fogler WE, Fidler IJ: Tumoricidal activity of human monocytes activated in vitro by free and liposome-encapsulated human lymphokines. J. Clin. Invest. 72:304-315, 1983.
18. Fidler IJ, Gersten DM, Bubmen MB: Characterization in vivo and in vitro of tumor cells selected for resistance to syngeneic lymphocyte medicated toxicity. Cancer Res. 36:3160-3165, 1976.
19. Hanna N, Fidler IJ: Relationship between metastatic potential and resistance to natural killer cell-mediated cytotoxicity in three murine tumor systems. J. Natl. Cancer Inst. 66:1183-1190, 1981.

20. Giavazzi R, Bucana CD, Hart IR: Correlation of tumor growth inhibitory activity of macrophages exposed to adriamycin and the adriamycin-sensitivity of the target tumor cells. J. Natl. Cancer Inst. (In press).

21. Giavazzi R, Miller L, Hart IR: Metastatic behavior of an adriamycin-resistant murine tumor. Cancer Res. 43:5081-5086, 1983.

22. Poste G, Kirsh R: Rapid decay of tumoricidal activity and loss of responsiveness to lymphokines in inflammatory macrophages. Cancer Res. 39:2582-2590, 1979.

23. Sone S, Pollack VA, Fidler IJ: Direct activation of tumoricidal properties in rat alveolar macrophages by Nocardia rubra cell wall skeleton. Cancer Immunol. Immunother. 9:227-232, 1980.

24. Lederer E: Synthetic immunostimulants derived from the bacterial cell wall. J. Med. Chem. 23:819-825, 1980.

25. Parant M, Parant L, Chedid L, Yapo A, Petit JF, Lederer E: Fate of the synthetic immunoadjuvant, muramyl dipeptide (14C-labelled) in the mouse. Int. J. Immunopharmacol. 1:35-41, 1979.

26. Ellouz FG, Adam A, Clorbaru R, Lederer E: Minimal structural requirements for adjuvant activity of bacterial peptidoglycan derivatives. Biochem. Biophys. Res. Commun. 59:1317-1324, 1974.

27. Fidler IJ, Sone S, Fogler WE, Smith D, Braun DG, Tarcsay L, Gisler RJ, Schroit AJ: Efficacy of liposomes containing a lipophilic muramyl dipeptide derivative for activating the tumoricidal properties of alveolar macrophages in vivo. J. Biol. Response Modifiers 1:43-55, 1982.

28. Gisler RH, Dietrich FM, Baschang G, Brownbill A, Schuman G, Staber FB, Tarcsay L, Wachsmuth ED, Dukor P: New developments in drugs enhancing the immune response: Activation of lymphocytes and accessory cells by muramyl-dipeptides. IN: Turk JL and Parker D (eds.) Drugs and Immune Responsiveness. MacMillan Press, London, pp. 133-160, 1979.

29. Fidler IJ, Sone S, Fogler WE, Barnes ZL: Eradication of spontaneous metastasis and activation of alveolar macrophages by intravenous injection of liposomes containing muramyl dipeptide. Proc. Natl. Acad. Sci. USA 78:1680-1684, 1981.

30. Knight CG: Liposomes: From Physical Structure to Therapeutic Applications. Elsevier/North-Holland, Amsterdam, 1981.

31. Ostro MJ: Liposomes. Marcel Dekker, New York, 1983.

32. Schroit AJ, Fidler IJ: Effect of liposome structure and lipid composition on the activation of the tumoricidal properties of macrophages by muramyl dipeptide liposomes. Cancer Res. 42:161-167, 1982.

33. Schroit AJ, Galligioni E, Fidler IJ: Factors influencing the in situ activation of macrophages by liposomes containing muramyl dipeptide. Biol. Cell 47:87-94, 1983.

34. Raz A, Bucana C, Fogler WE, Poste G, Fidler IJ: Biochemical, morphological, and ultrastructural studies on the uptake of liposomes by murine macrophages. Cancer Res. 41:487-494, 1981.

35. Scherphof G, Roerdink F, Dijkstra J, Ellens H, DeZander R, Wisse E: Uptake of liposomes by rat and mouse hepatocytes and Kupffer cells. Biol. Cell. 47:47-58, 1983.

226

36. Mehta K, Lopez-Berestein G, Hirst EM, Juliano SL: Uptake of liposomes and liposome-encapsulated muramyl dipeptide by human peripheral blood monocytes. J. Reticuloendothel. Soc. 32:155-164, 1982.
37. Key M, Talmadge JE, Fogler WE, Bucana C, Fidler IJ: Isolation of tumoricidal macrophages from lung melanoma metastasis of mice treated systemically with liposomes containing a lipophilic derivative of muramyl dipeptide. J. Natl. Cancer Inst. 69:1189-1198, 1982.
38. Sone S, Fidler IJ: Synergistic activation of lymphokines and muramyl dipeptide of tumoricidal properties in rat alveolar macrophages. J. Immunol. 125:2454-2458, 1980.
39. Fidler IJ: Therapy of spontaneous metastasis by intravenous injection of liposomes containing lymphokines. Science 208:1469-1471, 1980.
40. Fidler IJ, Schroit AJ: Synergism betwen lymphokines and muramyl dipeptide encapsulated in liposomes: In situ activation of macrophages and therapy of spontaneous cancer metastasis. J. Immunol. (In press).
41. Giavazzi R, Scholar E, Hart IR: Isolation and preliminary characterization of an Adriamycin-resistant fibrosarcoma cell line. Cancer Res. 43:2211-2222, 1983.

CHAPTER 15. BIOLOGICAL RESPONSE MODIFIERS AS ACTIVATORS OF NATURAL KILLER CELLS: POTENTIAL ROLE IN TREATMENT OF METASTASIS

RONALD B. HERBERMAN

I. INTRODUCTION

Until about five years ago, T-cell mediated immunity against tumor associated antigens was considered to be the main, if not the only, mechanism for host resistance against tumor growth. Then macrophages began to be increasingly considered as an alternative effector cell for host resistance (see Chapter 14). More recently, it has become increasingly appreciated that a diverse array of effector mechanisms may be involved in host resistance against tumor growth. In addition to classical, induced immune responses against tumor associated antigens, the host has a natural immune system, which may be particularly involved as a first line of defense (1). In addition to macrophages, a principal component of the natural immune system is the natural killer (NK) cell (2). NK cells represent a small subpopulation of lymphoid cells, distinct from typical T-cells or macrophages, and highly associated with a morphologic cell type, the large granular lymphocyte (LGL). Over the last several years there has been a rapid increase in our knowledge of the characteristics of NK cells, attributable largely to the ability to highly purify this cell population, either by Percoll density gradient centrifugation or by use of monoclonal or other antibodies against selective cell surface markers (2).

II. EVIDENCE FOR ROLE OF NK CELLS IN METASTASIS

A particular focus of research with NK cells has been exploration of their possible in vivo role in host resistance against tumor growth. Although some evidence has accumulated for involvement of NK cells in immune surveillance against the development of primary tumors (1), the strongest evidence has come from studies of the role of NK cells in resistance against systemic metastases. By intravenous inoculation of radiolabeled NK-susceptible tumor cells, and measurement of rapid clearance of the radiolabel from the lungs and other major organs, it was found that the levels of NK activity in the recipients correlated closely with the degree of rapid clearance, particularly from the lungs (3). These findings suggested that NK cells might be particularly involved in the interaction with tumor cells released into the circulation and, therefore, might help to prevent metastatic seeding in distant organs. In support of this possibility, Gorelik et al. found that pulmonary metastases are more resistant to NK activity than the parental tumor (4), suggesting that successful metastasis represents escape from this defense mechanism, and in vitro selected NK-resistant variants of a tumor are more metastatic then the unselected parental tumor (5). More direct evidence for a relationship between NK activity and resistance to metastases came from experiments in which the levels of NK activity were experimentally manipulated, and effects of such treatment on the extent of metastasis were evaluated (6,7). Depression of NK activity by various treatments, e.g., in vivo inoculation of an antiserum against asialo GM_1, or studies in beige mice which have a selective deficit in NK activity, is associated with a large increase in the number of pulmonary metastases and with the development of hepatic and other metastases, which ordinarily are not detectable. Conversely, mice with elevated NK activity are shown to be more resistant to metastases than mice with intermediate or low NK activity. Such an inverse correlation between levels of NK activity and the number of metastases is observed not only in mice with artificially induced metastases from intravenous inoculated tumor cells, but also in mice developing spontaneous metastases after amputation of locally growing tumors. Further, and the most direct, evidence for the central role of NK cells in resistance to metastases from NK-susceptible tumors has come from the observation that adoptive transfer of highly purified populations of LGL into rats whose NK activity had been depressed by anti-asialo GM_1 results in a reconstitution of resistance against metastases as well as a restoration of NK activity (8).

III. AUGMENTATION OF NK ACTIVITY BY BIOLOGICAL RESPONSE MODIFIERS
      (BRMs)

In addition to their spontaneous cytotoxic activity against tumor cells, the activity of NK cells has been found to be substantially augmented by treatment in vitro or in vivo with interferons, interleukin-2 or a variety of BRMs (2 and Chapter 13). In view of the above evidence for a role of NK cells in resistance to metastases, an attractive strategy for the prophylaxis and/or therapy of metastases is the augmentation of NK activity by administration of a BRM. Positive evidence in this direction has come particularly from studies related to the immunoprophylaxis of metastases by BRMs. A variety of agents known to augment NK activity have been shown to also substantially increase resistance against metastases, whereas BRMs lacking NK-boosting activity fail to prevent metastases (3,9). One BRM which has been used extensively to analyze the relationship between augmentation of NK activity and prevention of metastases has been MVE-2, a pyran co-polymer. Administration of MVE-2 to mice results in substantial augmentation of NK activity and increased resistance to the development of metastases. However, since MVE-2 and other NK boosting agents also activate macrophages for cytotoxic activity, it has been critical to determine the relative roles of these two effector mechanisms. A very useful approach has been the use of anti-asialo GM_1 administration around the time of MVE-2 treatment, which selectively depressed the augmented NK activity induced by MVE-2, but had little or no detectable effect on the levels of cytotoxicity of MVE-2-activated macrophages (R.H. Wiltrout, R.B. Herberman, S. Zhang, M.A. Chirigos,

J.R. Ortaldo, K.M. Green, Jr. and J.E. Talmadge, manuscript in preparation). In the initial experiments, it appeared as though NK cells were not required for resistance to pulmonary metastases since treatment of MVE-2-inoculated mice with anti-asialo GM_1 virtually eliminated splenic NK activity and rapid clearance of radiolabeled tumor cells from the lungs but had little or no effect on the strong resistance against the development of pulmonary or hepatic metastases. However, upon closer evaluation, it was found that the lungs and liver of MVE-2-treated mice contained large numbers of LGL with high NK activity (R.H. Wiltrout, B.J. Mathieson, J.E. Talmadge, C.W. Reynolds, S. Zhang, R.B. Herberman and J.R. Ortaldo, manuscript in preparation), and that the single treatment with anti-asialo GM_1 reduced but did not eliminate the tissue-associated NK activity. When two treatments with high concentrations of the antiserum were given, the NK activity in the lungs and liver of MVE-2-treated mice was completely abrogated and then a substantial increase in metastases was detected in the lungs, liver and other organs (R.H. Wiltrout, R.B. Herberman, S. Zhang, M.A. Chirigos, J.R. Ortaldo, K.M. Green, Jr. and J.E. Talmadge, manuscript in preparation). Thus, these data indicate that in addition to the important role that circulating NK cells or NK cells in the capillary beds play in the rapid elimination of tumor cells from the vasculature, NK cells induced in the tissues by a BRM can have a potent effect on the subsequent outgrowth of metastases. Such evidence lends encouragement to continuation of efforts to treat metastases by augmentation of NK activity with BRMs.

IV. RELATIONSHIP OF NK AUGMENTATION TO CLINICAL THERAPY OF TUMORS BY BRMs

In the last several years, considerable attention has been devoted to the possible role of NK cells in the therapeutic effects of various BRMs in the treatment of human cancers. One premise underlying such studies is that NK cells can have cytotoxic effects against autochthonous tumors as well as against the transplantable or cultured cell lines which are routinely utilized in the animal experiments. Although extensive studies on susceptibility of fresh tumor cells to autochthonous as well as allogenic NK cells have yet to be performed, the evidence to date supports the susceptibility, to at least some extent, of such tumor cells to attack by NK cells, particularly after augmentation of their reactivity by BRMs (10).

Since augmentation of NK activity has been considered to be a potentially important mechanism for therapeutic effects, NK activity has begun to be monitored during the course of clinical trials with various BRMs. In trials with interferon, the initial results are quite encouraging. Einhorn et al. (11) reported that administration of a partially purified natural interferon to patients with osteosarcoma results in strong and sustained augmentation of NK activity, which only returns to baseline levels after discontinuation of treatment. However, in most subsequent trials, interferon has been found to only induce a transient augmentation of NK activity, followed by a return to baseline levels or even depression below pretreatment levels, despite continued administration of interferon (12). This failure to sustain augmentation of NK activity by a BRM with known potent in vitro augmenting activity on NK cells has been quite surprising and has provided a considerable challenge to the investigators since sustained augmentation of NK activity might be important for optimal therapeutic benefits from interferon. Considerable efforts have been initiated to understand the basis for these paradoxical results and to develop strategies to circumvent this hyporesponsiveness to continued NK augmentation. In an attempt to provide animal models for this clinical situation, interferon or other BRMs have been administered daily to mice and the persistence of NK augmentation has been evaluated. Repeated administration to mice of a human recombinant hybrid interferon, one dose of which potently augments mouse-NK activity, results in hyporesponsiveness to continued augmentation (13). Repeated administration of MVE-2 or other BRMs induces even more clear-cut hyporesponsiveness (14), and my laboratory has therefore focused on studies with MVE-2 as a model system for this problem. In contrast to the efficacy of MVE-2 for the immunoprophylaxis of metastases from the B16 melanoma, treatment of mice bearing metastases from this tumor, by repeated inoculations of MVE-2, had little or no therapeutic effects (J. Talmadge, manuscript in preparation). In parallel with such negative results and in contrast to the considerable augmentation of NK activity by one dose of MVE-2, after two or more doses of MVE-2 no detectable augmentation of NK activity is seen (14). In a detailed examination of the possible mechanism underlying this effect (T. Saito, R.D. Welker, H. Fukui, R.B. Herberman and M.A. Chirigos, manuscript submitted for publication), several possible explanations were ruled out including generation of suppressor cells with the ability to inhibit the effector phase of reactivity, or increased production of prostaglandin E. Rather, the hyporesponsiveness was associated with a substantial decrease in the number of LGL recovered from the spleen, in contrast to the augmentation of LGL numbers in the spleens of mice treated once with MVE-2 or other BRMs (A. Santoni, M. Piccoli, J.R. Ortaldo and R.B. Herberman, manuscript submitted for publication). The hyporesponsivness to NK augmentation induced by multiple doses of MVE-2 could be reversed, at least in part, by further treatment with a different BRM, poly IC-LC, and this reinduction of augmented NK activity was accompanied by an increase in the number of splenic LGL (T. Saito, R.D. Welker, H. Fukui, R.B. Herberman and M.A. Chirigos, manuscript submitted for publication). Thus, a major factor influencing the degree of responsiveness to NK augmentation appears to be the regulation of the size of the effector cell population, and the expansion in LGL numbers after one dose of a BRM has been shown to be due to proliferation of the effector cell population, rather than to an increased distribution of these effector cells in the spleen at the expense of other organs (A. Santoni, M. Piccoli, J.R. Ortaldo and R.B. Herberman, manuscript submitted for publication). A clue to the mechanism underlying this regulation of numbers of effector cells has come from studies involving the administration of cyclophosphamide between the first and second doses of MVE-2 (E. Schlick, manuscript in preparation). Administration of cyclophosphamide at five days after the first dose of MVE-2 resulted in a substantial responsiveness to NK augmentation by a second dose of MVE-2 administered several days later.

These data suggest that cyclophosphamide has the ability to eliminate suppressor cells generated by the BRM, which can prevent the subsequent repeated augmentation of NK activity by the same BRM. Studies are now in progress to further understand the events underlying these observations.

Possible synergistic antimetastatic effects between BRMs and other agents and increased understanding of the mechanisms underlying the antimetastatic effects of various drugs may lead to an augmented ability to optimally treat metastatic disease. As described by others in this volume (see Chapters 9 and 11), treatment with various anticoagulants has been shown to increase resistance to the development and growth of metastases. As a possible alternative to the postulated ability of anticoagulants to interfere with attachment of circulating tumor cells to the vascular endothelium (see Chapter 9), our laboratory has evaluated the possibility that anticoagulants can increase the effective interactions between tumor cells and NK cells or other effector cells (15). In support of this hypothesis, we have found that the ability of heparin or other anticoagulants to interfere with metastases is abrogated by depletion of NK activity by administration of anti-asialo GM_1. Conversely, sequential treatment of mice with an anticoagulant and an NK-augmenting BRM like poly IC results in synergistic antimetastatic effects. Thus, it appears that the anti-metastatic effects induced by anticoagulants are dependent on the integrity of the NK mechanism and that augmentation of NK activity in addition to anticoagulation can lead to substantially enhanced anti-tumor effects than that conferred by either treatment alone. Further exploration of treatment protocols involving both types of agents therefore seems warranted and may have applications to the clinical therapy of metastases.

V. CONCLUSION

It is becoming increasingly clear that NK cells can play an important role in resistance against the development and growth of metastases. Such indications provide a major challenge to tumor immunologists to develop effective strategies for sustained augmentation of NK activity by BRMs, which in turn would be expected to lead to more effective treatment of cancer. The results to date in this area have been rather disappointing. Treatment of patients with metastatic disease by repeated administration of BRMs has usually not resulted in detectable antitumor effects. However, several explanations may be offered for such negative results. First, as discussed above, the protocols of administration of BRMs have been found not to cause the expected sustained augmentation of NK activity. It is hoped that a better understanding of the mechanism underlying this hyporesponsiveness to NK augmentation will lead to the development of optimal immunomodulatory schedules, in which sustained or repeated augmentation of NK activity as well as sustained augmentation of other effector functions can be produced. In addition, most of the clinical trials with BRMs have been with patients with advanced metastatic disease, with large tumor burdens. It seems likely that therapeutic

strategies based on augmentation of effector cell function will be more
likely to be successful in patients with micrometastases and minimal
tumor burdens. New Phase I clinical trials to determine the optimal
immunomodulatory doses of interferon and other BRMs, in patients with
minimal tumor burden, are now being organized by the Biological
Response Modifiers Program of the National Cancer Institute.

REFERENCES

1. Herberman RB: Immune surveillance hypothesis: Updated
    formulation and possible effector mechanisms. IN: Yamamura Y and
    Tada T (eds.) Progress in Immunology V. Academic Press, Tokyo,
    pp. 1157-1167, 1983.
2. Herberman RB: NK Cells and Other Natural Effector Cells. Academic
    Press, New York, pp. 1566, 1982.
3. Riccardi C, Santoni A, Barlozzari T, Puccetti P, Herberman RB: In
    vivo natural reactivity of mice against tumor cells. Int. J.
    Cancer 25:475-486, 1980.
4. Gorelik E, Fogel M, Feldman M, Segals S: Differences in
    resistance of metastatic tumor cells and cells from local tumor
    growth to cytotoxicity of natural killer cells. J. Natl. Cancer
    Inst. 63:1397-1404, 1979.
5. Gorelik E, Segal S, Feldman M: Selection of 3LL tumor subline
    resistant to natural effector cells concomitantly selected for
    increased metastatic potency.   Cancer Immunol. Immunother.
    12:105-109, 1982.
6. Hanna N, Fidler I: Relationship between metastatic potential and
    resistance to natural killer cell-mediated cytotoxicity in three
    murine tumor systems. J. Natl. Cancer Inst. 66:1183-1190,
    1981.
7. Gorelik E, Wiltrout RH, Okumura K, Habu S, Herberman RB: Role of
    NK cells in the control of metastatic spread and growth of tumor
    cells in mice. Int. J. Cancer 30:109-112, 1982.
8. Barlozzari T, Reynolds CW, Herberman RB: Reconstitution of NK
    activity and antitumor immunity in anti-asialo GM$_1$-treated rats by
    the adoptive transfer of LGL. IN: Hoshino T, Koren HS and Uchida
    A (eds.) Natural Killer Activity and Its Regulation. Excerpta
    Medica Ltd., Tokyo, pp. 378-381, 1984.
9. Talmadge JE, Lenz BF, Collins MS, Uithoven KA, Schneider MA, Adams
    JS, Pearson JW, Agee WJ, Fox RE, Oldham RK: Tumor models to
    investigate the therapeutic efficacy of immunomodulators. Behring
    Inst. Mitt., 1984.
10. Serrate SA, Vose BM, Timonen T, Ortaldo JR, Herberman RB:
    Association of human natural killer cell activity against human
    primary tumors with large granular lymphocytes. IN: Herberman RB
    (ed.) NK Cells and Other Natural Effector Cells. Academic Press,
    New York, pp. 1055-1060, 1982.
11. Einhorn S, Ahre A, Blomgren H, Johansson B, Mellstept H, Strander
    H: Enhanced NK activity in patients treated by interferon.
    Relation to clinical response. IN: Herberman RB (ed.) NK Cells
    and Other Natural Effector Cells. Academic Press, New York, pp.
    1259-1263, 1982.

12. Herberman RB, Thurman GB: Summary. Approaches to the immunological monitoring of cancer patients treated with natural or recombinant interferons. J. Biol. Response Modifiers 2:548-562, 1983.

13. Brunda MJ, Rosenbaum D: Modulation of murine natural killer cell activity in vitro and in vivo by recombinant human interferons. J. Immunol. (In press).

14. Piccoli M, Saito T, Chirigos MA: Bimodal effects of MVE-2 on cytotoxic activity of natural killer cell and macrophage tumoricidal activities. Int. J. Immunopharmacol. (In press).

15. Gorelik E, Bere WW, Herberman RB: Role of NK cells in the antimetastatic effects of anticoagulant drugs. Int. J. Cancer 33:87-94, 1984.

CHAPTER 16. BREAST CANCER DIAGNOSIS WITH HUMAN MAMMARY EPITHELIAL ANTIGENS AND THE PROSPECTIVE USE OF ANTIBODIES AGAINST THEM IN THERAPY

ROBERTO L. CERIANI, JERRY A. PETERSON AND EDWARD W. BLANK

I. INTRODUCTION

Antigens present in breast tumors can be separated into at least three categories: i) normal antigens which continue to be expressed in the tumors, ii) tumor antigens synthesized de novo, and iii) normal antigens expressed in the tumors but whose synthesis is incomplete or altered by the neoplastic process. Few examples exist of the latter two categories. The T antigen (1), being a clearly identified example of incomplete synthesis of a normal antigen, is found in tumors and its chemical structure has been elucidated. This latter antigen, however, is present in many neoplastic tissues other than breast tumors. In contrast, normal antigens of breast tissue, some of them with certain specificity, that remain present in their transformed counterpart are very prevalent (2) and they become useful in breast cancer diagnosis in direct relationship to their specificity and abundance in the original tissue. In the case of the human breast we were the first to describe a breast specific or characteristic antigenic system (2) which is called human mammary epithelial antigens (HME-Ags).

In 1977 our group at Bruce Lyon Memorial Research Laboratory reported these cell-type specific antigens of human mammary epithelial cells (HME-Ags; 2). These antigens are obtained from the human milk fat globule membrane (HMFGM). We also reported a similar system in the mouse, mouse mammary epithelial antigens (MME-Ags), which are also found in the mouse milk fat globule membrane (MMFGM; 3). Antisera were raised in rabbits against these membrane fractions and after repeated adsorptions were rendered breast specific, for they bind to mammary epithelial cells, but not to other cells of the gland, nor to any cells of other tissues tested to date. Thus, HME-Ags and MME-Ags are considered normal differentiation antigens of mammary epithelial cells.

The specificity of these antisera make them very useful in our hands in cell identification. With them, cells present in human milk (4) and epithelial cells in primary cultures prepared from breast tissue have been identified. An interesting feature we reported for HME-Ags is their persistence. Cultivation (5), in vivo transplantation of mouse mammary tumors in syngeneic mice (3) or of human breast carcinomas in nude mice (6) did not alter their expression; they always remain present.

236

Mechanically dispersed cells from human breast tumors also bind the anti-HME serum (7). HME-Ags are detected on the epithelial cells of every breast tumor or metastasis studied and in every benign dysplasia, while tumors of other tissue are always negative (7). The pattern of immuno-fluorescent staining of the neoplastic mammary epithelial cells is of the "ring type" and indicative of their presence on the cell surface. Pre-immune sera, duly adsorbed, is used as negative controls in every instance.

HME-Ags were also studied quantitatively and it was found that they are expressed to a lesser degree in the neoplastic cells than in their normal counterparts. Their levels were measured both by radioimmunoassay (RIA; 8) and flow cytofluorimetry (9). Deletions of up to 50% of HME antigens (8) in breast cancer cells are detected; these antigens comprise up to 5-10% of the membrane protein. With the advent of the hybridoma technique for the development of monoclonal antibodies, we applied our previous approach to the search for normal antigens (and their antibodies) on the HMFGM that are also expressed in breast neoplastic tissue, with the idea of creating monoclonal antibodies useful in breast cancer diagnosis and possibly in therapy.

Hybridomas recognizing specific components of the human milk fat globule membrane were first isolated by us (10). In these studies we prepared hybridomas by immunizing mice with HMFGM. The monoclonals produced have a narrow specificity. These monoclonals recognize mainly breast epithelial cells, and some other cells with secretory capacity. In other studies, they were proved by the immunoperoxidase technique to bind to breast epithelial tissue, sebaceous glands of the skin, lung epithelium and some cells of the kidney (11).

In new studies more hybridomas were isolated after fusion of mouse myeloma cells and spleen cells from BALB/c mice immunized with HMFGM. Screening for desirable hybridomas was performed against HMFGM and membranes of epithelial, lymphoid and fibroblastic cells in an effort to prepare hybridoma strains producing specific anti-breast epithelial cell antibodies. Two hybridomas were obtained initially and were assayed on a rudimentary plate assay for binding to the above mentioned human cell lines. Two of the hybridomas selected produce antibodies binding to most breast epithelial cell lines (12). Many fusions were later performed after immunization with HMFGM; from them, we obtained 56% antibody-secreting hybridomas out of which only 13.5% secrete antibodies against HMFGM, and out of which 1.3% secrete antibodies that bind to HMFGM and not to membranes of the other cells of the above panel.

The need for new techniques for producing monoclonal antibodies adapted to our requirements became urgent. We developed an appropriate solid phase screen, molecular weight determination and antigen quantification method in our laboratory which involved a successful and non-denaturing way of derivatizing antigens to plastic wells. The firm binding obtained allows for very reproducible results (12). With this solid phase procedure we designed a screening method wherein HMFGM, lymphoid (Bristol-8), colonic (HT-29), cervical epithelium (Hela) and fibroblast cell membranes are used to select the monoclonal antibody binding exclusively to HMFGM. The membranes are separated by a gradient centrifugation method with a vertical rotor SS-199 (12). With these techniques the original hybridomas were recloned and tested, and also several new hybridomas were developed. Four monoclonals remain stable and reclonable: BLMRL-HMFG-Mc$_1$, BLMRL-HMFG-Mc$_3$, BLMRL-HMFG-Mc$_5$ and BLMRL-HMFG-Mc$_8$.

With the solid phase methodology plus a radiolabeling method, a modification of the GELELISA technique, we determined the molecular weight of the antigens identified by the monoclonal antibodies. MC$_3$ binds to a component of 45,000 daltons in molecular weight (12). This component is apparently the one called component IV of those specific components, described by us, of the HMFGM (2). Another monoclonal Mc$_5$ binds to a component that does not penetrate a 10% concentration in acrylamide gel electrophoresis and in that is similar to BLMRL-HMFG-Mc$_1$ [previously referred to as 3.14A3 (10)]. When using a gradient acrylamide gel (4-25%) the component penetrates and seems to have an apparent molecular weight of 4 x 10^5 daltons. It was named non-penetrating glycoprotein (NPGP). This component is strongly PAS positive and stains poorly with Coomassie blue, so the likelihood is that it corresponds to a mucin-type glycoprotein since it can also be labeled with ^{125}I. These components seem to have several bands in the polyacrylamide gel profile. It is thought that the jagged peak could be the result of the way the gel fragments are cut, plus the microheterogeneity of the glycoprotein. Other authors have also studied this component with similar results (13). Further, Mc$_1$ and Mc$_5$ recognize the same molecule, however the cellular distribution of the antigen detected is different for each monoclonal, and since they do not compete for binding of HMFG on a solid phase they seem to recognize different NPGP epitopes. A monoclonal antibody detecting another epitope of the 45,000 dalton molecule identified by Mc$_3$ has been created. It was named Mc$_8$.

The first use that these anti-breast monoclonal antibodies were put to was to detect breast epithelial cells in paraffin-embedded sections of human tissues routinely studied by the pathologist. Both the immuno-fluorescence and the immunoperoxidase approaches were used; however, the latter was preferred since the preparations obtained are permanent. An array of tissues was stained and depending on the antibody used the breadth of the specificity changes. One phenomenon, however, became very outstanding: whenever breast epithelial cells are stained with these monoclonal antibodies, there is a cell to cell difference in expression of the breast epithelial antigens for both normal and neoplastic cells. Even with contiguous cells one can be positive and the next one negative; however, usually there are quantitative differences between them. This diversity could be attributed to fixation or handling of the tissues. However, ourselves like others (14) found that this heterogeneity exists in every breast epithelial tissue fixed and embedded and even in frozen sections of the same material. In fact, our previous experiments with flow cytofluorimetry clearly demonstrate the wide range of HME-Ags expressions for epithelial cell populations (9). Thus it seems that the heterogeneity of antigen expression can be found in every breast epithelial tissue, both normal and neoplastic, and could be an important factor weighing on every application of polyclonal and especially monoclonal antibodies for diagnostic and even therapeutic purposes.

In diagnostic methodology such as imaging, the variability in antigenic expression could affect the binding of labeled antibody to the tumor mass. If the expression of a given antigen were higher, the monoclonal binding to it would be the monoclonal of choice, or alternatively a "cocktail" of different anti-breast epithelial monoclonal antibodies could be used to adequately cover the antigenic range. In any case, a histopathological study of the primary tumor and, even better, of its metastatic tissue could be useful in choosing the monoclonal to be used in the imaging procedure.

In the field of therapy, this heterogeneity could reflect the partial heterogeneous therapeutic response to be found when giving one monoclonal antibody. With this in mind multiple antibodies could then produce an antibody mixture that would attack every (or almost every) cell in the tumor.

II. ANTIGENIC HETEROGENEITY IN BREAST EPITHELIAL CELLS

This heterogeneity of antigenic expression has been carefully studied by one of us (15); it is a random phenomenon that occurs in cells in tissue culture as well as in vivo. This heterogeneity could be at the basis of tumor progression and acquired refractoriness to cytotoxic drug therapy. To further explore this heterogeneous antigenic expression we have produced clonal colonies of normal breast epithelial cells (16,17), breast epithelial cell lines (16) and neoplastic breast epithelial cells from breast tumors (17) as well as from apparently normal breast epithelial cells surrounding a breast tumor (17). Colonies containing cells totally positive, totally negative and mixed (containing positive and negative cells) can be found (16,17). Using an approach already proposed by one of us (15), the rate at which the heterogeneity is generated could be quantitated and is at the level of 10^{-2}, which is a much higher rate than traditional mutation rates (16,17). This indicates that at any cell division there is a chance in one hundred that an asymmetric pair of daughter cells will be produced (i.e., cells with different levels of antigen expression).

Further, this quantitative approach to heterogeneity led us to determine the rate of phenotypic variability, the rate at which heterogeneity is generated in a given cell population. What we found was that neoplastic breast epithelial cells (be they from solid tumors or from cell lines) have a ten times higher rate of phenotypic variability than normal breast epithelial cells. In addition, and most surprisingly, breast epithelial cells peripheral to a breast tumor have values three to four fold higher than the normal breast epithelial cells (possibly indicating a pre-neoplastic stage). All these results establish for the first time a means of quantitating the rate of progression of a given tumor. Whether the rate of phenotypic variability for a breast tumor has prognostic significance remains to be seen. However, one could hypothesize that breast tumors having a higher rate of phenotypic variability could be those able to more rapidly produce populations of cells refractory to therapy.

III. CIRCULATING LEVELS OF MAMMARY EPITHELIAL ANTIGENS

A. In the Mouse

Since we have already demonstrated that MME antigens are present in normal and neoplastic mouse mammary cells in culture (18), and since cultured cells are known to release cell surface components in vitro, we started by quantitating the MME antigen level of spent media from mouse mammary cell cultures. Positive values for MME antigen are found in the used medium of normal mouse mammary epithelial (MME) cells and neoplastic MME cells (19). The neoplastic mammary cell lines used were 66cl, 68H and 410-39, which carry MME antigens on their cell surface as determined by immunofluorescence (20). Mouse fetal fibroblasts acting as controls are negative. This finding brought confidence to our RIA studies, so we decided to test sera of BALB/c mice grafted with our transplantable mammary tumor cell line 3910-30, derived from retired BALB/c mice not infected exogeneously with mouse mammary tumor virus (MTV); HOG, derived from a transformed transplantable preneoplastic lesion (it was also free of exogeneous MTV); and CfZ#3, derived from an exogeneously MTV-infected BALB/c retired breeder (19). Our control was sera from normal female mice. The values of MME-Ags in the sera obtained in these tumor-bearing mice is elevated. Mice were bled at da 21. These transplantable tumors, which usually kill the mouse in a month, are vascularized at 6 da and at 3 wk they are about 1 1/2 - 2 cm diameter. These results show that, associated with the presence of mammary tumors, components appear in the sera of mice that block the binding of our heterologous antiserum to the normal MME antigens (21). This blocking factor(s) can be considered to be normal MME antigens and not circulating immune complexes. In these studies, we found that ^{125}I-labeled MME antigens added to the same plasma that blocked the above mentioned binding can not be precipitated by 2.5% polyethylene-glycol. However, if anti-MME antisera was then added in excess to this same mixture of ^{125}I-MME antigen and plasma of tumor-bearing mice, an appreciable amount of the ^{125}I-MME antigen can be precipitated by 2.5% polyethyleneglycol (19).

These preliminary results support our hypothesis that normal breast epithelial cell components will be found in circulation in breast cancer patients.

B. In the Nude Mouse Grafted with Human Breast Tumors

The RIA system described above for the quantitation of HME-Ags on breast epithelial cells was used to determine levels of HME-Ags in the circulation of nude mice carrying human breast and non-breast tumors (21). The high values of circulating HME-Ags in nude mice with human breast tumors (38 - 687 ng/ml) decline sharply after tumor removal (38 - 82 ng/ml). The difference between the pre- and the post-operative group is statistically significant at the 1% level, when compared by the paired t-test. The plasma levels found in animals grafted with non-breast tumors do not change significantly. Healthy nude mice have levels (22 - 49 ng/ml) that do not differ statistically from non-breast tumor bearing animals. When the values are pooled, it was calculated that our RIA test has a sensitivity of 66.7% and a specificity of 98.6%. These results show that breast epithelial cell membrane components are released by breast cancer cells into the circulation.

The present RIA for circulating HME-Ags has an advantage over the other presently used RIAs for breast tumor-associated markers (such as CEA), in that our methodology not only detects the presence of a tumor, but it assures us of its mammary origin. That is, our RIA has the advantage of specificity, specificity determined for this RIA to be above the 98% level (max. 100).

Our immunological approach is a continuation of previous work in which researchers had found different types of cellular components (mainly enzymes due to the easiness of assay) in the circulation of cancer patients. Ultimately it has been recognized that these enzymes originate in the tumor and could either result from tumor destruction, or facilitated release, or enhanced peri-tumoral permeability. In nude mice grafted with human breast tumors, simultaneous determinations were made of HME-Ags and sialyltransferase (22). HME-Ags and sialyltransferase are high in nude mice with breast cancer; however, nude mice carrying non-breast cancers (lung, colon, melanoma) have high sialyltransferase but low HME-Ags. Once the nude mice have the tumor removed the HME-Ags levels fall in the mice carrying breast tumors. In contrast, sialyltransferase remains high in all the mice whether they carry breast or non-breast human tumors. Control tumor-free sham-operated mice also have high values of sialyltransferase, possibly as a result of wound healing. The sensitivity and the specificity of the HME-Ags assay is clearly shown by these experiments when it is compared to sialyltransferase (22). These results prove that components of the cell surface of breast tumors are released, as in any other tumor, in circulation (as represented by sialyltransferase) but that HME-Ags are a marker only for the material released by breast tumors, thus proving their specificity (22).

C. In the Human

Once we demonstrated the presence and high levels of HME-Ags in nude mice grafted with human breast tumors we turned our attention to the sera of human breast cancer patients. For this purpose new methodology had to be devised to suit the peculiarities of human serum and the lower levels of HME-Ags found in the patients. Please note that the ratio of tumor to body weight in the mice grafted with human tumors is much greater than that of the patients. Thus the levels of HME-Ags are expected to be, and are, lower. After some search, we developed a solid phase RIA in which an antibody against HME-Ags is bound to a solid phase of Sepharose-4B. The HME-Ags present in the breast cancer patients are then harvested by means of this solid phase. Then, the antigen bound to the beads is recognized by radiolabeled anti-HME (23). Once the background for this preparation is diminished to almost zero value, it is possible to detect in the sera of the breast cancer patients high levels of HME-Ags. The standard curves are reproducible and are sensitive to the level of 3 to 10 nanograms. A further improvement to this methodology has been the biotinization of the second antibody layer (anti-HME) of the sandwich and its further recognition with radioiodinated avidin, in an effort to increase sensitivity without loss of specificity.

With this methodology we were able for the first time to detect HME-Ags in circulation of 75% of breast cancer patients with disseminated disease (p < 0.05%) and 25% of those with primary breast cancer (p < 0.05%). These antigens are not found in the sera of a group of female patients with disseminated non-breast neoplasias used as controls (23). Both male and female normal controls are also negative. Patients with disseminated breast cancer exhibit values well above those of any of the other groups (23). These patients' response to therapy and its evaluation by means of HME-Ags values is an area of active research at present. Further, we are also involved in determining the level of HME-Ags in a longitudinal fashion in as many cancer patients as possible.

The present RIA by its non-competitive nature did not assure us completely on the presence of the antigens that we are looking at in the sample assays. A cross-contaminant of any nature could have been responsible for the positive results. Thus, we were forced to devise methodology to be able to demonstrate that HME-Ags are present in the circulation of breast cancer patients by parallel procedures. The methodology to be devised had to be extremely sensitive, even more so than radioimmunoassay to make us feel confident of later results. Thus, the same immunobeads that are used for the radioimmunoassay are used to fractionate the antigen from the sera of the cancer patient (23). Once the antigens are bound by the immunobeads they are then radioiodinated in situ. It is very likely, that due to the extremely sensitive step introduced by the radiolabeling, almost any antigen bound will be detected. The labeled antigen now bound to the beads is then released and the eluant concentrated. The concentrate is then run in electrophoresis accompanied by standards such as HMFG preparations, molecular weight markers, and immunoglobulin fractions. By this procedure we are able to recover the three components of HME-Ags from the sera of patients with disseminated breast cancer. As we have shown before, the heterologous antibody raised in rabbits against human milk fat globule, that we use in this procedure, after appropriate adsorption, recognizes these same three components (2,8). The sera of non-breast cancer patients, in its disseminated form, as well as the sera of normal controls does not contain any of the components of the human milk fat globule detected in the breast cancer patients.

In support of this finding, we were also able to detect human breast antigens in the sera of breast cancer patients using our recently prepared monoclonal antibodies against components of the HMFG. In experiments similar to those described above, a monoclonal antibody is bound to a solid phase and thus it can retrieve from the sera of breast cancer patients its corresponding antigen (46K; 23). After radioiodination in situ, the antigen is released and run in polyacrylamide gel electrophoresis where a single band of radioactivity corresponding to a molecular weight of 46,000

242

daltons can be noticed (23). The sera of non-breast cancers as well as the controls do not have this component. These results make us feel very confident that we are detecting levels of HME-Ags in the circulation of breast cancer patients. The present methodology can be of use in the follow up of breast cancer patients as well as of value in assessing the immunological status of these patients.

IV. IMAGING

A. Imaging of Mouse Mammary Tumors Implanted in Mice

Mouse mammary tumors grafted in mice were first localized by us with polyclonal anti-mouse mammary epithelial antibody (anti-MME) Fab-fragments (24,25). For this purpose, the IgG fraction of serum immunoglobulins from rabbits immunized with mouse milk fat globule is separated using Sephadex G-200. The IgG fraction is subjected to digestion and the Fab-fragments obtained are radioiodinated and injected into BALB/c mice carrying mouse mammary tumors known to have mouse mammary epithelial antigens on them (18).

In this study ^{131}I-anti MME-Fab is rapidly removed from circulation both by tumor binding and by renal excretion, 98% of the dose is cleared from the blood at 18 hr, thus very clear images of the mammary tumor are seen. Other non-breast tumors (lung, colon, melanoma) cannot be localized (24). After these pioneer studies that established for the first time that mammary tumors can be localized with fragments of anti-mouse milk fat globule polyclonal antibodies we focused our full attention on human breast tumors.

B. Imaging with Anti-HME Polyclonal Antibodies of Human Breast Tumors Implanted in Nude Mice

For our studies we implanted nude mice (with a BALB/c background) with human breast tumors (MX-1 and MX-2), human lung and colon carcinomas and a human melanoma.

To prepare Fab-fragments large amounts of antiserum against human milk fat globule (HMFG) produced in rabbits were assembled. The immunoglobulin fraction was obtained by an ammonium sulfate precipitation and subsequent dialysis. The IgG fraction was separated and then used to prepare the Fab-fragments. The latter were then iodinated, and adsorbed with human red blood cells, human colon carcinoma cells (HT-29), Hela cells and human breast fibrocytes. Throughout these adsorptions, cellular material could have contaminated the radioiodinated Fab material, therefore, they were affinity purified with HMFG on the solid phase before injection.

We first studied the distribution of the radioiodinated Fab-fragments in both nude mice with and without tumors. Good binding to the human breast tumor, far above the level of binding to liver, muscle and brain, is found when the tissues are removed and counted after injection of the non-chromatographed ^{125}I-anti-HME-Fab.

At 48 hr after injection of the labeled Fab fragments we can obtain appropriate imaging and good tumor to background ratios (26). Human breast tumors are clearly imaged with ^{131}I tagged anti-HME-Fab in nude mice, whereas tumors of other origin (lung, colon, melanoma) are not. The resolution and sensitivity obtained are similar to those already reported for the mouse system (24). Similar fast urinary clearance of the unbound ^{131}I-anti-HME fragments is found and the results support our prediction for the usefulness of such procedures in patients. A recent paper also supports our use of Fab-fragments of anti-breast epithelial antibodies in breast tumor imaging (27).

C. Imaging with Anti-Breast Epithelial Monoclonal Antibodies of Human Breast Tumors

An undesirable feature in the preparation of anti-HME and its use in imaging is represented by the adsorption steps required to give it specificity, since many cellular proteins are released into the antiserum. To remedy this we decided to use monoclonal antibodies that we had prepared against cell surface components of human breast epithelial cells. The antibody employed was Mc_5 (12), which is a mouse IgG_1 kappa light chain, and which is directed to a glycoprotein of the cell surface, against which we had already described another monoclonal preparation (10). Thus, monoclonal Mc_5 was radioiodinated and injected into nude mice carrying simulated metastases of human breast tumors and human non-breast tumors (lung, colon and melanoma). In distribution studies breast tumors concentrate ^{131}I-Mc_5 2-3 times above liver at 24-48 hr, other tumors have ratios approaching 1.0 (28). Other monoclonal antibodies (non-breast directed) do not concentrate in the breast tumor. Similar nude mouse preparations were imaged in the high-purity germanium camera (University of California San Francisco, Radiologic Imaging Laboratory) and clear-cut images of the breast tumor are obtained after the injection of ^{131}I-Mc_5, both by visual observation of the screen and film displays and by the quantitative values of the print-outs. Ratios of 2-3 times the contralateral disease-free side are obtained (28). No positive images are obtained with the non-breast tumors. These successful experiments using our intact monoclonal antibodies warrant the possible use of Mc_5 in clinical studies in the near future. With another monoclonal antibody that we had created (10,12) and that recognizes the same antigen as Mc_5, other researchers appear to have localized with moderate success breast tumors in patients (29). In the same vein, this time labeling with ^{111}In, another monoclonal antibody directed against the antigen of Mc_5 was used for imaging studies on breast cancer patients (30). Good images are obtained in bony metastasis but not in soft tissue. This discrepancy plus the local altered vascular conditions at the site of the bony metastases make these results quite uncertain as of yet.

In an attempt to use monoclonal antibody fragments to image breast tumors and test their specificity a new approach was developed since the nude mouse grafted with a breast tumor does not entirely satisfy criteria for specificity of a given monoclonal in the human subject. For this purpose 100 ml of serum free medium of Mc_5 hybridomas was lyophilized. This material was then redissolved, digested with mercuri-papain and chromatographed on a DEAE-cellulose column. In acrylamide electrophoresis the main fraction is a 55,000 dalton component, estimated to be Fab-fragments (25).

The Fab fragments were then concentrated and iodinated by the chloramine-T procedure, at less than one molecule of iodine per molecule of Fab-fragment. Nude mice carrying human breast tumors and human non-breast tumors were then injected with ^{125}I-Fab fragments. After 24 hr the animals were sacrificed and the kidneys, livers, spleen, brain, lung, muscle, blood and the tumor itself were collected. The radioactivity present in each of these tissues was recorded and then expressed as cpm/gm of tissue. Finally, the percentage of the total dose per gram of tumor tissue was calculated (Table 1). In nude mice implanted with different human tumors the antibody concentrated in the breast tumors 5 times above other human tumors of non-breast origin. This is the most valid comparison to establish specificity because it is human breast tissue against other human tissues. If enough human tissues are compared the composite picture will approximate what we would find in a human subject. When the breast tumor in similar distribution studies is compared to any of the nude mouse tissues the comparison is less valid since the possibility of cross reactivity is much smaller and clearly it is not the same as the situation in an imaging procedure in a human subject. We advocate this procedure for the testing of the distribution of monoclonal antibodies or their fragments in the nude mouse system when breast specificity is sought.

Table 1. Percent of Total Injected Dose of ^{125}I-Mc$_5$-Fab per gm of Human Tumor Implanted in Nude Mice.

	Tumor	Dose
MX-1	Human Breast Carcinoma	0.77%
CX-1	Human Colon Carcinoma	0.14%
LX-1	Human Lung Carcinoma	0.12%
DAN-G	Human Pancreatic Carcinoma	0.11%
MRI-H166	Human Renal Carcinoma	0.008%

245

In the search for stronger and clearer images and better tumor to background ratio two approaches were explored. One was the use of mixtures or "cocktails" of monoclonal antibodies instead of single monoclonal antibodies to enhance the amount of tracer targeted to the tumor. The other was to explore the choice between the use of intact immunoglobulin or the use of its fragments in imaging.

To explore the first of these issues, a monoclonal antibody "cocktail" was compounded with four of our monoclonal antibodies: BLMRL-HMFG-Mc$_1$, -Mc$_3$, -Mc$_5$ and -Mc$_8$. The IgG fraction from ascites fluid was obtained by Sephadex G-200 chromatography, titered and the different monoclonal antibodies mixed, radioiodinated and injected into nude mice carrying human breast tumors. After 24 hr the mice were sacrificed and samples of tumors and different tissues weighed and counted for radioactivity and the bound tracer expressed in percentage of the tracer dose injected per gram of tissue (Table 2). When the % dose of ^{125}I-Mc$_5$ incorporated per gram of breast tumor was compared to the similar incorporation by the monoclonal "cocktail," the former was two-fold lower. In contrast, background levels remained quite similar, proving the advantage of the monoclonal "cocktail" over a single monoclonal antibody.

Table 2.

Percent Total Injected Dose of ^{125}I-Cocktail (Mc$_1$, Mc$_3$, Mc$_5$, Mc$_8$) IgG per gm of Human Tumor Implanted in Nude Mice		
	Tumor	% Dose
MX-1	Human Breast Carcinoma	5.43%
CX-1	Human Colon Carcinoma	0.12%

Percent Total Injected Dose of ^{125}I-Normal Mouse Serum IgG per gm of Human Tumor Implanted in Nude Mice		
	Tumor	% Dose
MX-1	Human Breast Carcinoma	0.53%
CX-1	Human Colon Carcinoma	0.78%

Percent Total Injected Dose of ^{125}I-Mc$_5$ per gm of Human Tumor Implanted in Nude Mice		
	Tumor	% Dose
MX-1	Human Breast Carcinoma	3.70%
CX-1	Human Colon Carcinoma	1.25%

To analyze the second issue above, i.e., whether fragments are better than intact immunoglobulin, fragments of monoclonal antibody Mc$_5$ were obtained. First Fab fragments were prepared and then F(ab)'$_2$ as described elsewhere (31). Samples of the intact immunoglobulin and the fragments were then iodinated by the chloramine-T method, at less than one molecule of ^{125}I per molecule of IgG a,nd injected into nude mice carrying human breast tumors. Comparable values were obtained for the intact IgG and for its F(ab)'$_2$ preparation for binding to the human breast tumor (Table 3). However, the liver background was lower for the F(ab)'$_2$ fragment. In contrast, a much smaller uptake of the radioiodinated Fab fragments of the Mc$_5$ by the tumor was found. Also, these Fab fragments, as has already been shown by us (25), accumulated in the kidneys.

Table 3.   Distribution of the Labeled Monoclonal Antibody Mc$_5$ and its Fragments in Nude Mice Carrying MX-1 Human Mammary Tumor.

Tissue	Intact Antibody	F(ab)'$_2$	Fab
Tumor	3.70*	3.995	0.499
Spleen	0.878	0	0.812
Kidney	0	0	1.053
Liver	2.32	0.489	1.772
Muscle	1.86	0.773	0.079
Brain	0	0.343	0.119

*% of injected dose per gm of tissue.

As a result of this study, it became apparent that the Fab preparation was inferior in terms of uptake by the breast or for imaging when compared to the intact IgG and its F(ab)'$_2$ fragments. The latter two when compared to each other did not differ much in terms of their accumulation in the tumor; however, the F(ab)'$_2$ preparation showed lower liver binding which can be of value. From a practical point of view, however, if low liver uptake is not imperative, the choice of the intact immunoglobulin seems warranted. The extensive handling required for the preparation of the fragment decreases yield and increases the risk of introducing pyrogenicity in the preparation.

V. IMMUNOTHERAPY WITH ANTI-BREAST MONOCLONAL ANTIBODIES

Presently, approaches are being developed for immunotherapy with monoclonal antibodies. These antibodies will directly attach to tumor cells or they will be the vectors of toxins or radiotherapeutic agents to the tumor mass. In either case, monoclonal antibodies will be the choice due to their defined and permanent specificity and the unlimited amounts which can be produced.

We have demonstrated the ability of monoclonal antibodies to breast epithelium to bind to breast tumors (12) and breast epithelial cells. This binding is not without consequences since the supplementation of culture medium used to grow MDA-MB-157 cells with monoclonal antibody Mc_5 plus rabbit complement significantly arrested the growth of these cells in 72 hr (Table 4).

Table 4. Effect of Mc_5 on MDA-MD-157 Cell Line Protein Synthesis[*].

Supernatant Added	mg/Protein per Dish
None	77.7 ± 2.4[†]
X63A medium (13%)	81.7 ± 1.2
MC-5 medium (13%)	40.9 ± 13.0

[*]Thirteen parts of supernatants from cultures producing Mc_5 grown in RMPI + 10% Newborn Calf Serum (NCS) were added to 87 parts Waymouth's + 10% FBS. As controls, an equivalent amount of RPMI + 10% NCS or supernatant from X63A myeloma grown in RPMI + 10% NCS was added from the start of culture. Cells were cultured in 30 mm diameter culture dishes for 72 hr.

[†]$\bar{x} \pm$ SEM.

These encouraging results prompted our use of monoclonal antibodies to treat human breast tumors implanted in nude mice. In early experiments (32), we showed that each of four monoclonal antibodies tested has tumor growth arresting capabilities; however, their injection as a mixture or "cocktail" was even stronger (Figure 1). Injections were started at the moment of grafting the breast tumor in the nude mouse and continued every other day. At 8 wk the untreated breast tumors killed most of their hosts, while the hosts for the treated tumors were still alive, and remained alive for a good number of weeks afterwards. The size of the human breast tumors implanted in nude mice and treated with the monoclonal "cocktail" at the end of 8 wk was 10% of that of similar tumors in untreated host mice that

248

were still alive at 8 wk (Figure 1). Each one of the monoclonal antibodies injected by itself had effects ranging from 40% to 70% of that of the "cocktail" of four antibodies.

Nude mice carrying breast tumors were also injected with ascites of the X63A parent myeloma line with no effect on the tumor growth, which was similar to that of the untreated group. The size and growth of other human tumors (colon, lung) also implanted in nude mice and treated with the "cocktail" did not differ from their non-treated controls (Figure 2). These mice implanted with non-breast tumors were mostly deceased by 8 wk as a result of the large tumor mass they harboured. Other investigators have also demonstrated the ability of monoclonal antibodies against breast epithelial cells to arrest the short term growth of tumors implanted in nude mice. They also claim a complement dependent cell cytotoxicity for their system (33).

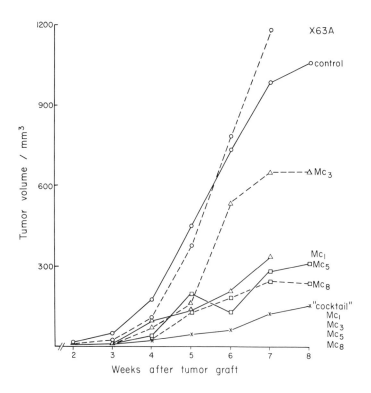

FIGURE 1. Comparison of Treatment of Human Breast Tumor MX-1 Grafted in Nude Mice with Different Monoclonal Antibodies Injected i.p. Singly and in "Cocktail" Form, and with X63A Myeloma Parent Cell Line Control Ascites. Injections were started the day of tumor grafting and continued every other day for 8 wk. Three mice per experimental group.

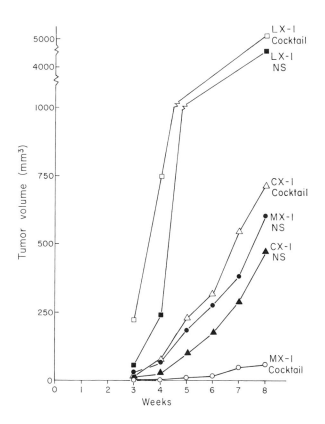

FIGURE 2. Effect of the Monoclonal Antibody "Cocktail" or Normal Mouse Serum on Human Breast (MX-1), Lung (LX-1) and Colon (CX-1) Carcinomas. Conditions as in Figure 1.

In view of the success obtained in arresting tumor growth with our monoclonal antibodies, a new model, testing a definitive pathophysiological situation, metastatic spread and early nidation of neoplastic micro-emboli, was used. Passive immunization was created in the nude mice by injection of the monoclonal "cocktail" before the implantation of the tumor. For this purpose, the mice were injected with a dose of the "cocktail" of monoclonals the day before grafting the breast and control tumors. By taking this approach, in three different experiments, it was found that in one of the experiments the "cocktail" injection managed to totally impair the implantation of the simulated metastases and further growth of the breast tumors and in two of the experiments the monoclonal "cocktail" reduced the tumor growth at 8 wk by 93%. The results of these last 3 experiments are shown in Figure 3. In addition, incomplete mixtures, such as monoclonals Mc_5 plus Mc_8, were less potent than the monoclonal "cocktail."

In other experiments different doses of monoclonal antibody "cocktail" were injected. Injections were given of 100, 200 and 400 μl of the "cocktail" of monoclonal antibodies represented by an equal mixture of ascites fluids of the different hybridomas. The weakest dose produced only a 40% reduction in tumor growth, while both higher doses obtained a maximal effect. The 200 μl dose inhibited 90% and the 400 μl dose 80%.

Note that depending on the experiment the "cocktail" totally inhibited the growth of 30 to 50% of the breast tumors implanted in nude mice. The remaining breast tumor-implanted mice treated with the monoclonal "cocktail" carried human breast tumors which were 9 to 10 times smaller than the non-treated or normal serum treated controls. These surviving tumors, after the injections were stopped, continued to grow at a faster pace than under the monoclonal "cocktail" treatment. The question then was: what is antigenically the make-up of the cell population of those tumors that survived the monoclonal "cocktail" treatment? To answer this, the tumors were excised 4 da after termination of the monoclonal "cocktail" treatment, fixed, embedded in paraffin, sectioned and stained by immuno-peroxidase using the monoclonal "cocktail" as the identifying antibody(ies). A surprising situation was found. The sections corresponding to the control tumors (human breast tumors implanted in nude mice treated for 8 wk with normal serum and the same tumors before any treatment) bound the monoclonal "cocktail" strongly producing very deeply stained cell populations. In contrast, those tumors that survived monoclonal "cocktail" treatment had very low monoclonal "cocktail" binding. These experiments demonstrate a cell population selection due to monoclonal antibody treatment in those tumors refractory to treatment (Table 5).

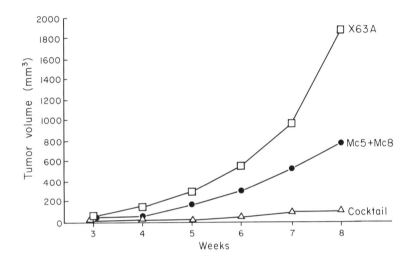

FIGURE 3. Effect of Passive Immunization on the Growth of Human Breast Tumor MX-1 in Nude Mice. For this purpose, nude mice were injected i.p. the day before tumor grafting and for 8 wk every other day with monoclonal antibody cocktail or X63A myeloma parent cell line control ascites. Nine mice per experimental group.

Table 5. MSA Determination of Anti-Breast Monoclonal Antibody Binding to MX-1 Human Breast Tumor Implanted in Nude Mice and Treated with Anti-Breast Monoclonal Antibody "Cocktail" for 8 wk.

Treatment to tumor bearing mouse	Reagent used in staining	MSA relative values
None	Monoclonal cocktail	0.91 ± 0.05*
Monoclonal cocktail	Monoclonal cocktail	0.17 ± 0.02
None	X-63A (control)	0.09 ± 0.02
Monoclonal cocktail	X-63A (control)	0.09 ± 0.00

*$\bar{x} \pm$ SEM

In summary, we have clearly demonstrated the ability of monoclonal antibodies against normal breast epithelium to arrest or inhibit human breast tumor growth in nude mice by direct injection into the host. The use of a mixture of antibodies, up to four of them, seems to be most effective as compared to any of the monoclonal antibodies alone or incomplete monoclonal "cocktails." An animal model simulating metastatic dissemination proved the effectiveness of passive immunization with monoclonal antibodies in arresting implantation of a considerable number of simulated metastases as well as significantly slowing the growth of all of those that developed. An important percentage of tumors that survived initial monoclonal "cocktail" treatment continued slow growth under continued monoclonal "cocktail" injections. The examination of the cell population refractory to this treatment showed that it was composed of cells showing very low expression of the antigens detected by the monoclonal "cocktail." Thus, the use of such "cocktails" seems warranted over the use of one single monoclonal antibody. Possibly the inclusion of an even larger number of monoclonal antibodies or the use of adjuvant therapy could make their effectiveness complete.

VI. CONCLUSION

If the HME-Ags and the antigens corresponding to the monoclonal antibodies we have developed against HMFG are useful in identifying breast epithelial tissue we have conceived an integral diagnostic and possible therapeutic approach to breast cancer using these immunoreagents (Figure 4). Briefly, the clinical identification of a breast tumor leads usually to a biopsy of the mass. At this time a serum sample will be

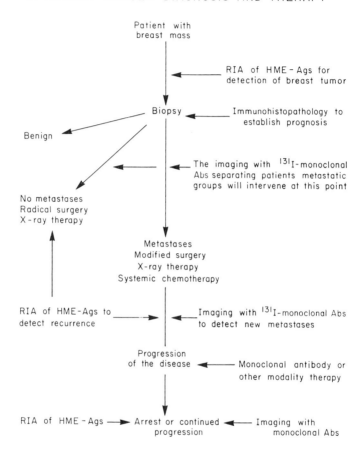

HUMAN MAMMARY EPITHELIAL ANTIGENS (HME-Ags)
IN BREAST CANCER DIAGNOSIS AND THERAPY

FIGURE 4. Scheme for Integral Diagnosis and Possible Therapy with Anti-Breast Epithelial Cell Antibodies.

obtained and the presence of considerable levels of HME-Ags will indicate the presence of a breast tumor and could possibly give an idea regarding its total mass. Once the biopsy is obtained an appropriate histopathological study using the different monoclonal antibodies that bind to breast tissue will be conducted and the differential expression of the antigens detected could provide an interpretation useful in establishing a prognosis. Then, before surgery, imaging with labeled anti-breast antibodies or their fragments could help rule out metastatic spread.

After tumor excision or the start of therapy the follow-up of the breast tumor can be accomplished in two ways using immunoreagents: i) serum levels of HME-Ags and ii) imaging of the tumor metastasis with labeled anti-breast epithelial antibodies or their fragments. Serum levels of HME-Ags will allow for a non-invasive and inexpensive follow-up of the breast cancer patient. Blood samples taken sequentially will monitor relapse and indicate success of therapy. In the case where a relapse is suspected by elevated serum values of HME-Ags, imaging studies could be requested to identify site of metastatic spread and perhaps tumor mass. A possible quantitative approach to monoclonal antibody imaging would be the quantitation of binding of the monoclonals to paraffin embedded sections of the original tumor and preferably its metastases. This approach could help choose the appropriate anti-breast monoclonal antibodies from a panel to compose an appropriate monoclonal "cocktail" to be labeled and injected into the patient for the imaging procedures.

If by the previous approach a metastatic dissemination is detected then therapy could be attempted, this time again choosing from a panel of anti-breast monoclonal antibodies after histopathological testing. This therapy with monoclonal antibodies will be direct or aided by cytotoxic or radioactive particle emitting conjugates. Again, the follow-up of the immune therapy could be performed by means of the circulating levels of the antigens and imaging with the labeled immunoreagents.

ACKNOWLEDGMENT

This investigation was supported by grants CA20286, CA26790 and CA34630 awarded by the National Cancer Institute, Department of Health and Human Services.

REFERENCES

1.   Springer G: Triple role of T and Tn antigens in cancer: as universal clonal carcinoma markers, in cancer cell adhesion, and as autoimmunogens. Surv. Synth. Pathol. Res. 2:141-164, 1983.
2.   Ceriani RL, Thompson KE, Peterson JA, Abraham S: Surface differentiation antigens of human epithelial cells carried on the human milk fat globule. Proc. Natl. Acad. Sci. USA 74:582-586, 1977.
3.   Ceriani RL, Peterson JA: Characterization of differentiation antigens of the mouse mammary epithelial cell (MME antigens) carried on the mouse milk fat globule. Cell Differentiation 7:355-366, 1978.

4. Ceriani RL, Taylor-Papadimitriou J, Peterson JA, Brown P: Characterization of cells cultured from early lactation milks. In Vitro 15:356-362, 1979.

5. Peterson JA, Buehring G, Taylor-Papadimitriou J, Ceriani RL: Expression of human mammary epithelial (HME) antigens in primary cultures of normal and abnormal breast tissue. Int. J. Cancer 22:570-575, 1978.

6. Sebesteny A, Taylor-Papadimitriou J, Ceriani RL, Millis R, Schmitt C, Trevan D: Primary human breast carcinomas transplantable in the nude mouse. J. Natl. Cancer Inst. 63:1331-1337, 1979.

7. Ceriani RL, Sasaki M, Peterson JA, Blank EW: Mammary epithelial cell identification by means of cell surface antigens. IN: McGrath C, Brennan MJ and Rich MA (eds.) Cell Biology of Breast Cancer. Academic Press, New York, pp. 33-56, 1980.

8. Sasaki M, Peterson JA, Ceriani RL: Quantitation of human mammary epithelial (HME) antigens in cells cultured from normal and cancerous breast tissues. In Vitro 17:150-158, 1981.

9. Peterson JA, Bartholomew JC, Stampfer M, Ceriani RL: Analysis of expression of human mammary epithelial (HME) antigens in breast cancer as measured by flow cytofluorimetry. Exp. Cell Biol. 49:1-14, 1981.

10. Taylor-Papadimitriou J, Peterson JA, Arklie J, Burchell J, Ceriani RL, Bodmer WF: Monoclonal antibodies to epithelial-specific components of the human milk fat globule membranes: Production and reaction with cells in culture. Int. J. Cancer 28:17-21, 1981.

11. Arkley J, Taylor-Papadimitriou J, Bodmer WF, Egan M, Millis R: Differentiation antigens expressed by epithelial cells in the lactating breast are also detectable in breast cancer. Int. J. Cancer 28:23-29, 1981.

12. Ceriani RL, Peterson JA, Lee JY, Moncada R, Blank EW: Preparation and characterization of monoclonal antibodies to normal human breast epithelial cells. Somatic Cell Genetics 9:415-427, 1983.

13. Burchell J, Durbin H, Taylor-Papadimitriou J: Complexity of expression of antigenic determinants recognized by monoclonal antibodies HMFG-1 and HMFG-2 in normal and malignant human mammary epithelial cells. J. Immunol. 131:508-513, 1983.

14. Colcher D, Hand H, Nuti P, Schlom J: A spectrum of monoclonal antibodies reactive with human mammary tumor cells. Proc. Natl. Acad. Sci. USA 78:3199-3203, 1981.

15. Peterson JA: Analysis of variability in albumin content of sister hepatoma cells and a model for geometric phenotypic variability ("Quantitative shift model"). Somatic Cell Mol. Genet. 10:345-357, 1984.

16. Peterson JA, Ceriani RL, Blank EW, Osvaldo L: Comparison of rates of phenotypic variability in surface antigens expression in normal and cancerous human breast epithelial cells. Cancer Res. 43:4291-4296, 1983.

17. Ceriani RL, Peterson JA, Blank EW: Variability in surface antigen expression of human breast epithelial cells cultured from normal breast, normal tissue peripheral to breast carcinomas, and breast carcinomas. Cancer Res. (In press).

256

18. Ceriani RL, Peterson JA, Abraham S: Immunologic methods for the identification of cell types. II. Expression of normal mouse mammary epithelial (MME) cell antigens in mammary neoplasia. J. Natl. Cancer Inst. 61:747-751, 1978.
19. Ceriani RL, Peterson JA, Blank E, Miller S: Use of mammary epithelial antigens as markers in mammary neoplasia. IN: Boelsma E and Rumke PH (eds.) Tumor Markers: Impact and Prospects. Elsevier/North-Holland Biomedical Press, Amsterdam, pp. 101-116, 1979.
20. Hager JC, Russo J, Ceriani RL, Peterson JA, Fligiel S, Jolly G, Heppner G: Epithelial characteristics of five subpopulations of a heterogeneous strain BALB/cfC3H mouse mammary tumor. Cancer Res. 41:1720-1730, 1981.
21. Sasaki M, Peterson JA, Wara W, Ceriani RL: Human mammary epithelial antigens (HME-Ags) in the circulation of nude mice implanted with breast and non-breast tumors. Cancer 48:2204-2210, 1981.
22. Sasaki M, Barber S, Ceriani RL: Breast cancer markers: Comparison between sialyltransferase and human mammary epithelial antigens (HME-Ags) for the detection of human breast tumors grafted in nude mice. Breast Cancer Res. Treat. (In press).
23. Ceriani RL, Sasaki M, Sussman H, Wara WE, Blank EW: Circulating human mammary epithelial antigens (HME-Ags) in breast cancer. Proc. Natl. Acad. Sci. USA 79:5420-5424, 1982.
24. Wilbanks T, Peterson JA, Miller S, Kaufman L, Ortendahl D, Ceriani RL: Localization of mammary tumors in vivo with ^{131}I labeled Fab fragments of antibodies against mouse mammary epithelial (MME) cells. Cancer 48:1768-1775, 1981.
25. Wilbanks T, Peterson JA, Miller S, Kaufman L, Ortendahl K, Ceriani RL: Imaging of mammary tumors with cell-type specific antibodies by a high purity germanium camera. IN: Burchiel S and Rhodes B (eds.) Tumor Imaging. Masson Publishing Co., New York, pp. 215-266, 1982.
26. Ceriani RL, Ortendahl D, Sasaki M, Kaufman L, Miller S, Wara W, Peterson JA: Use of mammary epithelial antigens (HME-Ags) in breast cancer diagnosis. IN: Nieburgs HE (ed.) Cancer Detection and Prevention: 1981, Volume 4, Marcel Dekker, Inc., New York, pp. 603-609, 1981.
27. Colcher D, Zalutsky M, Kaplan W, Kufe D, Austin F, Schlom J: Radiolocalization of human mammary tumors in athymic mice by 4 monoclonal antibodies. Cancer Res. 43:736-742, 1983.
28. Sasaki M, Ortendahl D, Kaufman L, Ceriani RL: Localization of human breast tumors grafted in nude mice with a monoclonal antibody directed against a defined cell surface antigen of human mammary epithelial cells. (Submitted).
29. Epenetos AH, Mather S, Granowska M, Taylor-Papadimitriou J, Bodmer WF: Targeting of iodine-123-labelled tumor-associated monoclonal antibodies to ovarian, breast and gastrointestinal tumors. Lancet 2:99-1006, 1982.
30. Rainsbury RM, Westwood JH, Coombes RC, Neville AM: Location of metastatic breast carcinoma by a monoclonal antibody chelate labelled with indium-111. Lancet 2:934-938, 1983.
31. Stanworth DR, Turner MW: Immunochemical analysis of immunoglobulins and their subunits. IN: Weir DM (ed.) Immunochemistry. Blackwell Scientific Publications, England, pp. 6.1-6.102, 1978.

32. Ceriani RL, Blank EW: Breast tumor growth inhibition by monoclonal antibodies against breast epithelial cell surface antigens. Hybridoma 3:86, 1984.

33. Capone PM, Papsidero LD, Crogham GA, Chu TM: Experimental tumoricidal effects of monoclonal antibody against solid tumors. Proc. Natl. Acad. Sci. USA 80:7328-7332, 1983.

CHAPTER 17. CHEMOTAXIS IN TUMOR CELLS: POSSIBLE MECHANISMS AND THEIR IMPLICATIONS FOR THERAPY

JAMES VARANI AND J. PHILIP MCCOY, JR.

I. INTRODUCTION

Studies carried out in several laboratories over the past 15 yr have clearly established that several types of non-leukocytic cells - both normal and malignant - are capable of responding to chemotactic factors. Chemotaxis is no longer thought to be limited to cells of leukocytic origin although leukocytes are clearly among the most responsive cells and are the most thoroughly investigated of the higher eukaryotic cells. The observation that several different types of tumor cells are capable of chemotactic responses goes back to the early 1970's. Studies published by Hayashi and his associates showed that extracts of solid tumors contain substances which specifically attract tumor cells (1-3). Following these studies, work in our laboratory showed that a fragment of the fifth component of complement (C5) is chemotactic for tumor cells (4). What made this of interest is that the C5-derived factor with tumor cell chemotactic activity is biochemically and immunochemically similar to the C5 (i.e., C5a) leukocyte chemotactic factor (5-7). This suggested that there might be similarities between leukocytes and tumor cells in their responses to chemotactic factors. We postulated that tumor cell trafficking during metastasis is influenced by chemotactic factors in much the same way as is leukocyte trafficking during response to inflammatory stimuli. This would not be too surprising because, in general terms at least, tumor cell movement during hematogenous spread and leukocyte movement in response to inflammatory conditions have several analogous features. The analogies are depicted in Table 1.

Following these initial observations, a number of factors were identified which have chemotactic activity for tumor cells. Among these are small molecular weight factors such as the N-formylated peptides and the biologically active phorbol esters (8-10) and a number of large molecular weight components of the extracellular matrix such as collagen, fibronectin and laminin (11-13) as well as an uncharacterized factor obtained from bone tissue during metabolic osteolysis (14,15). Along with these findings, several studies have begun to focus on the mechanism by which tumor cells respond to stimulation with these factors. As suggested above, our original finding with the C5-derived tumor cell chemotactic factor suggested similarities between leukocyte chemotaxis and chemotaxis in tumor cells. Obviously, the identification of a large and heterogenous group of factors with tumor cell chemotactic activity puts this simple concept in doubt. There may well be several mechanisms regulating the

260

directed movement of these cells. In tumor cells the response to small
molecular weight peptides may be similar to that of the more well-
studied leukocytes whereas the response to large molecular weight
glycoproteins such as laminin and fibronectin may be different.
Obviously, attempts to interfere with the response of the tumor cells
to chemotactic factors will depend on our understanding of the basic
cellular and molecular mechanisms involved. In this review, we will
summarize briefly what is known about the chemotactic mechanism (to the
small molecular weight chemotactic factors) in tumor cells. We will
then speculate on how an understanding of this mechanism may lead to
approaches for interfering with it.

Table 1. Similarities in Cell Traffic of Tumor Cells and Leukocytes.

Separation of tumor cells from the primary tumor	Release of leukocytes from the bone marrow
↓	↓
Entry of tumor cells into the circulation	Entry of leukocytes into the circulation
↓	↓
Dissemination	Dissemination
↓	↓
Exit of surviving cells from the circulation	Exit of surviving cells from the circulation
↓	↓
Invasion into the extravascular space	Localization of the leukocytes in the extravascular space
↓	↓
Proliferation of tumor cells	Local persistence, cell death or return to the circulation

---

II. TUMOR CELL RESPONSES TO PEPTIDE CHEMOTACTIC FACTORS AND TO PHORBOL
     ESTERS

A. The Leukocyte Model

Several small molecular weight substances such as the complement-
derived peptides, the N-formylated peptides and the phorbol esters are
chemotactic for several types of cells including both leukocytes and
non-leukocytic cells. The cellular and molecular basis of the leukocyte
response to these factors has been the subject of intense investigation
for several years; recent reviews on this topic are available (16,17).
The response to these agents follows the initial binding of the active
factor to high-affinity cell surface receptors. Receptors for both the
C5a and N-formylated peptide chemotactic factors have been identified
on leukocytes from various species (18-20). Phorbol ester receptors
have also been identified on cells of leukocytic origin (21,22).
Following the initial interaction between the receptors and the active
ligands, the cells undergo a very rapid membrane depolarization (16).
This is accompanied by an activation of membrane phospholipid
metabolism, alterations in calcium ion flux and changes in cyclic
nucleotide levels (16,17). How these metabolic events are brought
about and how they relate to the chemotactic response are not fully
understood. It is known, however, that the activation of phospholipid
metabolism results in the release of arachidonic acid and that the
released arachidonic acid can be metabolized to a variety of
lipoxygenase and cyclooxygenase products (23,24). Many of these
products, especially those of the lipoxygenase pathway such as
5-hydroxyeicosatetraenoic acid (5-HETE) and 5,12-dihydroxyeicosa-
tetraenoic acid (leukotriene B_4), are known to be potent chemotactic
factors (25,26). It is thought that these agents are essential
intermediates in the leukocyte chemotactic response. How the various
metabolic events which occur in the cells upon stimulation relate to
one another is not known with certainty. However, it is likely that
they are related (27).

Accompanying these metabolic events there is a rapid alteration in
cytoskeletal structure and a change in cell shape. Within 30 sec of
exposure to the chemotactic factors, leukocytes start to become
polarized (16), developing a broad lamellipodium at the front of the
cell (relative to the source of the chemotactic factor) and a long,
trailing uropodium. Bundles of microfilaments can be seen to form
immediately below the surface and are most prevalent in the
lamellipodium (28). Studies in our laboratory and others have shown
that the changes in cytoskeletal structure are associated with
molecular changes in the cytoskeletal proteins. Specifically, it has
been shown that the monomeric actin within the cell rapidly undergoes
polymerization upon stimulation (29,30). The triggering mechanism for
the polymerization of the actin in the chemotactic-stimulated cells is
not known. However, the relative amounts of actin in the monomeric and
polymeric form are a function of the environmental conditions and vary
in response to ionic changes in the internal environment (31). This

suggests, therefore, possible relationships between the metabolic events and the structural changes that occur rapidly during stimulation of leukocytes with chemotactic factors.

Finally, these changes in leukocyte physiology lead to the functional responses that result from chemotactic stimulation. In addition to the stimulation of directed motility (chemotaxis), activated cells also demonstrate an increase in random motility, cell to cell and cell to substrate adherence, release of lysosomal enzymes and the production of reactive oxygen metabolites (32,33). These functional responses are necessary for the localization of leukocytes at sites of inflammation and no doubt also contribute to the expression of the bactericidal (and tissue destructive) activities at these sites.

B. Chemotactic Mechanisms in Non-Leukocytic Cells

The mechanisms of chemotaxis in tumor cells, and in non-leukocytic cells in general, have not been investigated as extensively as in leukocytes. However, this is beginning to change as more and more work with these cells is undertaken. Studies in our laboratory have focused on the response of tumor cells to the small molecular weight factors which are identical to or similar to the factors which have chemotactic activity for leukocytes. Specifically, these include the C5-derived tumor cell chemotactic factor (which is similar to, and derived from, C5a), the synthetic N-formyl peptide, N-formyl-methionyl-leucyl-phenylalanine (FMLP) and the biologically-active phorbol ester, 12-O-tetradecanoyl phorbol acetate (TPA). These agents all stimulate motility and adhesiveness in the Walker 256 carcinosarcoma cells and in certain other established tumor cell lines (4-8,10,34).

We have begun to characterize the cellular response to these agents. Our studies have, for the most part, been carried out using Walker 256 carcinosarcoma cells as the target cells and the adherence response as the indicator of biological activity. Our findings thus far are summarized in the following paragraphs. The adherence response to all three agents is rapid and transient (35,36). With TPA and FMLP at least, the response appears to follow binding of the active ligands to high affinity receptors on the cells (37 and unpublished). At present, there is no evidence for receptors for the C5-derived chemotactic factor on the Walker cells. This is due to the fact that insufficient quantities of the tumor cell chemotactic peptide from C5 have not been available in a radiolabeled, biologically-active form which would allow receptor characterization. Hopefully, this will change once the reagent becomes available. The stimulated cells attach to a variety of substrates including dishes coated with collagen or with intact endothelial cells (36). In Figure 1 is shown the sequence of morphological changes seen in the Walker 256 carcinosarcoma cells upon exposure to TPA. The adherence response is followed rapidly by cell spreading. Maximum attachment and spreading occur within 45 min; following that, the cells gradually round up and detach. After they have been stimulated and responded, they undergo a period of 48-72 hr during which they are refractory to restimulation. If the cells are

stimulated and then maintained in suspension so that they cannot
attach, after 30 min to two hours they no longer respond. They still
undergo a period of non-responsiveness just as if they had been allowed
to attach (38).

The stimulated adherence response appears to be an energy-
dependent process since it is temperature-dependent and can be
completely inhibited by sodium azide, iodoacetate and 2-deoxyglucose.
An intact cytoskeleton is also important as the response is blocked by
both colchicine and cytochalasin B. On the other hand, stimulated
adherence does not appear to require protein synthesis since it is
unaffected by high concentrations of cycloheximide (10,36). In these
respects, the tumor cell response is analogous to the leukocyte
response.

The cellular response to the small peptide factors and phorbol
esters requires the presence of both Ca^{2+} and Mg^{2+}. In the absence of
either, the cells cannot respond optimally to the chemotactic factors.
Basal adherence requires only a source of divalent cation (either Ca^{2+}
or Mg^{2+}) with perhaps a trace of the other cation (38). When cells
which have been preequilibrated with $^{45}Ca^{2+}$ are stimulated with FMLP,
there is a rapid influx of $^{45}Ca^{2+}$ into the cells. Inhibitors which
block the biological response to chemotactic factors prevent the influx
of the $^{45}Ca^{2+}$ into the cells. These agents also prevent $^{45}Ca^{2+}$ uptake
by unstimulated cells so the effect may not be specific (38). In these
respects, the Walker cells are quite similar to leukocytes. However,
there is at least one difference. In leukocytes TPA stimulation
proceeds in the absence of extracellular Ca^{2+} (39) - possibly because
TPA can release sufficient quantities of Ca^{2+} from internal stores. In
the tumor cells, both extracellular Ca^{2+} and Mg^{2+} are necessary for
optimal response.

Is phospholipid and arachidonic acid metabolism important in the
tumor cell chemotactic response? Indirect evidence suggests that it is
since inhibitors which block the release of arachidonic acid from
phospholipids, or which prevent arachidonic acid metabolism via the
lipoxygenase pathway, prevent the Walker cells from responding to the
chemotactic factors (10,36). In contrast, inhibitors such as
indomethacin, which block cyclooxygenase metabolism, potentiate the
response (10). While these inhibitor studies do not prove the
involvement of phospholipid and arachidonic acid metabolism in tumor
cell chemotaxis, they are compatible with this idea. It has also been
shown that the Walker cells are capable of synthesizing lipoxygenase

A   B

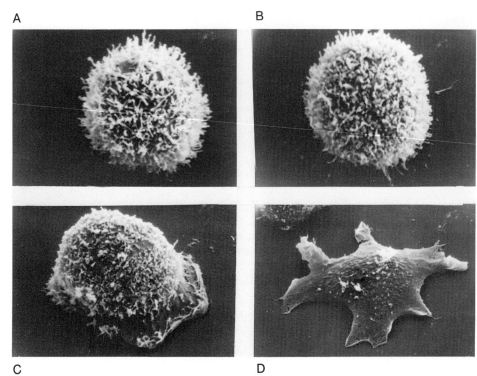

C   D

FIGURE 1.   Adherence and Spreading in Stimulated Walker 256 Carcinosarcoma Cells.   A) Cells in suspension are round and covered with short
microvilli. B) Cells initially adhere to the substratum through long,
slender filopodia. C) Some of the cells begin to undergo spreading. D)
Within 15-30 min, the cells have completely spread on the substratum.

metabolites and that at least one metabolite of the lipoxygenase
pathway (i.e., leukotriene B_4) can duplicate the adherence stimulating
effects of the peptide chemotactic factors (40).   Leukotriene B_4 has
also been shown by Mensing and Czarnetski (41) to stimulate chemotactic
motility in normal fibroblasts.   Though far from complete, these data
suggest that in non-leukocytic cells, as in leukocytes, an
important - though as yet not well-defined - role for arachidonic acid
metabolites will emerge.   In summary then, the observations made with
the Walker 256 carcinosarcoma suggest that in these cells the response
to chemotactic stimulation has many similarities to the response in
leukocytes.

C. Chemotactic Responses to Peptide Factors and Phorbol Esters:
    Targets for Intervention

From a theoretical standpoint, it may be possible to interdict the
chemotactic response either by interfering with the generation or
activity of the chemotactic factors or by blocking the cellular
response to the active factors. Obviously, the first approach requires
an understanding of the relevant chemotactic factors in vivo. While
this information is not readily available with most of the potentially
important chemotactic factors, we understand, in some detail, the
biology of the C5-derived chemotactic peptides. As with other
biologicallly active peptides, the complement chemotactic peptides are
closely regulated in vivo. A serum-derived factor termed the
"chemotactic factor inactivator" prevents the existence of biologically
active levels of complement-related chemotactic activity in plasma
under normal conditions (42). Likewise, cells that respond to the
complement-derived chemotactic factors (in this case leukocytes) also
have a mechanism for inactivating these factors. Specifically, the
potent proteolytic enzymes which are responsible for much of the tissue
destruction seen in inflammatory conditions also inactivate the peptide
chemotactic factors for leukocytes (42). This may contribute to
limiting the inflammatory condition. Whether it will be possible to
therapeutically manipulate the natural chemotactic factor inactivators
to alter their effects on tumor cells is not known. Another approach is
the development of synthetic agents which inhibit the generation or
activity of the complement peptides. One such inhibitor, K-76COONa,
has been developed and in a recent study was shown to block the
generation of the tumor cell chemotactic factor derived from the fifth
component of complement (43).

In addition to these approaches, which are based on an understanding of the chemotactic factors, it may also be possible to
interfere with the chemotactic response by directly inhibiting the
cellular response to the active factors. One group of agents which
show promise in this regard are the cyclooxygenase metabolites of
arachidonic acid. These agents, specifically the E-series prostaglandins, block stimulus-coupled responses in both platelets (44) and
leukocytes in vitro (45,46). Studies by Kunkel et al. (47,48) have
shown that treatment of animals with these agents can inhibit a variety
of experimentally-induced inflammatory conditions. In vitro studies of
cells from animals treated in vivo indicate that these cells have the
same chemotactic defects as cells treated in vitro. How the E-series
prostaglandins evoke the inhibition of stimulus-coupled responses is
not known. A report by Rivkin et al. (45) showed that treatment of
rabbit leukocytes with prostaglandins produces an elevation of cAMP
levels and a recent study by Fantone et al. (49) showed that prostaglandins suppress the expression of chemotactic receptors on
neutrophils.

Studies in our laboratory have investigated the modulating role of cyclooxygenase metabolites in various tumor cell functions. These studies (50,51) have shown that agents such as prostaglandin E_1 (PGE_1) and prostacyclin (PGI_2) inhibit the adherence response in the Walker cells induced by either FMLP or TPA (Table 2). In contrast, prostaglandin $F_{2\alpha}$ is much less effective and thromboxane B_2 has no effect, or perhaps stimulates the response slightly (51). Mokashi et al. (52) showed that E-series prostaglandins block the stimulated motility response to the complement-derived chemotactic peptide in the same cells. We also have demonstrated inhibition of stimulated motility in murine fibrosarcoma cells (53). Both our studies and those by Mokashi et al. (52) have demonstrated that these metabolites are effective down to a concentration of 10 nM. This compares favorably with concentrations reported to be effective in neutrophils (45,46).

Although there is no evidence to suggest that the chemotactic peptides are mitogens (54), the biologically active phorbol esters are known to stimulate growth in some cells. As part of our effort to characterize the chemotactic response, we examined TPA for mitogenic effects on several chemotactically-responsive and non-responsive cells. Interestingly, those cells which responded to TPA mitogenically were the cells which did not respond in the chemotactic assays for stimulated adherence and motility. In contrast, chemotactically-responsive cells did not proliferate in response to TPA. These cells all showed a marked, temporary inhibition of proliferation (53). The cells which underwent proliferation when stimulated with TPA also responded to $PGF_{2\alpha}$. $PGF_{2\alpha}$ was effective at concentrations as low as 10 nM. The kinetics of the response and the magnitude of the response to $PGF_{2\alpha}$ paralleled those of the response to TPA. In spite of this, it is not likely that $PGF_{2\alpha}$ is an essential intermediate in the TPA-induced mitogenic response. Rather it is more likely that both TPA and $PGF_{2\alpha}$ work through a common pathway. $PGF_{2\alpha}$ did not duplicate the growth-inhibiting effects of TPA in the chemotactically responsive cells. However, PGE_1, at concentrations as low as 10 nM, inhibited both TPA-induced proliferation and serum-induced proliferation of all the cells tested (53). These results indicate that certain cyclooxygenase metabolites - notably PGE_1 and PGI_2 - can suppress a variety of stimulus-coupled responses in tumor cells. These agents are effective at concentrations as low as 10 nM (~ 3 ng/ml) and exhibit structural specificity since agents such as $PGF_{2\alpha}$ or thromboxane B_2 cannot duplicate their effects.

Table 2. Inhibition of Chemotactic Factor-Induced Adherence of Walker 256 Carcinosarcoma Cells by Cyclooxygenase Metabolites.

Treatment Adherence	Percent Inhibition of TPA-Induced Adherence	Percent Inhibition of FMLP-Induced
10^{-4} M 15-M-PGE$_1$	108 ± 4	71 ± 6
10^{-5} M 15-M-PGE$_1$	80 ± 10	90 ± 7
10^{-6} M 15-M-PGE$_1$	24 ± 6	14 ± 3
10^{-8} M 15-M-PGE$_1$	17 ± 1	ND
10^{-4} M PGI$_2$	123 ± 7	104 ± 7
10^{-5} M PGI$_2$	110 ± 11	84 ± 4
10^{-6} M PGI$_2$	11 ± 1	24 ± 1
10^{-4} M 15-M-PGF$_{2\alpha}$	45 ± 6	ND
10^{-5} M 15-M-PGF$_{2\alpha}$	30 ± 1	ND
10^{-6} M 15-M-PGF$_{2\alpha}$	25 ± 3	ND
10^{-4} M TXB$_2$	16 ± 1	-69 ± 12
10^{-5} M TXB$_2$	-10 ± 1	-35 ± 15
10^{-6} M TXB$_2$	-20 ± 3	-79 ± 12

15-M-PGE$_1$ and 15-M-PGF$_{2\alpha}$ are 15-methyl-derivatives of the natural metabolites. ND = not done. See references 50,51 for complete details.

Because the prostanoid metabolites are effective inhibitors of the tumor cell chemotactic responses and because these agents are produced by many types of cells, we wondered if endogenous prostaglandins might be a part of the mechanism regulating these responses. To probe this question, we examined the production of various prostaglandin metabolites in chemotactically-responsive and non-responsive cells. The chemotactically-responsive cells consisted of a line of highly-malignant murine fibrosarcoma cells (designated as 1.0/L1). Swiss 3T3 cells were used as a non-responsive control. The 3T3 cells are not chemotactically responsive to TPA although TPA is a potent mitogen for these cells. The cells were incubated in serum-free medium and either kept as controls or stimulated with 16 nM TPA. Four hours later, the supernatant fluids were harvested and analyzed for PGE$_2$ and 6-keto-PGF$_{1\alpha}$ (a prostacyclin metabolite) by radioimmunoassay (53). As seen in Figure 2, both cells produce cyclooxygenase metabolites in response to TPA stimulation. However, the levels are much higher in the non-responsive 3T3 cells than in the chemotactically-responsive 1.0/L1 cells.

We next examined the production of these metabolites in the Walker cells. It is interesting that these cells, which are highly chemo-tactically-responsive (4-8,10,11,14, 15,35-38) produce virtually no cyclooxygenase metabolites either when left unstimulated or treated with a variety of potent stimulating agents (Table 3 and 40). Four hour data is shown in this Table but the same trends are also seen at

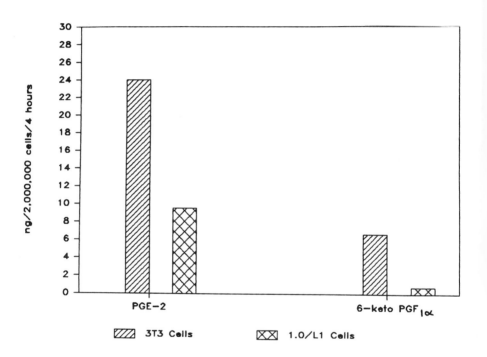

FIGURE 2. Production of Cyclooxygenase Metabolites by Chemotactically-Responsive 1.0/L1 Cells and Chemotactically Non-Responsive 3T3 Cells. See reference 53 for complete details.

Table 3. Production of Cyclooxygenase Metabolites by Walker 256 Carcinosarcoma Cells.

Stimulating Factor	Picograms per 2×10^6 cells per 4 hr		
	PGE_2	6-keto-$PGF_{1\alpha}$	$PGF_{2\alpha}$
None	277 ± 30	<30	18 ± 4
1.6×10^{-8} M TPA	295 ± 32	<30	19 ± 4
1.0×10^{-6} M FMLP	72 ± 15	<30	10 ± 4
2.0×10^{-6} M A23187	94 ± 17	<30	6 ± 3

24 hr. We routinely maintain these cells as suspension cells in culture and discovered quite by accident that when these cells were injected intraperitoneally and allowed to grow as an ascites tumor, they became refractory to TPA in vitro. Non-responsiveness appeared to be temporary since the cells regained their ability to respond when they were recultured in vitro. By two days, they regained partial responsiveness and by 5-7 da, they were indistinguishable from the cells maintained continuously in culture. As can be seen from Table 4, immediately upon removal from the animals, the non-responsive cells produced significant amounts of PGE_1 and 6-keto-$PGF_{1\alpha}$. However, as responsiveness was reacquired, levels of prostaglandins decreased. Thus, there was an inverse association between response to TPA in the adherence assay and production of cyclooxygenase metabolites. As with the cells maintained continuously in culture, TPA did not stimulate significant prostaglandin production in the the non-responsive cells from the ascites tumors.

Table 4. Comparison of Walker Cells Maintained in Culture and as
Ascites Tumors for Production of Cyclooxygenase Metabolites.

Condition of Maintenance	Picograms per 2 x 10^6 cells per 4 hr		
	PGE_2	6-keto-$PGF_{1\alpha}$	$PGF_{2\alpha}$
Suspension culture	116 ± 35	<35	14 ± 12
As ascites tumors, then in culture			
0 da	1600 ± 136	3500 ± 410	127 ± 20
5 da	450 ± 78	<35	26 ± 8

While this inverse association between prostaglandin levels and
responsiveness is consistent with the interpretation that endogenous
cyclooxygenase metabolites regulate chemotactic responsiveness, it
certainly does not prove it. To probe this relationship further, cells
were placed in culture from ascites tumors and treated with 1-100 µM
indomethacin. Eighteen hours later, the treated and control cells were
stimulated with TPA. As expected, the cells not pretreated with
indomethacin showed no response. In contrast, the indomethacin-treated
cells responded to TPA stimulation. The effects of indomethacin were
dose-responsive and at the highest concentration, the response was
nearly as great as that of the cells which were continuously maintained
in culture. This data further suggests that endogenous prostaglandins
may play a role as modulators of chemotactic responses. If this turns
out to be the case, then it may be possible to modulate these responses
by manipulating the metabolism of arachidonic acid in these cells.

III.   SUMMARY AND CONCLUSIONS

Our studies suggest that the metabolism of arachidonic acid may
play a physiological role in the chemotactic responses of tumor cells
and that it may be possible to modulate chemotactic responses by use of
appropriate cyclooxygenase metabolites. It has already been shown that
cyclooxygenase metabolites have antimetastatic activity (55) and it may
be that the ability of these agents to alter the physiology of the
tumor cells, themselves, contributes to their antimetastatic activity.
Additionally, it may be possible to use agents which alter arachidonic
acid metabolism to achieve the same ends.

REFERENCES

1. Hayashi H, Yoshida K, Ozaki T, Ushijima K: Chemotactic factor
    associated with invasion of cancer cells. Nature (London)
    226:174-175, 1970.
2. Yoshida K, Ozaki T, Ushijima K, Hayashi H: Studies on the
    mechanism of invasion in cancer. I: Isolation and purification
    of a factor chemotactic for cancer cells. Int. J. Cancer
    6:123-132, 1970.
3. Ozaki T, Yoshida K, Ushijima K, Hayashi H: Studies on the
    mechanism of invasion in cancer. II: In vivo effects of a factor
    chemotactic for cancer cells. Int. J. Cancer 7:93-100, 1971.
4. Romualdez AG, Ward PA: A unique, complement-derived chemotactic
    factor for tumor cells. Proc. Natl. Acad. Sci. USA 72:4128-4132,
    1975.
5. Romualdez AG, Ward PA, Torikata T: Relationship between the C5
    peptides chemotactic for leukocytes and tumor cells. J. Immunol.
    117:1762-1766, 1975.
6. Orr W, Varani J, Ward PA: Characteristics of the chemotactic
    response of neoplastic cells to a factor derived from the fifth
    component of complement. Am. J. Pathol. 93:405-422, 1978.
7. Orr W, Phan S, Varani J, Ward PA, Kreutzer DL, Webster RO, Henson
    PM: Chemotactic factor for tumor cells derived from the C5a
    fragment of complement component 5. Proc. Natl. Acad. Sci. USA
    76:1986-1989, 1979.
8. Wass JA, Varani J, Ward PA: Size increase induced in Walker
    ascites cells by chemotactic factors. Cancer Lett. 9:313-318,
    1980.
9. Thorgeirsson UP, Liotta LA, Kalebic T, Margulies IMK, Thomas K,
    Rios-Candelore M, Russo RG: Effect of natural protease inhibitors
    and a chemoattractant on tumor cell invasion in vitro. J. Natl.
    Cancer. Inst. 69:1049-1058, 1982.
10. Varani J: Chemotaxis of metastatic tumor cells. Cancer
    Metastasis Rev. 1:17-28, 1982.
11. Mundy GR, DeMartino S, Rowe DE: Collagen and collagen-derived
    fragments are chemotactic for tumor cells. J. Clin. Invest.
    68:1102-1105, 1981.
12. Gauss-Muller V, Kleinman HK, Martin GR, Schiffmann E: Role of
    attachment factors and attractants in fibroblast chemotaxis. J.
    Lab. Clin. Med. 96:1071-1080, 1980.
13. McCarthy JB, Palm SL, Furcht LT: Migration by haptotaxis of a
    Schwann cell tumor line to the basment membrane glycoprotein,
    laminin. J. Cell Biol. 97:772-777, 1983.
14. Orr W, Varani J, Gondek MD, Ward PA, Mundy GR: Chemotactic
    responses of tumor cells to products of resorbing bone. Science
    203:176-179, 1979.
15. Orr FW, Varani J, Gondek MD, Ward PA, Mundy GR: Partial
    characterization of a bone-derived chemotactic factor for tumor
    cells. Am. J. Pathol. 99:43-52, 1980.
16. Snyderman R, Goetzel EJ: Molecular and cellular mechanisms of
    leukocyte chemotaxis. Science 213:830-836, 1981.

272

17. Keller HU, Till GO: Leukocyte Locomotion and Chemotaxis. Agents and Actions Supplements Volume 12. Birkhauser Verlag, Basel, 1983.
18. Aswanikumar S, Corcoran B, Schiffmann E, Day AR, Freer RJ, Showell HJ, Becker EL, Pert CB: Demonstration of a receptor on rabbit neutrophils for chemotactic peptides. Proc. Natl. Acad. Sci. USA 74:1204-1208, 1977.
19. Snyderman R, Pike MC: N-formyl-methionyl peptide receptors on equine leukocytes initiate secretion but not chemotaxis. Science 209:493-495, 1980.
20. Sullivan SJ, Zigmond SH: Chemotactic peptide receptor modulation in polymorphonuclear leukocytes. J. Cell Biol. 85:703-711, 1980.
21. Sando JJ, Hilfiker ML, Salomon DS, Farrar JJ: Specific receptors for phorbol esters in lymphoid cell populations: Role in enhanced production of T-cell growth factor. Proc. Natl. Acad. Sci. USA 78:1189-1193, 1981.
22. Chang J: Characterization of a high-affinity receptor for phorbol esters in rat alveolar macrophages. Inflammation 7:15-23, 1983.
23. Samuelsson B: The leukotrienes: A new group of biologically-active compounds including SRS-A. Trends Pharmacol. Sci. 1:227-230, 1980.
24. Smith MHJ: Prostaglandins and the polymorphonuclear leukocytes. IN: Ford-Hutchinson AW and Rainsford KD (eds.), Prostaglandins and Inflammation. Birkhauser Verlag, Basel, pp. 91-103, 1980.
25. Goetzl EJ, Woods JM, Gorman RR: Stimulation of human eosinophil and neutrophil polymorphonuclear leukocyte chemotaxis and random migration by 12-L-hydroxy-5,8,10,14-eicosatetrenoic acid. J. Clin. Invest. 59:179-183, 1977.
26. Goetzl EJ, Brash AR, Tauber AI, Oates JA, Hubbard WC: Modulation of human neutrophil function by mono-eicosatetraenoic acids. Immunol. 39:491-501, 1980.
27. Becker EL, Naccache PH, Sha'afi RK: Some early ionic events in neutrophil activation by chemotactic factors. IN: Keller HU and Till GO (eds.) Leukocyte Locomotion and Chemotaxis. Agents and Actions Supplements Volume 12, Birkhauser Verlag, Basel, pp. 338-352, 1983.
28. Malech HL, Root RK, Gallin JI: Structural analysis of human neutrophil migration: Centriole, microtubule and microfilament orientation and function during chemotaxis. J. Cell Biol. 75:606-616, 1977.
29. Rao KMK, Varani J: Actin polymerization induced by chemotactic peptide and concanavalin A in rat neutrophils. J. Immunol. 129:1605-1607, 1982.
30. Fechheimer M, Zigmond SH: Changes in cytoskeletal proteins of polymorphonuclear leukocytes induced by chemotactic peptides. Cell Motility 3:349-361, 1983.
31. Clark M, Spudich JA: Nonmuscle contractile proteins: The role of actin and myosin in cell motility and shape determination. Ann. Rev. Biochem. 46:797-822, 1977.

32. Kreutzer DL, O'Flaherty JT, Orr W, Showell HJ, Ward PA, Becker EL: Quantitative comparisons of various biological responses of neutrophils to different active and inactive chemotactic factors. Immunopharmacol. 1:39-47, 1978.

33. Simchowitz L, Mehta J, Spilberg I: Chemotactic factor-induced superoxide radical generation by human neutrophils: Requirement for protease (esterase) activity. J. Lab. Clin. Med. 94:403-407, 1979.

34. Orr FW, Varani J, Delikatny J, Jain N, Ward PA: Comparison of the chemotactic responsiveness of fibrosarcoma subpopulations of differing malignancy. Am. J. Pathol. 102:160-167, 1981.

35. Varani J, Wass JA, Piontek J, Ward PA: Chemotactic factor-induced adherence of tumor cells. Cell Biol. Int. Rep. 5:525-530, 1981.

36. Varani J, Fantone JC: Phorbol myristate acetate-induced adherence of Walker 256 carcinosarcoma cells. Cancer Res. 42:190-197, 1982.

37. Clarke PRH, Varani J: Phorbol ester binding to chemotactically-responsive and non-responsive Walker 256 carcinosarcoma cells. Cancer Res. (In press).

38. Grimstad IA, Wass JA, Spirnak J, Fantone JC, Varani J: Chemotactic factor-induced adherence of tumor cells: Involvement of Ca^{2+} and Mg^{2+}. Invasion Metastasis 2:274-288, 1982.

39. O'Flaherty JT, DeChatelet LR, McCall CE, Bass DA: Neutrophil aggregation: Evidence for a different mechanism of action by phorbol myristate acetate. Proc. Soc. Exp. Biol. Med. 165:225-232, 1980.

40. Varani J: Chemotaxis. IN: Honn K and Marnett L (eds.) Prostaglandins, Leukotrienes and Cancer Volume 1. Basic Biochemical Processes. Martinus Nijhoff, The Hague, (In press).

41. Mensing H, Czarnetski BM: Leukotriene B_4 induces in vitro fibroblast chemotaxis. J. Invest. Dermatol. 82:9-12, 1984.

42. Ward PA: Natural inhibitors of leukotaxis. IN: Greenwalt TJ and Jamieson GA (eds.), The Granulocyte: Function and Clinical Utilization. Alan R. Liss, Inc., New York, pp. 77-81, 1977.

43. Bumpers HL, Baum J: The effect of a novel C5 inhibitor (K-76 COONa) on tumor cell chemotaxis. J. Lab. Clin. Med. 102:421-427, 1983.

44. Feinstein MB, Becker EL, Fraser C: Thrombin, collagen and A23187-stimulated endogenous platelet arachidonate metabolism: Differential inhibition of PGE_1, local anesthetics and a serum protease inhibitor. Prostaglandins 14:1075-1093, 1977.

45. Rivkin I, Rosenblatt J, Becker EL: The role of cyclic AMP in the chemotactic responsiveness and spontaneous motility of rabbit peritoneal neutrophils. The inhibition of neutrophil movement and the elevation of cyclic AMP levels by catecholamines, prostaglandins, theophylline and cholera toxin. J. Immunol. 115:1126-1134, 1975.

46. O'Flaherty JT, Kreutzer DL, Ward PA: Effect of prostaglandins E_1, E_2, and $F_{2\alpha}$ on neutrophil aggregation. Prostaglandins 17:201-210, 1979.

47. Kunkel SL, Thrall RS, Kunkel RG, McCormick JR, Ward PA, Zurier RB: Suppression of immune complex vasculitis in rats by prostaglandins. J. Clin. Invest. 64:1525-1529, 1979.

48. Kunkel SL, Chensue SW, Plewa M, Higashi GI: Macrophage function in the Schistosoma mansoni egg-induced pulmonary granuloma. Role of arachidonic acid metabolites in macrophage Ia antigen expression. Am. J. Pathol. 114:240-249, 1984.

49. Fantone JC, Marasco WA, Elgas LJ, Ward PA: Anti-inflammatory effects of prostaglandin E_1: In vivo modulation of the formyl peptide chemotactic receptor on the rat neutrophil. J. Immunol. 130:1495-1497, 1983.

50. Fantone JC, Elgas LJ, Weinberger L, Varani J: Modulation of tumor cell adherence by prostaglandins. Oncology 40:421-426, 1983.

51. Fantone JC, Kunkel SL, Varani J: Inhibition of tumor cell adherence by prostaglandins. IN: Mundy GR (ed.), Prostaglandins and Cancer: First International Conference. Alan R. Liss, Inc., New York, pp. 673-677, 1982.

52. Mokashi S, Delikatny J, Orr FW: Relationships between chemotaxis, chemotactic modulators and cyclic nucleotide levels in tumor cells. Cancer Res. 43:1980-1983, 1983.

53. Lee EC, Situ R, Fantone JC, Varani J: Functional responses of tumor cells to phorbol esters: Role for prostaglandins. Oncology (In press).

54. Orr FW, Lam WC, Delikatny EJ, Mokashi S, Varani J: Localization of intravenously injected tumor cells in the rat mesentery after intraperitoneal administration of chemotactic stimuli. Invasion Metastasis 1:239-247, 1981.

55. Honn KV, Cicone B, Skoff A: Prostacyclin: A potent antimetastatic agent. Science 212:1270-1272, 1981.

CHAPTER 18.   INVASION OF VASCULAR ENDOTHELIUM AND ORGAN TISSUE IN VITRO BY B16 MELANOMA VARIANTS

GARTH L. NICOLSON, MOTOWO NAKAJIMA AND TATSURO IRIMURA

I.   INTRODUCTION

When cancer cells become blood-borne, they have the potential to form secondary tumor foci at distant sites. In a variety of cancers, as well as animal tumor models, blood-borne metastasis occurs often to particular secondary sites (1-4). Although most regional metastases can be explained strictly on anatomic circulatory pathways or on mechanical lodgment of blood-borne tumor emboli in the first capillary bed encountered, distant blood-borne organ colonization by metastatic tumor cells does not always follow this pattern. There are numerous examples where malignant tumors tend to metastasize to unusual secondary locations. For example, prostatic carcinoma often metastasizes to bone, small cell carcinoma of the lung spreads at high frequency to the brain, and neuroblastoma to adrenal glands and liver (1,2).

It has been known for some time that the mere presence of cancer cells in the blood does not necessarily determine that metastatic disease will occur (5). The initial distribution of blood-borne tumor cells does not always reflect the distribution of metastatic foci that ultimately form (6,7). Thus, events other than simple mechanical lodgment of blood-borne tumor cells must be important in determining the locations of metastatic disease.

Blood-borne metastasis formation has as a requirement that the blood-borne tumor cells arrest or implant within the microcirculation. This can be strictly by mechanical means if the blood-borne embolus is of sufficient size to lodge nonspecifically in the capillaries (8). Alternatively, implantation could occur by adhesion to blood vessel walls in the capillaries and post-capillary venules (9-11). Malignant cells must penetrate the endothelial cell layer and the vessel wall to reach the extravascular tissue, suggesting that hematogenous metastasis formation has a number of important requirements. These are that the circulating tumor cells recognize endothelial cells or their subendothelial stroma within an organ, that they undergo extravasation and invade into surrounding tissues and that they selectively survive or grow at specific distant sites, or combinations of these processes, to form gross metastases (2,4,12).

Most malignant cells die rapidly in the circulation; only a small fraction of these tumor cells survive to yield metastatic foci (13-15). Circulating tumor cells can die due to random processes, such as mechanical factors and hydrodynamic trauma, or they can be killed by host cells in the circulation, such as natural killer (NK) cells (16,17).

In some cases metastatic tumor cells specifically implant, survive and grow at particular organ sites, such as the lung. This has been shown by implanting lung tissue intramuscularly into the thighs of syngeneic mice and examining whether lung-colonizing tumor cells can recirculate to and form metastatic colonies in ectopic organ tissues (1,18,19). In just such an experiment, Hart and Fidler (19) examined the kinetic distribution of radiolabeled, lung-colonizing B16 melanoma cells in mice bearing ectopic lung or kidney implants. They did not find differences in the kinetic distribution patterns of lung-colonizing B16 melanoma cells between animals without organ implants and those bearing ectopically implanted lung or kidney tissue. These results suggest that the events subsequent to implantation, such as invasion, survival, vascularization and growth may be more important in determining lung tissue colonization in this system. However, it should be noted that a substantial portion of the vascular system in the ectopic implants may be derived from surrounding tissues. Also, the mere localization of radiolabeled cells in the ectopic implants does not signify their exact location, and most of these cells would not be expected to extravasate and survive to form gross tumor lesions. Hart and Fidler (19) found that similar numbers of lung-colonizing B16 melanoma cells are localized in ectopically implanted lung or kidney tissue, but tumor foci fail to subsequently form in the kidney implants.

II. HETEROGENEITY OF METASTATIC NEOPLASMS

Neoplastic cells isolated from tumors growing at primary or secondary sites show considerable diversity in cellular properties, such as histologic structure, growth patterns, tissue responses, invasion and metastasis. They also differ in their sensitivities to drugs, heat, radiation and host immunologic mechanisms, and they contain differing quantities of cell surface glycoproteins, glyco-lipids, antigens, enzymes and cellular recognition components (2,4,7,20-23). Cell population diversity also occurs in normal cells within tissues, although the heterogeneity of cells in normal tissues is less pronounced compared to malignant neoplasms (24,25).

Since it is well established that most neoplasms develop from single cells (26,27), the cellular heterogeneity of malignant neoplasms has been explained by a process of tumor evolution or progression (26,28). Tumor progression is thought to occur by a combination of cellular phenotypic diversification and sequential host selection which together results in neoplastic cell populations that ultimately possess altered autonomy, survival, growth and malignant characteristics.

The microenvironment of proliferating tumor cells may be important in generating phenotypic diversity, as well as in selecting variant cells for enhanced survival and growth characteristics, or alternatively, poor survival and growth characteristics (29,30). To survive and proliferate within a competitive cell population, tumor cells must have selective survival, growth and other advantages over the remaining cells in the tumor, and they must also circumvent host defenses. Thus, certain tumor cell subpopulations may eventually become dominant, and such dominant subpopulations could evolve with particular phenotypic characteristics. Since alterations in the cellular composition of tumors may occur with changes in micro-environment and host response, the result is a dynamically heterogeneous tumor which contains multiple cell subpopulations with varying properties (29,30). As a tumor progresses, its overall properties may gradually change by the acquisition or loss of certain characteristics (31).

Different experimental approaches have been used in vivo or in vitro to obtain tumor cell subpopulations with different phenotypic characteristics. The use of in vitro or in vivo selection procedures and in vitro cloning techniques to obtain subpopulations of highly malignant cells has been particularly advantageous for studies on the role of tumor and host properties in metastasis formation. However, the success of such procedures in certain tumor systems does not guarantee that in every tumor analyzed differences in phenotypic properties will be found, nor does it guarantee that particular cell phenotypes will remain stable during cell propagation in vivo or in vitro. Several studies have shown that great care must be taken in the propagation of tumor cell subpopulations for further study, due to problems in phenotypic variability in metastatic and other properties, as discussed above (2,7,20,22,32). The utility of using tumor cells of known metastatic potentials derived from the same neoplasm is that this allows tumor cell properties essential in certain steps of metastasis to be identified and eventually studied in detail. As long as investigators know that such malignant cells are potentially unstable in their phenotypic properties, parallel studies on low and high metastatic cell subpopulations are likely to yield important informa-tion on the properties involved in various steps of metastasis (4,22).

III. METASTATIC TUMOR CELL INTERACTIONS DURING BLOOD-BORNE TRANSPORT

The interactions of malignant cells with their environment, and particularly their interactions with host cells and tissues, are mediated by cell surface constituents (2,4,20-22). Several lines of evidence have underscored the involvement of cell surface components in certain aspects of metastasis formation, such as blood-borne tumor cell implantation and invasion. Early experiments demonstrated that modification of cell surface glycoproteins can alter tumor cell implantation properties in the microcirculation without altering tumor cell viability and growth properties (33,34). Modification in the specific biosynthesis of cell surface glycoproteins has also been shown to inhibit blood-borne implantation and metastasis formation (35,36).

The role of the plasma membrane in implantation and organ colonization has been studied by the transfer of portions of plasma membranes from highly metastatic B16 melanoma cells to B16 cells of lower metastatic potential (37). Taking advantage of the fact that B16 melanoma cells spontaneously shed closed plasma membrane vesicles in vitro, as well as in vivo, Poste and Nicolson (37) harvested, purified and subsequently used these plasma membrane vesicles in cell fusion experiments to introduce plasma membrane components into the surface membranes of recipient cells. When vesicles from the high lung-colonizing B16F10 cells are fused into the surfaces of the low lung-colonizing B16F1 cells, the ability of the vesicle-modified B16F1 cells to colonize lung is increased significantly. The changes induced by the fusion of plasma membrane vesicles are reversible over a one day period, correlating with the natural turnover of B16 cell membrane components (37). It is now well accepted that highly metastatic cells show differences in the display, dynamics, contents or structures of cell surface proteins, glycolipids and glycoproteins which may be involved in various cellular interactions during the metastatic process (2,4,22).

Metastatic tumor cells are involved in several types of interactions during their dissemination in the blood, including homotypic interactions to form multicellular tumor emboli and heterotypic interactions with a variety of host cells or blood components. Such interactions can result in the formation of multicellular tumor emboli which implant in the microcirculation at higher efficiencies than single metastatic cells (38,39). As mentioned above, certain mechanical factors, such as the size and deformability of the circulating tumor cells and their multicellular emboli, as well as host capillary deformability, can modify blood-borne malignant cell lodgment properties (40,41). However, even tumor cell emboli of large size can often pass through the first capillary bed encountered and recirculate to other sites (40,42).

The homotypic interactions of malignant cells with themselves to form multicellular emboli enhances blood-borne implantation. This has been shown in the B16 melanoma system where the B16 cells of highest lung implantation and colonization potentials possess the highest rates of homotypic adhesion, when measured in cell aggregation type assays (43,44). Similar results have been obtained in a murine sarcoma system (45). Although the constituents involved in homotypic adhesion, for the most part, have not been elucidated, Raz and Lotan (46) have found that human and murine tumor cells contain cell surface lectins capable of binding galactosyl-containing glycoconjugates. Their results suggest that cell surface lectins or other adhesion components may be responsible for mediating at least some of the intercellular interactions of blood-borne tumor cells.

During blood-borne transport malignant cells can interact with normal host cells, such as platelets and lymphocytes. For example, the interactions of tumor cells with platelets can result in the enhancement of implantation in the microcirculation via the formation of platelet-tumor cell emboli which arrest better in the microcirculation. In fact, over ten years ago Gasic et al. (47) found that B16 melanoma cells of high lung colonization potential induce platelet aggregation at higher rates than B16 cells of low lung colonization potential. Various tumor cell systems have been found to induce platelet aggregation (48,49), and experimental metastasis has been inhibited in certain systems by the induction of thrombocytopenia or by administration of anti-platelet agents (47,50,51). However, Warren (14) has reviewed the literature in this area and has concluded that not all tumor cells induce platelet aggregation during blood-borne transport and after implantation. In some metastatic systems there is no correlation between platelet aggregation potential and metastatic behavior (52,53).

Heterotypic interactions of tumor cells with host lymphocytes can also occur in the blood. Fidler (54) studied the interactions of B16 melanoma cells with syngeneic lymphocytes and found that B16 cells of high lung colonization potential bind to syngeneic lymphocytes to form heterotypic cell aggregates at higher rates than B16 sublines of low lung colonization behavior (55). Evidence for the involvement of lymphocyte-tumor cell interactions in B16 melanoma implantation has also been obtained by sequential selection of B16 sublines in vitro for resistance to lymphocyte-mediated cytolysis (56). Lymphocyte-resistant B16 sublines have been found to be less adhesive to lymphocytes in vitro and possess lower rates of blood-borne implantation and experimental metastasis formation than parental B16 cells (55).

During malignant cell dissemination, tumor cells are exposed to natural host defense mechanisms. These defense mechanisms include: natural antibodies and NK cells (57-59). NK cells seem to be extremely effective against certain metastatic cells during their transport (16 and Chapter 15). In the B16 metastatic cell system the effectiveness of NK cells in eliminating blood-borne tumor cells correlates inversely with the formation of experimental metastases (16,60). Hanna and Fidler (17) have utilized young nude mice with low NK activities to demonstrate that certain tumor cells can potentially form large numbers of experimental metastases. However, in older (> 6 wk) nude mice with higher NK activities, these same tumor sublines display low metastatic potential. Not all malignant cells are equally susceptible to NK-mediated cytolysis; it is often found that highly metastatic tumor cells are not very sensitive to NK-mediated cytolysis, and cell variants have been selected sequentially for resistance to NK-mediated cytolysis resulting in increased potential for metastasis formation (60). Similar results have been obtained by Hanna and Fidler (61) using B16 melanoma sublines. After several in vitro selections for resistance to NK-mediated cytolysis, the NK-resistant B16 subline possesses increased lung colonization potential and gains the capacity to metastasize in adult nude mice, in contrast to the parental B16 cells which are quickly killed in the circulation of adult nude mice (61).

The interactions of blood-borne malignant cells with plasma components during their transport can also affect metastasis formation. Tumor cells are often thromboplastic and elicit formation of fibrin during blood-borne transport or after implantation in the micro-circulation (14,62). Fibrin clots can form at the sites of tumor cell implantation; however, the arrest of multicellular tumor emboli can result from damage to the endothelium and accumulation of platelets and fibrin clots at the exposed basal lamina surface. Warren (14) has reviewed the evidence for fibrin clot formation in metastasis and concluded that it is nonessential for blood-borne tumor cell implantation. For example, Kinjo et al. (63) could not demonstrate a correlation between tumor thromboplastic levels, fibrin formation and metastatic potential.

Once blood-borne tumor cells have undergone implantation in the microcirculation, they usually extravasate by invading blood vessel walls (64-67). Malignant cells can invade out of the vessel between adjacent endothelial cells (9,68,69) or by penetrating the endothelial cells (70,71). Once malignant cells have penetrated the endothelial cell layer, they adhere tightly to the underlying endothelial basal lamina.

IV. THE INTERACTIONS OF METASTATIC TUMOR CELLS WITH ENDOTHELIAL BASAL LAMINA

During blood-borne implantation, circulating malignant cells interact with endothelial cells lining the microcirculation. In some cases these interactions are thought to be specific (2). Vascular endothelial cells present in different organs appear to possess unique properties, such as cell surface antigens (72) and proteins (73) which may determine their tissue of origin. Recognition of unique endothelial cell or subendothelial basal lamina determinants by blood-borne malignant cells could be important in determining organ colonization properties (2).

Once malignant cells attach to the apical surfaces of endothelial cells, they can induce endothelial cell junction breakage and cell retraction (2,69,73,74). After the endothelial cells are retracted, the malignant cells can migrate through the endothelial cell layer and attach to the underlying basal lamina. Differential adhesion of malignant cells to endothelial basal lamina probably sets up a haptotactic gradient that drives metastatic cells to basal lamina and eventually extravasation (75,76). Using an in vitro model for the vascular endothelium, we have found that many types of cells can bind to endothelial cell monolayers and stimulate retraction, but only a few of these cells can migrate under the endothelial cell layer (69,74). Similar events have been found to occur in vivo (9,14,77). After invasion endothelial cells can reseal their disrupted junctions to reform an intact endothelium.

Heterogeneity exists in the abilities of individual tumor cells to attach to and invade endothelial cell monolayers (2,69,73,74,78). This has also been noted in vivo, and tumor cell populations have been found to display heterogeneity in their abilities to extravasate (77,79). Using the B16 melanoma system we have studied the interactions of B16 cells with endothelial basal lamina-like matrix and with the purified components of basal lamina immobilized on polyvinyl surfaces (Figure 1). The basal lamina matrix contains the glycoproteins, fibronectin (75,76) and laminin (80,81), collagens (82-84) and sulfated proteoglycans (85-88). Metastatic tumor cells can adhere to various isolated components of the endothelial basal lamina matrix (Figure 1), and we have proposed that different metastatic systems may utilize different parallel adhesive mechanisms to adhere to intact basal lamina (76). For example, B16 melanoma cells adhere rapidly to immobilized-fibronectin, -laminin and subendothelial basal lamina-like matrix synthesized by endothelial cells (Figure 1). Whereas adhesion to immobilized-fibronectin can be completely blocked by an affinity purified antibody to fibronectin, adhesion to basal laminia-like matrix can be only partially inhibited by this same antibody (76). These results suggest that metastatic cells use several different adhesive mechanisms to attach to endothelial basal lamina. It follows that the most metastatic tumor cells may have the capacity to attach to virtually all of the components of the endothelial basal lamina which should increase the affinity of their interactions with this matrix and decrease the chance that they could be mechanically detached by circulatory shear forces.

V.   THE INTERACTIONS OF METASTATIC TUMOR CELLS WITH ORGAN PARENCHYMAL CELLS

Once malignant cells have extravasated, they can interact with parenchymal cells and extracellular tissue stroma. These interactions have been studied in vitro using singly suspended organ cells, reconstructed organoid cell aggregates and small pieces of organ tissue (89). B16 melanoma cells have been found to adhere heterotypically to suspended organ cells, and this has been used as a model for tumor cell-parenchymal cell interactions. In such studies B16 cells of high lung colonization potential adhere at faster rates to suspended lung cells than do B16 cells of low lung colonization potential. However, substitution of other organ cells for lung cells abolishes such selectivity (90). Phondke et al. (91) found that spleen-colonizing leukemia cells adhere at high rates to spleen cells but not to suspended lung cells, and Schirrmacher et al. (92) have noted that mouse lymphoma cells of high liver-colonization potential bind to mouse hepatocytes at higher rates than does a parental lymphoma line of low liver colonization potential.

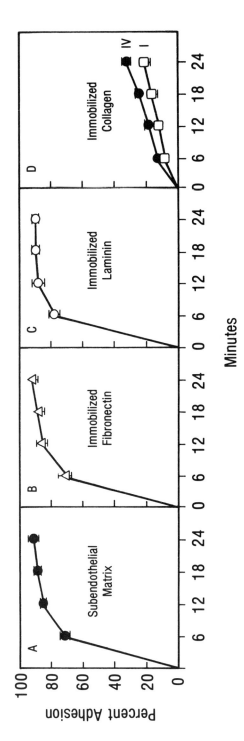

FIGURE 1. Attachment of Radiolabeled Murine B16-F10 Melanoma Cells to Subendothelial Basal Lamina-like Matrix and Immobilized Basal Lamina Matrix Components in Vitro. (For methods see 76).

Since suspending organ cells in vitro results in tremendous cell loss and low viability, small pieces of intact organ tissue have been used for tumor cell binding and invasion studies. Various organ colonizing variants of B16 melanoma were found to possess differing abilities to attach to and eventually invade into organ tissues such as lung, ovary and heart (Table 1). In this series of experiments high lung-colonizing B16 sublines bound better to lung tissue and invaded this tissue at higher rates in vitro. Conversely, ovary-colonizing B16 cells attached at higher rates and invaded ovary tissue more quickly than the other B16 sublines (Table 1). Thus, there appears to be some specificity in the ability of various selected B16 sublines to preferentially adhere to and invade target organ tissue, a finding which may explain the experiments of Hart and Fidler (19) using ectopic implants of organ tissue.

VI. THE DEGRADATION OF ENDOTHELIAL BASAL LAMINA BY METASTATIC TUMOR CELLS

In most cases metastatic tumor cells must breach the endothelial basal lamina and invade into surrounding parenchyma to form secondary tumor foci, and mechanical disruption and enzymatic degradation have both been postulated as important in the penetration of basal lamina. However, using in vitro models for vascular invasion, mechanical disruption can be eliminated entirely without affecting the ability of metastatic cells to penetrate basal lamina structures.

Several degradative enzymes have been considered important in basal lamina destruction (2,93,94). Among these are the enzymes that degrade collagens, particularly type IV collagen, proteinases which degrade matrix glycoproteins, such as fibronectin and laminin, and endoglycosidases which cleave glycosaminoglycan side chains from matrix proteoglycans (2,85-88,93,94,95; Figure 2).

Metastatic tumor cells solubilize essentially all the major components of the endothelial basal lamina, but only some of these molecules are released in degraded forms. Utilizing biosynthetically-labeled basal lamina-like matrix synthesized by endothelial cells it is possible to determine the susceptibility of different matrix components to enzymatic solubilization by tumor cells and to identify which components are degraded (74,85,88). Seeding metastatic tumor cells onto biosynthetically-labeled, cell free endothelial matrix results in a solubilization of macromolecules that are precipitable with trichloroacetic acid. B16 melanoma sublines of high organ colonization and metastatic properties release [^{3}H]leucine-labeled molecules from subendothelial matrix at higher rates than B16 cells of lower metastatic potential (74,88,94). In this case the most obvious glycoproteins solubilized by B16 melanoma cells are fibronectin and laminin, the former being released into the media in a slightly lower molecular weight form, suggesting that solubilized fibronectin is modified by B16 melanoma cell proteinases or glycosidases (85). In contrast, laminin appears to be released in an essentially undegraded form.

Table 1. The Interactions of Various Organ-Colonizing B16 Variant Cells with Isolated Syngeneic Organ Tissue*.

| | Attachment to Tissue (hr)† | | | | | | | | | Invasion of Tissue (hr)† | | | | | | | | | | | |
| | Lung | | | Heart | | | Ovary | | | Lung | | | | Heart | | | | Ovary | | | |
B16-	0.5	1.0	3.0	0.5	1.0	3.0	0.5	1.0	3.0	6	12	18	24	12	24	36	48	12	24	36	48
F1	0	+	+	+	+	+	0	0	+	-	-	+	+	0	0	0	+	0	0	0	+
F10	+	++	++	+	+	+	0	+	+	+	++	++	+++	0	0	+	+	0	0	+	+++
O10	0	+	+	0	+	+	+	+	++	0	0	+	+	0	0	0	0	+	++	++	+++
BL6	0	+	+	+	+	+	0	0	+	0	+	+	++	+	+	++	++	0	0	+	++
B14b	0	+	+	0	+	+	0	0	+	0	+	+	++	0	0	0	0	0	0	0	+

*Organ tissues were removed from C57BL/6 mice, cut into 1 mm³ pieces and suspended in complete medium in vials on a rotary shaker at 37°C for 18 hr. Tumor cells were then added at a concentration of 1×10^6 cells/ml and the incubation continued for various times until the tissue pieces were removed, washed, fixed and processed for light microscopy.

†Degree = +, 0–10 cells/field; ++, 10–20 cells/field; +++, > 20 cells/field.

285

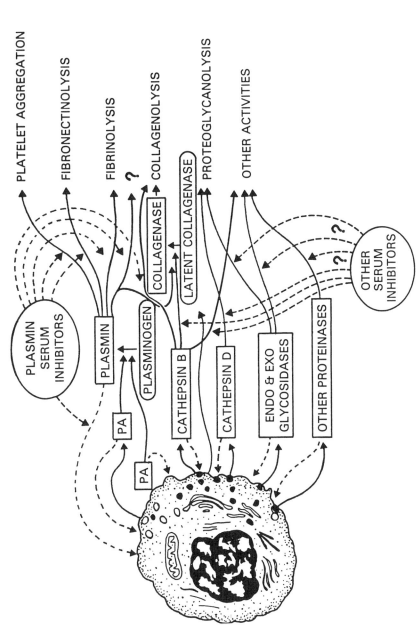

FIGURE 2. Release or Cell Surface Display of Tumor-Associated Degradative Enzymes and Their Possible Roles in Metastatic Processes. The solid lines represent the possible direct or indirect effects of tumor-associated enzymes on biologic substrates that form part of the barriers to malignant cell invasion. The broken lines represent possible feedback inhibitory or autolysis mechanisms. [From Nicolson (2) with permission.]

Metastatic tumor cells can also solubilize sulfated glycosamino-glycans from biosynthetically-labeled subendothelial matrix. Experiments with [^{35}S]sulfate-labeled subendothelial matrix indicate that metastatic tumor cells degrade matrix proteoglycan resulting in the release of lower molecular weight glycosaminoglycan fragments which are greater than 95% heparan sulfate (HS) in composition. These studies indicate that metastatic cells have an endoglycosidase capable of cleaving heparan sulfate molecules from matrix proteoglycans. The degradation of subendothelial matrix HS and its solubilization occurs at higher rates when B16 melanoma sublines of high organ colonization and metastatic potential are seeded onto biosynthetically-labeled subendothelial matrix than when B16 sublines of low colonization and metastatic potentials are seeded (74,88,94).

In addition, metastatic tumor cells are known to have collagenases which can degrade basal lamina collagen. Liotta et al. (84,93) found that B16 cells of high metastatic potential have higher activities against type IV collagen than B16 cells of low metastatic potential (see also Chapter 19). Examination of several different B16 sublines for activities against type IV collagen supports the findings of Liotta et al. (84; Table 2). Thus, B16 sublines selected for blood-borne implantation, invasion, survival and growth possess the correct type of collagenase to penetrate subendothelial basal lamina.

Other proteinases and glycosidases may also be important in basal lamina digestion. Sloane et al. (96,97) found that B16 melanoma cells of high lung-colonization potential have higher levels of certain lysosomal enzymes, such as cathepsin B. This cysteine proteinase can activate latent collagenase to active collagenase and it can, under certain conditions, directly degrade some of the other basal lamina components (see also Chapter 22).

We have studied the enzymes involved in solubilizing basal lamina proteoglycans. This followed from our development of assays to directly measure endoglycosidase and exoglycosidase activities against purified glycosaminoglycans in vitro (86-88, 95). In such assays, we measure the appearance of glycosaminoglycan degradation products by high performance liquid chromatography (86,95). Using these techniques we have found that HS from several sources, such as lung tissue, subendothelial matrix and EHS sarcoma (Figure 2), is degraded into intermediate molecular weight fragments by a heparanase of B16 melanoma cells (Figure 3). In these experiments exoglycosidase activities could be inhibited by D-saccharic acid 1,4 lactone (SAL), a potent inhibitor of lysosomal β-glucuronidase. Of the glycosaminoglycans examined, only HS is significantly degraded at pH 6.0 during a 6 hr incubation at 37°C (Figure 3). Examination of several B16 sublines indicates that B16 cells of high organ colonization and metastatic potential possess higher heparanase activities than B16 cells of low metastatic potential (Table 2).

Table 2. Degradation of Type IV Collagen and Heparan Sulfate by Living
B16 Melanoma Variant Cells.

| B16 subline | Degradation Rate (pg/cell/hr) | |
	Type IV Collagen[*]	Heparan Sulfate[†]
F1	0.98 ± 0.07	1.39 ± 0.08
F10	1.31 ± 0.03	2.08 ± 0.19
BL6	1.42 ± 0.10	3.50 ± 0.28
O13	0.79 ± 0.02	0.89 ± 0.08
B15b	1.88 ± 0.08	3.33 ± 0.29

[*]Type IV collagen degradation was determined by use of [^{3}H]proline-
labeled type IV collagen purified from EHS sarcoma tissue according to
Liotta et al. (84). Cells (2×10^4) suspended in 200 µl of a 1:1
mixture of Dulbecco-Modified Eagle's and Ham's F12 medium were placed
on a type IV collagen film (6 µg, 3000 cpm) and incubated at 37°C in a
humidified atmosphere of 95% air - 5% CO_2 for various times. Incubation
was terminated by chilling to 4°C and addition of 1/5 volume of a 10%
TCA, 0.5% tannic acid solution. After removal of insoluble materials
by centrifugation, radioactivity in the supernatant was measured.
Degradation rates were calculated from results during the first 12 hr
of incubation.

[†]Heparan sulfate degradation was assessed according to Nakajima et al.
(88). Cells (1×10^5) were incubated with 50 µg of purified heparan
sulfate from bovine lung in 200 µl of DMEM/F12 medium containing 20 mM
Tricine buffer, pH 7.3. Degradation products were analyzed by polyacrylamide gel electrophoresis (88). Degradation rates were calculated
from results during the first 6 hr of incubation.

     The interactions of the B16 melanoma heparanase with various
glycosaminoglycans could be examined using an enzyme inhibition assay
where glycosaminoglycans are added to a B16 cell extract mixture
containing an equal amount of [^{3}H]labeled HS. The effects of glycosaminoglycans on HS fragmentation are then determined by high-speed gel
permeation chromatography. The only glycosaminoglycan that affects the
B16 heparanase is heparin (95). The addition of porcine intestinal
mucosa heparin almost completely inhibits the appearance of
intermediate molecular weight HS fragments (Figures 3 and 4),
indicating that B16 heparanase can bind, but not cleave, the major
components of heparin. Other glycosaminoglycans tested show no
significant inhibitory effects on the B16 heparanse degradation of HS
(95). That HS could be degraded by B16 cell extracts into specific

288

high molecular weight fragments in the presence of SAL, an inhibitor of exo-β-glucuronidase, indicates that the B16 heparanase may recognize a specific sequence in the HS chain (95).

The cleavage products produced by B16 melanoma heparanase action on HS have been examined. HS fragments derived from bovine lung HS previously reduced with NaBH₄ at the reducing termini have been isolated and labeled at their newly formed reducing termini with [³H]NaBH₄, and the labeled, reducing-terminal sugars analyzed after acid hydrolysis or nitrous acid deamination followed by mild acid hydrolysis using paper chromatography and high voltage paper electrophoresis. Greater than 90% of that reducing terminal sugar of the HS fragments where glucuronic acid, indicating that this enzyme is a β-endoglucuronidase (heparanase).

It is likely that similar enzymes could also be important in restructuring endothelial basal lamina, for example, during angiogenesis and leukocyte extravasation. Indeed, HS endoglycosidases have been found in normal tissues (98-100). The cleavage of heparan sulfate by B16 heparanase may require the recognition of N-acetyl groups, as well as sulfate groups, since heparanase can distinguish HS from heparin and cleave the former at specific intrachain sites (95). HS differs from heparin by its higher content of D-glucuronic acid residues and N-acetyl groups and its lower sulfate content (101). These differences, and the fact that HS has been described as a 'block-type' structure with areas low in sulfate, high in N-acetyl groups and intermediate or high in O- and N-sulfate, suggests that B16 heparanase may recognize one or more block-type structures, and cleave HS into specific intermediate molecular weight fragments (95).

ACKNOWLEDGMENTS

Supported by Research Grant RO1-CA28844 and RO1-CA28867 from the National Institutes of Health U.S. Public Health (to G.L. Nicolson), American Cancer Society Institutional Grant IN-34 (to M. Nakajima) and IN-121B (to T. Irimura).

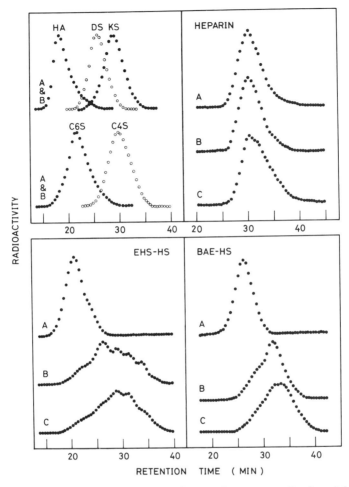

FIGURE 3. Analysis of Glycosaminoglycan Fragments Produced by B16 Melanoma Glycosidases. Incubation products were analyzed by high-speed gel permeation chromatography according to Irimura et al. (86). HA, hyaluronic acid from human umbilical cord; DS, dermatan sulfate from porcine mucosal tissue; KS, keratan sulfate from bovine cornea; C6S, chondroitin 6-sulfate from shark cartilage; C4S, chondroitin 4-sulfate from rock; heparin from porcine intestinal mucosa; EHS-HS, heparan sulfate from EHS sarcoma; BAE-HS, heparan sulfate from BAE subendothelial matrix. A, glycosaminoglycans incubated with heat-inactivated B16-BL6 cell extracts; B, glycosaminoglycans incubated with B16 extracts in the presence of 20 mM SAL; C, glycosaminoglycans incubated with B16 cell extracts without SAL [From Nakajima et al. (95) with permission.]

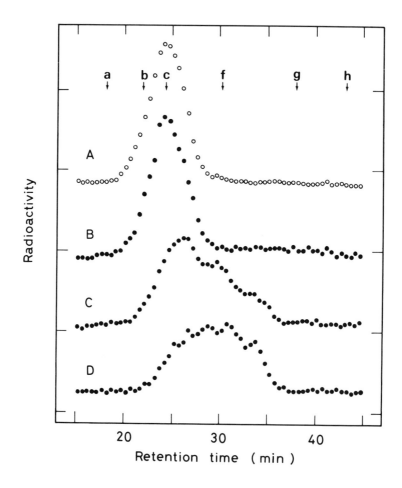

FIGURE 4. Effect of Heparin on Heparan Sulfate (HS) Degradation by B16 Heparanase. HS from bovine lung was incubated with B16-BL6 cell extracts containing 20 mM SAL for 6 hr at 37°C in the presence or absence of porcine intestinal mucosa heparin. Samples were analyzed by high-speed gel permeation chromatography. A, HS incubated with heat-inactivated B16 cell extract; B, HS incubated with B16 cell extract in the presence of 10 µg heparin; C, HS incubated with cell B16 extract in the presence of an additional 10 µg of HS; D, HS incubated with B16 cell extract. Arrows at a,b,c,f,g and h indicate the elution positions of standard glycans [From Nakajima et al. (95) with permission.]

REFERENCES

1. Sugarbaker EV: Cancer metastasis: A product of tumor-host interactions. Curr. Prob. Cancer 3:3-59, 1979.
2. Nicolson GL: Cancer metastasis: Organ colonization and the cell surface properties of malignant cells. Biochim. Biophys. Acta 695:113-176, 1982.
3. Sugarbaker EV: Patterns of metastasis in human malignancies. Cancer Biol. Rev. 2:235-278, 1981.
4. Nicolson GL, Poste G: Tumor implantation and invasion at metastatic sites. Int. Rev. Exp. Pathol. 25:77-181, 1983.
5. Salsbury AJ: The significance of the circulating cancer cells. Cancer Treatment Rev. 2:55-72, 1975.
6. Fidler IJ, Nicolson GL: Organ selectivity for implantation, survival and growth of B16 melanoma variant tumor lines. J. Natl. Cancer Inst. 57:1199-1201, 1976.
7. Hart IR, Fidler IJ: The implications of tumor heterogeneity for studies on the biology and therapy of cancer metastasis. Biochim. Biophys. Acta 651:37-50, 1981.
8. Zeidman I, Buss JM: Transpulmonary passage of tumor cell emboli. Cancer Res. 12:731-733, 1952.
9. Sindelar WF, Tralka TS, Ketcham AS: Electron microscopic observations on formation of pulmonary metastases. J. Surg. Res. 18:137-161, 1975.
10. Roos E, Dingemans KP, Van De Pavert IV, Van Den Bergh-Weerman M: Invasion of lymphosarcoma cells into the perfused mouse liver. J. Natl. Cancer Inst. 58:399-407, 1977.
11. Kawaguchi T, Kawaguchi M, Lembo TM, Nicolson GL: Influence of splenectomy on brain meninges tumor formation by murine melanoma variants. (In preparation).
12. Hart IR: Seed and soil revisisted. Mechanism of site specific metastasis. Cancer Metastasis Rev. 1:5-16, 1982.
13. Fidler IJ: Patterns of tumor cell arrest and development. IN: Weiss L (ed.) Fundamental Aspects of Metastasis. North-Holland Publishing Co., Amsterdam, pp. 275-289, 1976.
14. Warren BA: Origin and fate of blood-borne tumor emboli. Cancer Biol. Rev. 2:95-169, 1981.
15. Weiss L: Random and non-random processes in metastasis and metastatic efficiency. Invasion Metastasis 3:193-208, 1983.
16. Hanna N: Expression of metastatic potential of tumor cells in young nude mice is correlated with low levels of natural killer cell-mediated cytotoxicity. Int. J. Cancer 26:675-680, 1980.
17. Hanna N, Fidler IJ: Role of natural killer cells in the destruction of circulating tumor emboli. J. Natl. Cancer Inst. 65:801-809, 1980.

292

18. Kinsey DL: An experimental study of preferential metastasis. Cancer 13:674-676, 1960.

19. Hart IR, Fidler IJ: Cancer invasion and metastasis. Q. Rev. Biol. 55:121-142, 1980.

20. Nicolson GL, Poste G: Tumor cell diversity and host responses in cancer metastasis. I. Properties of metastatic cells. Curr. Prob. Cancer 7(6):1-83, 1982.

21. Nicolson GL, Poste G: Tumor cell diversity and host responses in cancer metastasis. II. Host immune responses and therapy of metastases. Curr. Prob. Cancer 7(7):1-43, 1983.

22. Nicolson GL: Cell surface molecules and tumor metastasis. Regulation of metastatic diversity. Exp. Cell Res. 150:3-22, 1984.

23. Heppner GH, Miller BE: Tumor heterogeneity: Biological implications and therapeutic consequences. Cancer Metastasis Rev. 2:5-23, 1983.

24. Peterson JA, Bartholomew JC, Stampfer M, Ceriani RL: Analysis of expression of human mammary epithelial antigens in normal and malignant breast cells at the single cell level by flow cytofluorimetry. Exp. Cell Biol. 49:1-14, 1981.

25. Peterson JA, Ceriani RL, Blank EW, Osvaldo L: Comparison of rates of phenotypic variability in surface antigen expression in normal and cancerous breast epithelial cells. Cancer Res. 43:4291-4296, 1983.

26. Nowell PC: The clonal evolution of tumor cell populations. Science 194:23-28, 1976.

27. Fialkow PJ: Clonal origin of human tumors. Ann. Rev. Med. 30:135-176, 1979.

28. Nowell PC: Tumor progression and clonal evolution: The role of genetic instability. IN: German J (ed.) Chromosome Mutation and Neoplasia. Alan R. Liss, Inc., New York, pp. 413-432, 1983.

29. Nicolson GL: Generation of phenotypic diversity and progression in metastatic tumors. Cancer Metastasis Rev. 3:25-42, 1984.

30. Nicolson GL: Tumor progress, oncogenes and the evolution of metastatic phenotypic diversity. Clin. Exp. Metastasis (In press).

31. Foulds L: Neoplastic Development. Academic Press, New York, 1975.

32. Heppner GH, Loveless SE, Miller FR, Mahoney KH, Fulton AM: Mammary tumor heterogeneity. IN: Nicolson GL and Milas L (eds.) Cancer Invasion and Metastasis: Biologic and Therapeutic Aspects. Raven Press, New York, pp. 209-221, 1984.

33. Hagmar B, Norrby K: Influence of cultivation, trypsinization and aggregation on the transplantibility of melanoma B16 cells. Int. J. Cancer 11:663-675, 1973.

34. Fidler IJ: General considerations for studies of experimental cancer metastasis. Meth. Cancer Res. 15:399-439, 1978.

35. Irimura T, Gonzalez R, Nicolson GL: Effects of tunicamycin on B16 metastatic melanoma cell surface glycoproteins and blood-borne arrest and survival properties. Cancer Res. 41:3411-3418, 1981.

36. Irimura T, Nicolson GL: The role of glycoconjugates in metastatic melanoma blood-borne arrest and cell surface properties. J. Supramol. Struct. Cell. Biochem. 17:325-336, 1981.
37. Poste G, Nicolson GL: Arrest and metastasis of blood-borne tumor cells are modified by fusion of plasma membrane vesicles from highly metastatic cells. Proc. Natl. Acad. Sci. USA 77:399-403, 1980.
38. Fidler IJ: The relationship of embolic homogeneity, number, size and viability to the incidence of experimental metastasis. Eur. J. Cancer 9:223-227, 1973.
39. Liotta LA, Kleinerman J, Saidel GM: The significance of hematogenous tumor cell clumps in the metastatic process. Cancer Res. 36:889-894, 1976.
40. Zeidman I, Buss JM: Experimental studies on the spread of cancer in the lymphatic system. I. Effectiveness of the lymph node as a barrier to the passaage of embolic tumor cells. Cancer Res. 14:403-405, 1954.
41. Sato H, Suzuki M: Deformability and viability of tumor cells by transcapillary passage, with reference to organ affinity of metastasis in cancer. IN: Weiss L (ed.) Fundamental Aspects of Metastasis. North-Holland Publishing Co., Amsterdam, pp. 311-317, 1976.
42. Fisher B, Fisher ER: Anticoagulants and tumor cell lodgment. Cancer Res. 27:421-425, 1967.
43. Winkelhake JL, Nicolson GL: Preparation of protease-free neuraminidase by affinity adsorption on fetuin derivatized cellulose. Anal. Biochem. 71:281-289, 1976.
44. Nicolson GL, Irimura T, Nakajima M, Updyke TV, Poste G: The cellular interactions of metastatic tumor cells with special reference to endothelial cells and their basal lamina-like matrix. IN: Honn KV and Sloane BF (eds.) Hemostatic Mechanisms and Metastasis. Martinus Nijhoff, The Hague, pp. 295-318, 1984.
45. Nicolson GL: Experimental tumor metastasis: Characteristics and organ specificity. Bioscience 28:441-447, 1978.
46. Raz A, Lotan R: Lectin-like activities associated with human and murine neoplastic cells. Cancer Res. 41:3642-3647, 1981.
47. Gasic GJ, Gasic TB, Galanti N, Johnson T, Murphy S: Platelet-tumor cell interaction in mice. The role of platelets in the spread of malignant disease. Int. J. Cancer 11:704-718, 1973.
48. Gasic GJ, Boettiger D, Catalfamo JL, Gasic TB, Stewart GJ: Aggregation of platelets and cell membrane vesiculation by rat cells transformed in vitro by Rous sarcoma virus. Cancer Res. 38:2950-2955, 1978.
49. Pearlstein E, Salk PL, Yogeeswaran G, Karpatkin S: Correlation between spontaneous metastatic potential, platelet-aggregating activity of cell surface extracts, and cell surface sialylation in 10 metastatic-variant derivatives of rat renal sarcoma cell line. Proc. Natl. Acad. Sci. USA 77:4336-4339, 1980.
50. Fisher B, Fisher ER: Experimental studies of factors which influence hepatic metastasis. VIII. Effect of anticoagulants. Surgery 50:240-247, 1961.

51. Brown JM: A study of the mechanism by which anticoagulation with Warfarin inhibits blood-borne metastasis. Cancer Res. 33:1217-1224, 1973.

52. Nicolson GL, Irimura T, Nakajima M, Estrada J: Metastatic cell attachment to and invasion of vascular endothelium and its underlying basal lamina using endothelial cell monolayers. IN: Nicolson GL and Milas L (eds.) Cancer Invasion and Metastasis: Biologic and Therapeutic Aspects. Raven Press, New York, pp. 145-167, 1984.

53. Estrada J, Nicolson GL: Tumor cell-platelet aggregation does not correlate with metastatic potential of rat 13762NF mammary adenocarcinoma tumor cells clones. Int. J. Cancer (In press).

54. Fidler IJ: Activation in vitro of mouse macrophages by syngeneic, allogeneic, or xenogeneic lymphocyte supernatants. J. Natl. Cancer Inst. 55:1159-1163, 1975.

55. Fidler IJ, Bucana C: Resistance of tumor cells to lysis by syngeneic lymphocytes: A possible mechanism. Cancer Res. 37:3945-3956, 1977.

56. Fidler IJ, Gersten DM, Budmen MB: Characterization in vivo and in vitro of tumor cells selected for resistance to syngeneic lymphocyte-mediated cytotoxicity. Cancer Res. 36:3160-3165, 1976.

57. Vaage J, Agarwal S: Stimulation or inhibition of immune resistance against metastatic or local growth of a C3H mammary carcinoma. Cancer Res. 36:1831-1836, 1976.

58. Gorelik E, Fogel M, Segal S, Feldman M: Tumor-associated antigenic differences between the primary and the descendant metastatic tumor cell populations. J. Supramol. Struct. 12:385-402, 1979.

59. Hanna N: Inhibition of experimental tumor metastasis by selective activation of natural killer cells. Cancer Res. 42:1337-1342, 1982.

60. Gorelik E, Segal S, Shapiro J, Katsav S, Ron Y, Feldman M: Interactions between the local tumor and its metastases. Cancer Metastasis Rev. 1:83-94, 1982.

61. Hanna N, Fidler IJ: Relationship between metastatic potential and resistance to NK cell-mediated cytotoxicity in three murine tumor systems. J. Natl. Cancer Inst. 66:1183-1190, 1981.

62. Chew EC, Josephson RK, Wallace AC: Morphologic aspects of the arrest of circulating cancer cells. IN: Weiss L (ed.) Fundamental Aspects of Metastasis. North-Holland Publishing Co., Amsterdam, pp. 121-150, 1976.

63. Kinjo M, Oka K, Naito S, Kohga S, Tanaka K, Oboshi S, Hayata Y, Yasumoto K: Thromboplastic and fibrinolytic activities of cultured human cancer cell lines. Br. J. Cancer 39:15-23, 1979.

64. Dingemans KP: Invasion of liver tissue by blood-borne mammary carcinoma cells. J. Natl. Cancer Inst. 53:1813-1819, 1974.

65. Nakamura K, Kawaguchi T, Asahina S, Sakurai T, Ebina Y, Yokoya S, Morita M: Electron microscopic studies on extravasation of tumor cells and early foci of hematogenous metastases. Gann Monogr. Res. 20:57-71, 1977.

66. Kawaguchi T, Kawaguchi M, Miner KM, Lembo TM, Nicolson GL: Brain meninges tumor formation by in vivo-selected metastatic B16 melanoma variants in mice. Clin. Exp. Metastasis 3:247-259, 1983.

67. Kawaguchi T, Kawaguchi M, Dulski K, Nicolson GL: Cellular behavior of metastatic B16 melanoma in experimental blood-borne implantation and cerebral invasion: An electron microscopy study. Invasion Metastasis (In press).

68. Kramer RH, Nicolson GL: Interactions of tumor cells with vascular endothellial cell monolayers: A model for metastatic invasion. Proc. Natl. Acad. Sci. USA 76:5704-5708, 1979.

69. Nicolson GL: Metastatic tumor cell attachment and invasion assay utilizing vascular endothelial cell monolayers. J. Histochem. Cytochem. 30:214-220, 1982.

70. Dingemans KP: Behavior of intravenously injected malignant lymphoma cells: A morphologic study. J. Natl. Cancer Inst. 51:1883-1897, 1973.

71. Roos E, Dingemans KP: Infiltration of metastasizing tumor cells into liver and lungs. IN: Schweiger HS (ed.) International Cell Biology 1980-1981. Springer-Verlag, Berlin, p. 774, 1981.

72. Joseph J, Miao T, Alby L, Grieves J, Houser B, Kubai L, Morrissey L, Sidky YA, Watt SL, Auerbach G: Immunological probes for the study of endothelial cell diversity. IN: Thilo D (ed.) Endothelial Cell Identification and Culture Methods. Karger, Basel, pp. 25-29, 1984.

73. Belloni PN, Nicolson GL: In situ cell surface radiolabelling of various organ vascular endothelium. An analysis and localization by tissue autoradiography and SDS-PAGE. IN: Biology of the Vascular Endothelial Cell, Third International Symposium (Abstract), p. 38, 1984.

74. Kramer RH, Nicolson GL: Invasion of vascular endothelial cell monolayers and underlying matrix by metastatic human cancer cells. IN: Schweiger S (ed.) International Cell Biology 1980-1981. Springer-Verlag, Heidelberg, pp. 794-799, 1981.

75. Kramer RH, Gonzalez R, Nicolson GL: Metastatic tumor cells adhere preferentially to the extracellular matrix underlying vascular endothelial cells. Int. J. Cancer 26:639-645, 1980.

76. Nicolson GL, Irimura T, Gonzalez R, Ruoslahti E: The role of fibronectin in adhesion of metastatic melanoma cells to endothelial cells and their basal lamina. Exp. Cell Res. 135:461-465, 1981.

77. Ludatsher RM, Luse SA, Suntseff V: An electron microscopic study of pulmonary tumor emboli from transplanted Morris hepatoma 5123. Cancer Res. 27:1939-1952, 1967.

78. Poste G, Nicolson GL: In vitro systems for studying the interaction of metastatic tumour cells with endothelial cells and subendothelial basement membranes. IN: Jaffe EA (ed.) The Biology of Endothelial Cells, (27) of Development in Cardiovascular Medicine. Martinus Nijhoff, The Hague, pp. 438-449, 1983.

79. Wood S, Jr: Experimental studies of the intravascular dissemination of ascitic V2 carcinoma cells in the rabbit, with special reference to fibrinogen and fibrinolytic agents. Bull. Schweiz. Akad. Med. Wiss. 20:92-121, 1964.

80. Terranova VP, Rohrbach DH, Martin GR: Role of laminin in the attachment of PAM212 (epithelial) cells to basement membrane collagen. Cell 22:719-726, 1980.

81. Gospodarowicz D, Greenburg G, Foidart JM, Savion N: The production and localization of laminin in cultured vascular and corneal endothelial cells. J. Cell. Physiol. 107:171-183, 1981.

82. Howard BV, Macarak EJ, Gunson D, Kefalides NA: Characterization of the collagen synthesized by endothelial cells in culture. Proc. Natl. Acad. Sci. USA 73:2361-2364, 1976.

83. Murray CJ, Liotta LA, Rennard SI, Martin GR: Adhesion characteristics of murine metastatic and non-metastatic tumor cells in vitro. Cancer Res. 40:347-351, 1980.

84. Liotta LA, Tryggvason S, Garbisa S, Hart I, Foltz CM, Shafie S: Metastatic propensity correlates with tumor cell degradation of basement membrane collagen. Nature (London) 284:67-68, 1980.

85. Kramer RH, Vogel KG, Nicolson GL: Tumor cell interactions with vascular endothelial cells and their extracellular matrix. IN: Jamieson GA (ed.) Interaction of Platelets and Tumor Cells. Alan R. Liss, Inc., New York, pp. 333-351, 1982.

86. Irimura T, Nakajima M, DiFerrante N, Nicolson GL: High-speed gel permeation chromatography of glycosaminoglycans: Its application to the analysis of heparan sulfate of embryonic carcinoma and its degradation products by tumor cell derived heparanase. Anal. Biochem. 130:461-468, 1983.

87. Irimura T, Nakajima M, Nicolson GL: Metastatic tumor cell attachment to vascular endothelial cells and destruction of their basal lamina-like matrix. Gann Monogr. Cancer Res. 29:35-46, 1983.

88. Nakajima M, Irimura T, DiFerrante DT, DiFerrante N, Nicolson GL: Heparan sulfate degradation correlates with tumor invasive and metastatic properties of B16 melanoma sublines. Science 220:611-613, 1983.

89. Mareel MM: Recent aspects of tumor invasiveness. Int. Rev. Exp. Pathol. 22:65-129, 1980.

90. Nicolson GL, Winkelhake JL: Organ specificity of blood-borne tumour metastasis determined by cell adhesion? Nature (London) 255:230-232, 1975.

91. Phondke GP, Madyastha KR, Madyastha PR, Barth RF: Relationship between concanavalin A-induced agglutin-ability of murine leukemia cells and their propensity to form heterotypic aggregates with syngeneic lymphoid cells. J. Natl. Cancer Inst. 66:643-647, 1981.

92. Schirrmacher V, Cheinsong-Popov R, Arnheiter H: Hepatocyte-tumor cell interaction in vitro. I. Conditions for rosette formation and inhibition by anti-H-2 antibody. J. Exp. Med. 151:984-989, 1980.

93. Liotta LA, Thorgeirsson UP, Garbisa S: Role of collagenases in tumor cell invasion. Cancer Metastasis Rev. 1:277-317, 1982.

94. Vlodavsky I, Aviva Y, Fucks Z, Altevogt P, Schirrmacher V: Lymphoma cell-mediated degradation of sulfated proteoglycans in the subendothelial extracellular matrix: Relationship to tumor cell metastasis. Cancer Rev. 43:2704-2711, 1983.

95. Nakajima M, Irimura T, DiFerrante N, Nicolson GL: Metastatic melanoma cell heparanase. Characterization of heparan sulfate degradation fragments produced by B16 melanoma endoglucuronidase. J. Biol. Chem. 259:2283-2290, 1984.

96. Sloane BF, Dunn JR, Honn KV: Lysosomal cathepsin B: Correlation with metastatic potential. Science 212:1151-1153, 1981.

97. Sloane BF, Honn KV, Sadler JG, Turner WA, Kimpson JJ, Taylor JD: Cathepsin B activity in B16 melanoma cells: A possible marker for metastatic potential. Cancer Res. 42:980-986, 1982.

98. Hook M, Wasteson A, Oldberg A: A heparan sulfate degrading endoglycosidase from rat liver tissue. Biochem. Biophys. Res. Commun. 67:1422-1428, 1975.

99. Wasteson A, Glimelius B, Bush D, Westermark B, Heldin C-H, Norling B: Effect of a platelet endoglycosidase on cell surface associated heparan sulfate of human cultured endothelial and glial cells. Thromb. Res. 11:309-311, 1977.

100. Klein U, von Figura K: Partial purification and characterization of a heparan sulfate specific endoglucuronidase. Biochem. Biophys. Res. Commun. 73:569-576, 1976.

101. Linker A, Hovingh P: The heparitin sulfates (Heparan Sulfate). Carbohydrate Res. 29:41-62, 1973.

CHAPTER 19. DOMAINS OF LAMININ AND BASEMENT MEMBRANE COLLAGEN WHICH PLAY A ROLE IN METASTASES

LANCE A. LIOTTA, NAGESWARA C. RAO, SANFORD H. BARSKY AND TAINA M. TURPEENNIEMI-HUJANEN

I. DOMAINS OF LAMININ WHICH ALTER METASTASES

Metastasis is a complex multistep process in which interaction of tumor cell surface components with the extracellular matrix may play a role (1-7). An important type of matrix traversed by tumor cells at multiple stages of metastases is the continuous basement membrane. Metastasizing tumor cells traverse endothelial basement membranes during both entrance into and egress from the circulation (8). The initial step of this traversal is thought to be attachment (9), which may be mediated in part through tumor cell surface receptor binding to laminin, a glycoprotein uniquely localized to basement membranes (1-4). We have previously demonstrated that human carcinoma cells and murine BL6 melanoma cells bind laminin with high affinity and that they possess a cell surface plasma membrane laminin receptor with a M_r of approximately 67,000 (1-3). A similar receptor has been identified on murine fibrosarcoma cells (4). Murine melanoma cells can be selected for metastatic propensity based on their ability to use laminin to attach to type IV collagen in vitro (10). Those tumor cells which preferentially utilize laminin for attachment exhibit a ten fold increase in metastatic propensity (10). By electron microscopy the laminin molecule has the structure of a "cross" with one long arm (75 nm) and three short arms (37 nm), each containing globular end regions (1,5,11). The carbohydrate composition of laminin is heterogeneous. Specific sugar moieties are enriched on the globular end regions compared to the rod shaped portions of the molecule (11). Digestion of laminin with alpha thrombin will remove the long arm but leave the short arms intact (12). Cathepsin G or chymotrypsin will produce a laminin fragment devoid of the long arm and the globular end regions of the short arms (12). The C_1 fragment is "T" shaped and contains the disulfide "knot" where the three short arms are joined together.

We have developed an experimental model to study the domains of the laminin molecule which alter experimental metastases. We have investigated the effect of whole laminin and its two purified proteinase fragments on the production of pulmonary metastases by BL6 melanoma cells (10,13) injected intravenously.

Syngeneic laminin was extracted from the C57 black mouse Engelbreth-Holm-Swarm (EHS) tumor in 50 mM Tris, 0.5 M NaCl, pH 7.6, and purified by DEAE-cellulose and agarose A-5 column chromatography as described previously (1). The alpha fragment and the C_1 fragment of laminin were purified and characterized by rotary shadowing electron microscopy as described previously (1,2,13). The alpha fragment was produced by complete digestion of the subunit of laminin by thrombin and verified by SDS polyacrylamide slab gel electrophoresis. The C_1 fragment was produced in an analogous manner by digestion of laminin with cathepsin G. Complete digestion of the subunit was achieved and verified by SDS polyacrylamide gel electrophoresis.

Cultured BL6 cells were removed with EDTA and washed in serum-free RPMI media. The suspended cells were then incubated in serum-free media with either whole laminin or the purified fragments. The incubation was carried out under gentle agitation for 30 min at room temperature. After incubation and cell washing, a single cell suspension ($0.5 - 2.0 \times 10^5$ cells) was injected via the tail vein into 3 wk old C57 black female mice. Viability of $> 95\%$ (by Trypan blue dye exclusion) and the absence of cell clumps was verified by hemocytometer inspection of the cells, after incubation and immediately prior to injection (14).

All mice were sacrificed 3 wk after injection. The lungs were removed, inflated with Bouin's fixative and the number of metastases determined by inspecting separated lung lobes with a dissecting microscope. As an additional control for viability, tumor cells which had undergone preincubation with whole laminin or the laminin fragments were injected into the subcutaneous tissue and tumorigenicity assessed.

BL6 tumor cells were harvested using EDTA or trypsin and suspended in 0.05 M Tris/saline buffer, pH 7.4, with calcium (5 mM) and magnesium (1 mM). BL6 tumor cells (2×10^5) were incubated for 60 min at 25°C in a volume of 1 ml with ^{125}I labeled with or without 100x ligand excess competitor (3). Additional binding experiments were performed with ^{125}I labeled alpha fragment and ^{125}I labeled C_1 fragment. Scatchard analysis was performed.

To study the effect of laminin on tumor cell retention in the lung, tumor cells were labeled with $[^{125}I]UdR$ as described previously (15). The labeled cells were preincubated with the ligands as described in Table 1. The number of mice in each group was 8 with 25,000 cpm (0.75 cpm/10^5 cells) injected per mouse. At various time intervals after injection the mice were sacrificed and the total radioactivity in each lung counted (16).

We also investigated the effect of laminin domains on tumor cell attachment to whole basement membranes. Intact native amnion membrane surfaces were prepared as described previously (17). The basement membrane surface was verified to contain both abundant laminin and type IV collagen by immunohistology. Attachment was conducted in serum-free media at 37°C using amnion chambers containing a surface area of 1.5 cm^2. Labeled tumor cells were placed in these chambers. The basement membrane surface was washed at a series of time intervals and the number of attached cells was determined by counting the bound radioactivity.

EFFECT OF WHOLE LAMININ OR ITS C1 FRAGMENT
ON PULMONARY METASTASES FORMATION

EXP.	NO. CELLS INJECTED	N	PULMONARY METASTASES MEDIAN (Range)		
			CONTROL	+ LAMININ 10 μg/ml	+ C1 10 μg/ml
1.	0.5×10^5	10	12(3-22)	72(38-90)	—
2.	0.5×10^5	10	15(5-18)	65(33-80)	—
3.	0.75×10^5	10	28(15-30)	110(45-130)	1(0-6)
4.	0.75×10^5	10	18(6-26)	80(30-110)	2(0-5)
5.	1.0×10^5	10	75(25-90)	165(80-240)	5(0-10)
6.	1.0×10^5	5	85(30-100)	122(24-162)	6(0-16)
7.	2.0×10^5	10	98(50-106)	210(150-290)	40(28-55)

Table 1. Effect of Whole Laminin or its C_1 Fragment on Pulmonary Metastases Formation. Murine BL6 melanoma cells were trypsinized and allowed to regenerate cell surface laminin receptors. The cells were preincubated for 30 min at 25°C in serum free media containing whole laminin or the C_1 fragment at a concentration of 10 μg/ml. Control cells were incubated in media alone. The washed cells were injected via tail vein. In all groups, at least 90% of the cells were in single cell form. The number of cells injected per mouse and the number of mice (N) in each group is listed. Three weeks after injection all mice were sacrificed and the number of pulmonary metastases were counted in separated lung lobes. Significant differences between the treatment groups and the control (p < 0.05) were noted for all experiments except No. 7 (+ C_1 group) using both Student's t test and the Mann-Whitney test.

The suspended BL6 cells demonstrate saturable binding for laminin. Scatchard analysis demonstrates 90-115,000 binding sites/cell with high affinity (K_d = 2 nM). The C_1 fragment and the alpha fragment compete for the laminin receptor as well as the whole laminin molecule (18). Collagen, denatured laminin, and fibronectin do not compete for binding. The K_d for the binding of the fragments is similar to that found for whole laminin (18). Therefore, these data indicate that the long arm and the globular end regions of the laminin molecule are not required for binding to the tumor cell receptor. Binding of laminin to the tumor cell surface was verified by immunofluorescence studies utilizing the addition of exogenous laminin to a monolayer of cultured BL6 cells followed by rabbit anti-laminin and fluorescein-conjugated goat anti-rabbit. In the absence of exogenous laminin, surface immunofluorescence was absent.

Tumor cells labeled with [^{125}I]UdR displayed significant differences _in vivo_ in lung retention at 60 min, 5 hr and 20 hr depending on whether they were incubated with whole laminin or the C_1 fragment (Figure 1). The C_1 fragment markedly decreased retention of BL6 cells in the lungs whereas whole laminin increased retention. The attachment of tumor cells _in vitro_ to native basement membrane of human amnion was significantly altered by the addition of exogenous laminin or the C_1 laminin fragment. The time course of attachment reached a plateau in all three groups at 3 hr. Whole laminin stimulated attachment. In contrast the C_1 fragment reduced attachment (Figure 1 insert).

The effect of laminin and the C_1 fragment on the number of metastases paralleled the lung retention data. The C_1 fragment markedly decreased or abolished pulmonary metastases in a dose-dependent fashion whereas whole laminin or the alpha fragment markedly increased metastatic number (Table 2). The laminin fragments or whole laminin had no effect on the percent take or growth rate of tumors produced by BL6 cells injected subcutaneously. BL6 cells incubated with denatured laminin, and BL6 cells alone injected 15 min after intravenous laminin infusion showed no change in metastatic number.

We can hypothesize that tumor cells with free laminin receptors may utilize these receptors to interact with the laminin in vascular basement membrane. Saturating these receptors with added laminin results in an increase rather than a decrease in lung retention and metastasis because BL6 tumor cells with added laminin utilize the globular end regions of this molecule to interact with basement membrane type IV collagen or proteoglycan. In a similar manner, other tumor cells which may already have on their surface self-secreted laminin may utilize this molecule to promote their attachment to basement membranes. This argument has been supported by the study of Varani et al. (19) demonstrating an endogenous laminin-like substance on the cell surface of highly metastatic fibrosarcoma cells. This substance is absent from low metastatic cells derived from the same parent. The addition of laminin to these low metastatic cells promotes metastasis.

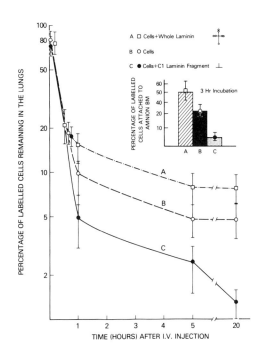

FIGURE 1. Pulmonary Retention of Labeled BL6 Tumor Cells Injected Intravenously. Whole laminin increased pulmonary retention whereas the C_1 fragment produced a significant decrease in retention which became more pronounced at later times. Insert: Amnion basement membrane attachment in vitro. $[^{125}I]$Udr labeled tumor cells attached were measured. The plateau of attachment was reached at 3 hr. The data shown is the percent attached cells: a) cells treated with whole laminin (10 μg/ml), b) untreated cells, and c) cells treated with the C_1 fragment (10 μg/ml).

However, the C_1 laminin fragment, a fragment of laminin which lacks the globular end regions but binds to the cell, can inhibit metastasis because it can block the laminin receptor without increasing the cell's ability to interact with other basement membrane components.

DOSE DEPENDENT EFFECT OF LAMININ FRAGMENTS
ON PULMONARY METASTASES FORMATION

EXPERIMENTAL GROUP	PULMONARY METASTASES MEDIAN (Range)	PERCENT CHANGE
A. BL6 Tumor Cells Alone	19(10-30)	—
B. BL6 Tumor Cells + Laminin		
1 μg/ml	34(22-68)	100% Increase
10 μg/ml	80(39-120)	300% Increase
100 μg/ml	102(55-141)	400% Increase
C. BL6 Tumor Cells + Alpha Fragment		
10 μg/ml	72(58-130)	280% Increase
100 μg/ml	114(42-138)	400% Increase
D. BL6 Tumor Cells + C1 Fragment		
1 μg/ml	18(12-29)	No Change
10 μg/ml	8(6-9)	50% Decrease
100 μg/ml	2(0-10)	90% Decrease

Table 2. Dose Dependent Effect of Laminin Fragments on Pulmonary Metastases Formation. The experiments were conducted as described in the legend to Table 1, except that the tumor cells were incubated with a series of different concentrations of the ligand. The structure of the laminin molecule or the fragment is depicted. The number of cells injected was 0.5×10^5 with 10 mice in each experimental group. Aliquots of the same cell suspension were injected subcutaneously. 100% tumorigenicity was observed in all groups with no differences in subcutaneous tumor growth rate.

II. DOMAINS OF TYPE IV COLLAGEN CLEAVAGE

Following attachment, the next step in tumor cell invasion of the basement membrane is degradation of this matrix. The basement membrane is an insoluble meshwork with type IV collagen comprising the major structural supporting scaffold. Thus a limiting factor in the degradation of the basement membrane is lysis of type IV collagen. Classic collagenases which cleave interstitial collagens fail to degrade basement membrane type IV collagen. Type V collagen which is associated with the basement membrane interface with the stroma is also resistant to classic interstitial collagenase. Therefore, separate classes of proteinases are required to degrade basement membrane associated collagens.

III. BASEMENT MEMBRANE DEGRADING COLLAGENASES

Type IV collagenase is inhibited by EDTA, and is thus a metallo proteinase. It specifically degrades basement membrane collagen, and cleaves procollagen IV into two segments which comprise $\frac{1}{4}$ and $\frac{3}{4}$ of the total length of the molecule (20,21; Figure 2). The cleavage site is

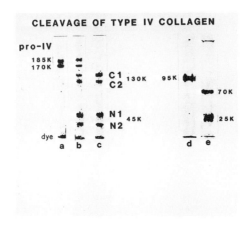

FIGURE 2. Type IV Collagen Degradation Products Identified by Sodium Dodecyl Sulfate Polyacrylamide Gel Electrophoresis (after reduction). The EHS mouse tumor type IV procollagen (22): (a) was incubated with enzyme 5 hr; (b) and 18 hr; (c) at 30°C. The cleavage yields peptides corresponding to $\frac{3}{4}$ (C_1 and C_2) and $\frac{1}{4}$ (N_1 and N_2) of the procollagen molecule; (d) pepsin digested placenta type IV collagen (12); (e) the placenta type IV collagen plus enzyme. Two cleavage products are produced consistent with a single site of cleavage.

located near the N-terminal end of the collagen molecule and the cleavage produces a complex containing the highly disulfide-linked "7-S region" joined with the residual parts of the four procollagen IV N-terminal ends (Figure 3). Type IV collagenase has been found in

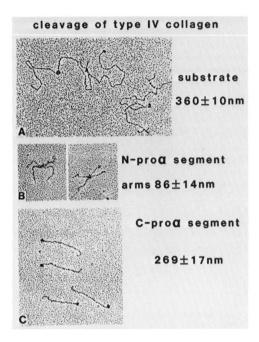

cleavage of type IV collagen

substrate
360±10nm

N-proα segment
arms 86±14nm

C-proα segment
269±17nm

FIGURE 3. Rotary Shadowing Electron Microscopy of Type IV Collagen Cleavage Products. Panel A: Type IV procollagen substrate. Four molecule are linked together to form a "7-S" bow tie shaped unit at the N-terminal end. The globular regions on the C-terminus link together at the other end of the molecule. Panel B: N-terminal segment of type IV cleavage product after treatment with the tumor type IV collagenase. Panel C: C-terminal cleavage product. The enzyme cleaves at a single site located 25% of the distance from the N-terminus.

normal migrating cells and metastatic tumor cells (23,24). The enzyme is secreted into the culture media in a latent form which can be activated with trypsin and plasmin. Type IV collagenase has been purified from a mouse tumor (pulmonary metastasis of the T241 sarcoma; 21), and from supernatants of cultured human sarcoma (HT-1080) and metastatic melanoma (A2058) cells (T. Turpeenniemi-Hujanen et al., unpublished). The enzyme migrated as a doublet on polyacrylamide gel with molecular weights of approximately 62,000 and 68,000. Type IV collagenase activity of culture supernatants or cell lysates is assayed using biosynthetically labeled, acid extracted EHS sarcoma type IV collagen substrate. Vascular dissemination of tumor cells is critical in the cascade of events that lead to metastases. Therefore, type IV collagenase might be one of the most important factors, although not sufficient, for metastasis formation. Type IV collagenolytic activity of many metastatic tumor cell lines studied has been shown to correlate with their malignancy (23). Nevertheless, it is unlikely that there is a strict quantitative relationship between the enzyme level and the metastatic capacity in all types of malignant tumors since there are many other cellular and host factors that are involved in the metastatic process (25). For example, tumor cells that secrete large amounts of collagenase but are also highly susceptible to host defense factors could be poorly metastatic.

REFERENCES

1. Rao CN, Margulies IM, Tralka TS, Terranova VP, Madri JA, Liotta LA: Isolation of a subunit of laminin and its role in molecular structure and tumor cell attachment. J. Biol. Chem. 257:9740-9744, 1982.
2. Terranova VP, Rao CN, Kalebic T, Margulies IM, Liotta LA: Laminin receptor on human breast carcinoma cells. Proc. Natl. Acad. Sci. USA 80:444-448, 1983.
3. Rao NC, Barsky SH, Terranova VP, Liotta LA: Isolation of a tumor cell laminin receptor. Biochem. Biophys. Res. Commun. 111:804-808, 1983.
4. Malinoff HL, Wicha MS: Isolation of a cell surface receptor protein for laminin from murine fibrosarcoma cells. J. Cell Biol. 96:1475-1479, 1983.
5. Engel J, Odermott E, Engel A, Madri JA, Furthmayr H, Rohde H, Timpl R: Shapes, domain, organization, and flexibility of laminin and fibronectin, two multifunctional proteins of the extracellular matrix. J. Mol. Biol. 150:97-120, 1981.
6. Nicolson GL, Poste G: The cancer cell: Dynamic aspects and modifications in cell-surface organization. N. Engl. J. Med. 295:197-203; 253-258, 1976.
7. Poste G, Nicolson GL: Biomembranes. Plenum Publishing Corp., New York, pp. 341-364, 1983.
8. Liotta L, Hart IR: Tumor Invasion and Metastasis. Martinus Nijhoff, The Hague, 1982.
9. Nicolson GL, Irimura T, Nakajima M, Estrada J: Metastatic cell attachment to and invasion of vascular endothelium and its underlying basal lamina using endothelial cell monolayers. IN: Nicolson GL and Milas L (eds.) Cancer Invasion and Metastasis: Biologic and Therapeutic Aspects, Raven Press, New York, pp. 145-167, 1984.
10. Terranova VP, Liotta LA, Russo RG, Martin GP: Role of laminin in the attachment and metastasis of murine tumor cells. Cancer Res. 42:2265-2269, 1982.
11. Rao CN, Goldstein IJ, Liotta LA: Lectin binding domains on laminin. Arch. Biochem. Biophys. 227:118-124, 1983.

308

12. Rao CN, Margulies IMK, Goldfarb RH, Madri JA, Woodley DT, Liotta LA: Differential proteolytic susceptibility of laminin alpha and beta subunits. Arch. Biochem. Biophys. 219:65-70, 1982.
13. Hart IR, Fidler IJ: The role of organ selectivity in the determination of metastatic patterns of the B16 melanoma. Cancer Res. 40:2281-2287, 1980.
14. Liotta LA, Kleinerman J, Saidel GM: The signifcance of hematogenous tumor cell clumps in the metastatic process. Cancer Res. 36:889-894, 1976.
15. Fidler IJ: Metastasis: Quantitataive analysis of distribution and fate of tumor emboli labelled with ^{125}I-5-iodo-2'-deoxyuridine. J. Natl. Cancer Inst. 45:773-782, 1970.
16. Liotta LA, Delisi C: Method for quantitating tumor cell removal and tumor cell invasive capacity in experimental metastases. Cancer Res. 37:4003-4008, 1977.
17. Russo RG, Foltz CM, Liotta LA: Preparation of whole surfaces of human intact basement membrane for tumor invasion studies. Clin. Exp. Metastasis 1:115-127, 1983.
18. Barsky SH, Rao NC, Williams J, Liotta LA: Domains of laminin which alter metastases in a murine model. J. Clin. Invest. (In press).
19. Varani J, Lovett EJ, McCoy JP, Garbisa A, Maddox DE, Goldstein IJ, Wicha M: Differential expression of a laminin-like substance by high and low metastatic tumor cells. Am. J. Pathol. 111:27-34, 1983.
20. Liotta LA, Tryggvason K, Garbisa S, Gehron-Robey P, Abe S: Partial purification and characterization of neutral protease which cleaves type IV collagen. Biochemistry 20:100-104, 1981.
21. Salo T, Liotta LA, Tryggvason K: Purification and characterization of a murine basement membrane collagen-degrading enzyme secreted by metastatic tumor cells. J. Biol. Chem. 258:3058-3063, 1983.
22. Timpl R, Martin GR, Buckner P, Wick G, Wiedemann H: Nature of the collagenous protein in a tumor basement membrane. Eur. J. Biochem. 84:43-52, 1978.
23. Liotta LA, Tryggvason K, Garbisa S, Hart I, Foltz CM, Shafie S: Metastatic potential correlates with enzymatic degradation of basement membrane collagen. Nature (London) 284:67-68, 1980.
24. Kalebic T, Garbisa S, Glaser B, Liotta LA: Basement membrane collagen: Degradation by migrating endothelial cells. Science 221:281-283, 1983.
25. Dabbous MK, El-Torky M, Haney L, Brinkley Sr. B., Sobhy N: Collagenase activity in rabbit carcinoma: Cell source and cell interactions. Int. J. Cancer 31:357-364, 1983.

CHAPTER 20. INTERACTION OF MALIGNANT CELLS WITH SUBSTRATA: ADHESION, DEGRADATION AND MIGRATION

JAMES QUIGLEY, EVA CRAMER, SANDRA FAIRBAIRN, RHONDA GILBERT, JANIS LACOVARA, GEORGE OJAKIAN and RANDI SCHWIMMER

I. INTRODUCTION

The experimental analysis of cultured malignant cells, although far removed from the natural environment in vivo, nevertheless has provided some basic and fundamental information on the biochemical and biological properties that appear to characterize oncogenic cells. Their proliferative ability, their surface membrane alterations, their morphological deviations, their aberrant metabolism, and their unique expression of specific genes were all discovered (and analyzed) in cell culture systems that have served as models for transformed cell behavior. The analysis of metastasis, however, requires a new and challenging approach to that property of malignant cells that usually spells disaster for the host. In the past five or six years imaginative and clever experimental approaches to metastasis have been initiated in an attempt to determine when and how tumor cells break away from their primary site, travel to distant tissues and establish themselves as secondary tumor growths. Selected isolation of tumor cells, the employment of unique animal models, and the use of complex whole organ cultures have made inroads into the mechanistic analysis of the metastatic cascade. Nevertheless, there still remain some basic properties of malignant cells, which are related to their metastatic potential, that can be examined and probed in cell culture.

One such feature of malignant cells is their interaction with biological substrata. Normal tissue substratum, whether it be connective tissue matrix or basement membrane, provides a restrictive barrier for normal cells that in part maintains tissue integrity. Malignant cells appear to circumvent this restriction and are able to alter the substratum they encounter and migrate into and through these rather formidable barriers. A malignant cell's initial and possibly highly specific interaction with substratum and its ability to migrate over and through it is a phenomenon that can be examined in culture on a biological and biochemical basis. Our laboratory in the past few years has been involved in two separate and distinct projects, one involves the directed migration of established tumor cells and the other involves the proteolytic activity of retrovirus transformed cells. In this chapter we will describe these two systems and establish a link between the two based on the theme that a malignant cell's encounter with a biological substratum involves the sequential processes of adhesion, degradation and migration.

II. EXPERIMENTAL RESULTS

A. The Role of Fibronectin as a Substratum for the Directed
    Migration of B16 Melanoma Cells

1. Fibronectin enhancement of directed migration of B16 melanoma
cells. When a suspension of B16 cells was placed in the upper
compartment of a chemotactic chamber, the directed migration of these
cells into a 12 μm pore nitrocellulose filter was stimulated by the
presence of fibronectin in the lower compartment (Table 1A). Fibonectin
placed in the upper compartment or equal concentrations of fibronectin
in both compartments, had little or no effect on B16 cell migration as
compared to controls (no fibronectin in either chamber). Other plasma
proteins placed in the lower compartment had only a minimal effect on
B16 cell migration (Table 1B). The specificity of the response was
further indicated by the absence of enhanced migration when the
incubation was carried out with trypsin-digested fibronectin or reduced
and alkylated fibronectin. The response to a positive gradient of
fibronectin was not due to low molecular weight chemotactic peptides
that might be present in the fibronectin preparation since exhaustive
dialysis of fibronectin did not diminish its stimulatory effect on cell
migration (Table 1B).

Table 1. Effect of Fibronectin on the Directed Migration of B16
Melanoma Cells in Chemotactic Chambers[*].

Protein Present in		Cell Migration into Filter (% of cell population)		
Upper	Lower	0-20 μm	20-40 μm	40-60 μm
A. None	None	35	65	0
None	Fibronectin	18	60	22
Fibronectin	None	34	62	2
Fibronectin	Fibronectin	36	64	0
B. None	None	26	71	3
None	Fibronectin	27	68	5
None	γ Globulin	27	67	6
None	Dialyzed Fibronectin	20	57	23
None	Trypsinized Fibronectin	29	67	4
None	Reduced Fibronectin	32	63	5

[*]Proteins were added to the chemotactic chambers at 300 μg/ml and were
prepared as described in Section III. Cell migration into cellulose
nitrate filters fitted between the upper and lower compartments of
chemotactic chambers was carried out and analyzed as described in
Section III.

A light micrograph further illustrating the effect of fibronectin is shown in Figure 1. After 5 hr, very few B16 cells migrated more than 20 to 30 μm from the surface of the filter when buffer only was in the lower compartment of the chemotactic chamber (Figure 1A). However, when fibronectin was present in the lower compartment, B16 cells were seen to have migrated considerably farther into the filter (Figure 1B).

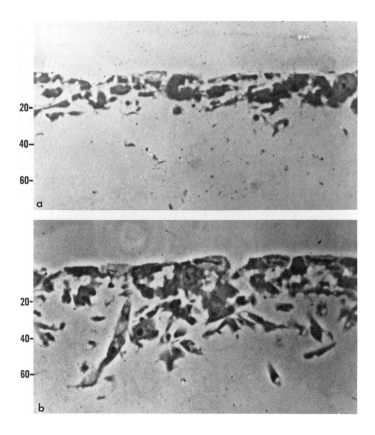

FIGURE 1. Light Micrograph of B16 Cells Migrating into Nitrocellulose Filters. B16 cell migration into filters was carried out for 5 hr. A, filter from a chemotactic chamber which contained buffer in the lower compartment. Very few cells have migrated more than 20 μm. B, filter from a chemotactic chamber which contained fibronectin in the lower compartment. Extensive migration away from the surface of the filter has occurred, and some cells have migrated as much as 60 μm (x 450).

The stimulation of B16 cell migration by a positive gradient of fibronectin exhibits a dose-response to fibronectin concentration and is time dependent, increasing between 1 and 5 hr, with overall cell migration slowing down between 5 and 10 hr (1). The observed stimulation of B16 cell migration is not due to fibronectin increasing the rate or extent of cell attachment to the filter, thereby giving rise to an apparent enhanced cell penetration into the filter. If cells are allowed to attach to filters in the absence of fibronectin and then filters containing equal numbers of cells are transferred to chemotactic chambers containing either buffer or fibronectin in the lower compartment, fibronectin still causes a 5 to 10-fold stimulation of cells migrating 40 μm or more into the filter (1). This indicates that the enhancing effect of fibronectin is on cell movement and is independent of cell attachment.

2. <u>Nature of the fibronectin response</u>. Fibronectin may exert its directed cell locomotory effect either as a soluble chemotactic agent, diffusing upward through the filter toward the migratory cells, or as a haptotatic agent, bound to the filter and mediating enhanced cell-substratum interaction along a concentration gradient of substratum-bound fibronectin. This was examined by pretreatment of the substratum (nitrocellulose filter) with fibronectin. Filters were incubated in the absence of cells in chemotactic chambers containing fibronectin above and/or below the filter in order to preestablish a fibronectin gradient within the filter. The filters were extensively washed to remove any unbound fibronectin within the filter pores. The washed filters were placed into a second set of chemotactic chambers. B16 cell migration across the pretreated filters was carried out in chambers containing only buffer in the upper and lower compartments. A standard migration assay was performed in parallel using untreated filters and a solution of fibronectin in the lower compartment. The results (Table 2) indicate that filters pretreated with fibronectin in the lower compartment significantly increased B16 cell migration as compared to filters that had been preincubated with buffer only in both compartments. The extent of B16 cell migration in a fibronectin-pretreated filter was equal to or greater than that observed when fibronectin was added directly to the lower compartment in the standard migration assay across an untreated filter. The pretreatment of filters in a homogeneous environment of fibronectin or with fibronectin in the upper compartment caused little or no migration beyond 40 μm.

These results suggested that fibronectin becomes bound to the filter and stimulates B16 cell migration as a haptotactic agent. To examine this, a migration assay was conducted with ^{125}I-labeled fibronectin in the lower compartment. After 1, 2.5, 5 and 10 hr of incubation, the lower compartments, the upper compartments and the filters were analyzed for radioactivity. The filters were washed extensively to remove any unbound radioactivity. The results (Figure 2) indicate that the disappearance of radioactivity from the lower compartment with time of incubation was not accompanied by a compensatory amount of radioactivity appearing in the upper compartment

Table 2. B16 Cell Migration into Filters Pretreated with Fibronectin.

Pretreatment Conditions*		Migration Conditions†		Migration (% cells migrating > 40 μm)
Fibronectin Present		Fibronectin Present		
Upper	Lower	Upper	Lower	
0	0	0	0	2.6
0	75 μg	0	0	25.3
75 μg	0	0	0	3.4
75 μg	75 μg	0	0	0
No pretreatment		0	0	2.4
No pretreatment		0	75 μg	22.1

*Cellulose nitrate filters were incubated for 5 hr in chemotactic chambers in the absence of cells and in the presence or absence of 75 μg of fibronectin placed in the upper or lower compartment. The filters were then removed, washed extensively and placed into a 2nd set of chambers for migration.

†B16 cells (2.5 x 10⁵) migrating for 5 hr into either pretreated or untreated filters in the presence or absence of 75 μg of fibronectin placed in the lower compartment.

due to simple diffusion. Instead a large portion of the radioactivity became progressively bound to the filter, manifesting a gradient of fibronectin from lower to upper compartments. Visualization of the gradient is illustrated in autoradiographs of filters from a parallel experiment in which the filters were removed, washed and fixed at the corresponding times of incubation, 1, 2.5, 5 and 10 hr (Figure 3). The grains, representing localized radioactive fibronectin, were present in the lower portions of the filter at the early time point and became progressively distributed in upper portions of the filters with time. By the late time point (10 hr) the grains had become more evenly distributed and the gradient was not as pronounced. Independent grain counts across separate sections from a number of filters have confirmed this distribution (data not shown). These results and the data in Table 2 indicate that when fibronectin was placed in the lower compartment of of a chemotactic chamber, a gradient of fibronectin becomes firmly bound to the filter. Only those filters containing a gradient of bound fibronectin were sufficient to cause enhanced migration of B16 cells (Table 2). The apparent dissipation of the

314

fibronectin gradient by 5-10 hr (Figures 2 and 3) correlates with the observed diminishment of cell migration that occurs between 5 and 10 hr (1).

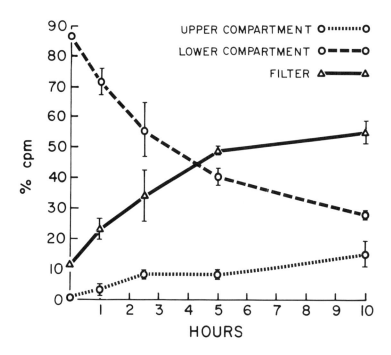

FIGURE 2. Distribution of ^{125}I Fibronectin in Chemotactic Chambers During Various Times of Cell Migration. ^{125}I-labeled fibronectin (see Section III) was placed in the lower compartments of chemotactic chambers. B16 cells (2.5×10^5) were added to the upper compartments. The chambers were then incubated at 37°C. At the indicated times, the upper and lower compartments and filters were analyzed for radioactivity. The filters were washed extensively before counting.

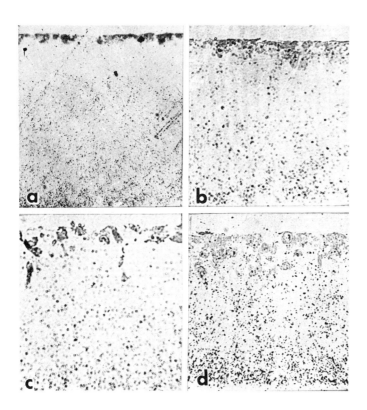

FIGURE 3. Autoradiographic Analysis of Filters Removed at Various Times from Chemotactic Chambers that Contained ^{125}I Fibronectin in the Lower Compartment. A cell migration assay was carried out in chemotactic chambers containing B16 cells in the upper compartment as described in Figure 2. At 1 (a), 2.5 (b), 5 (c) and 10 (d) hr the filters were removed and processed for light microscopy and nuclear emulsion autoradiography as described in Section III.

3. Possible role of proteolytic enzymes in cell migration. When B16 cells migrated into filters containing a gradient of ^{125}I-labeled fibronectin, a small amount of radioactivity (8-10%) was released from the filters. This radioactivity represented, in part, fragments of fibronectin and some intact fibronectin. Since the area of the filter occupied by migrating cells only represented approximately 20% of the total radioactivity in the filter (by grain count), release of 8-10% of the radioactivity indicates a significant removal of fibronectin in the path of migrating cells. In order to examine whether proteolysis of filter-bound fibronectin might be involved in B16 cell migration, a number of proteinase inhibitors were added to the upper compartment of a B16 cell migration assay. Table 3 indicates that the serine proteinase inhibitor DFP, at concentrations that did not affect cell viability or cell adhesion, inhibited migration by 80%. Proteinase inhibitors that are arginine analogs (leupeptin, benzamidine) also inhibited cell migration substantially, whereas a proteinase inhibitor that is a lysine analog (ε aminocaproic acid) had little effect on cell migration. This apparently selective effect of proteinase inhibitors on cell migration, coupled with the release of radioactivity in the path of the migrating cells, suggests a role for proteolytic enzymes in cell migration.

Table 3. Migration of B16 Cells in Response to Fibronectin in the Presence of Proteinase Inhibitors*.

Fibronectin in Lower Compartment	Inhibitor (conc)	B16 Migration (% cells migrating > 40 μm)	% of Control
-	-	0	0
+	-	25.4	100
+	DFP (0.2 mM)	4.5	18
+	leupeptin (100 μg/ml)	6.7	26
+	benzamidine (1.0 mM)	1.7	7
+	ε aminocaproic acid (10 mM)	20.4	80

*B16 cells were placed in the upper compartment of chemotactic chambers in the absence of fibronectin (75 μg) in the lower compartment. Proteinase inhibitors at the indicated concentrations were placed in the upper compartment. The chambers were incubated for 5 hr at 37°C and cell migration was analyzed on fixed and stained filters.

The effectiveness of specific proteinase inhibitors in diminishing cell migration is consistent with a serine proteinase of arginine specificity being involved in cell migration. Previous studies from this laboratory had demonstrated that plasminogen activator (PA), elevated in a number of malignant cells, is a serine proteinase of arginine specificity that is inhibited by DFP, leupeptin, and benzamidine, but not inhibited by ε aminocaproic acid (2). Table 4 indicates that PA activity was enhanced when B16 cells were placed in migration chambers (over control values when the same number of cells were placed in stationary culture) and further enhanced when the cells were placed under conditions where directed migration can occur. This by no means proves that PA is involved in directed cell migration, but does indicate that elevated levels of PA were secreted at the time of migration and that specific inhibitors of that class of enzymes diminished cell migration. A mono-specific antibody, that inhibits the catalytic activity of B16 PA, would be a reagent that might be extremely useful in examining this aspect of cell migration. Procurement of such a reagent is ongoing at this time.

Table 4. PA Secretion by Migrating and Stationary B16 Cells[*].

Number of Cells	Conditions	PA Activity (Units/2.5×10^5 Cells)
2.5×10^5	Stationary	200
2.5×10^5	Random Migration	825
2.5×10^5	Directed Migration	1510

[*]B16 cells in serum-free MEM were plated into tissue culture dishes (Stationary), into Boyden chambers with buffer in the lower compartment (Random Migration) or into Boyden chambers with fibronectin (300 µg/ml) in the lower compartment (Directed Migration). Five hours later the culture and chamber supernatants were harvested and assayed for PA activity. A unit of activity is 2000 cpm of ^{125}I fibrin released/2 hr.

B. Extracellular Matrix (ECM) as a Substratum for Rous Sarcoma Virus (RSV) Transformed Chick Embryo Fibroblasts (CEF)

1. Preparation and characterization of ECM from monolayer cultures of CEF. Growing cultures of CEF were incubated with ^{35}S-methionine to biosynthetically radiolabel the protein components of the extracellular matrix. After the cultures had reached confluency and an extensive matrix had been deposited underneath the monolayer, the cells were removed by four different methods employing either detergent-, hypotonic- or ammonium hydroxide-mediated cell lysis. The resulting cell-free matrices were examined by polyacrylamide gel electrophoresis. Autoradiographic visualization of cellular and matrix polypeptides shown in Figure 4 reveals that the major protein component of the

318

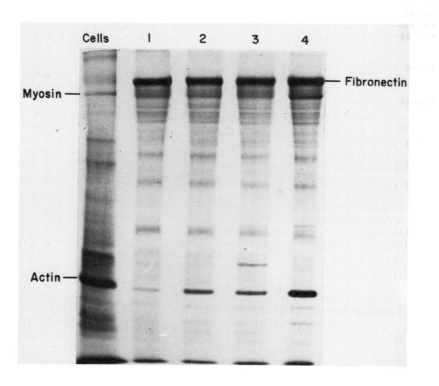

FIGURE 4. Preparation of Extracellular Matrix (ECM) from Chick Embryo Fibroblasts (CEF) by Four Different Methods. Cultures of CEF, radio-labeled with ^{35}S-methionine for 24 hr, were washed with PBS and incubated for 10 min in PBS-5 mM EDTA. The cells were lysed and ECM prepared in parallel cultures by four different methods employing: 1. 0.025 M NH_4OH according to Jones and DeClerk (3), 2. 0.2% NP40 according to Kramer et al. (4), 3. 0.5% sodium deoxycholate according to Keshi-Oja and Vaheri (5) or 4. 0.5% Triton X-100 according to Vlodavsky et al. (6). The ECM were removed from the dishes by scraping in 1% SDS and analyzed by polyacrylamide gel electrophoresis and autoradiography. Intact cells were dissolved directly in 1% SDS and run in a parallel lane in the gel. Purified preparations of chicken myosin, actin and cellular fibronectin were also run in parallel lanes and their positions in the gel are indicated.

matrices was a 220,000 dalton polypeptide that co-migrated with chick fibronectin. Protein bands corresponding to chick myosin and actin, not normally present in ECM, were present to varying degrees in the different matrix preparations and represent apparent contamination of the ECM by cellular components. The method of preparation using 0.025 M NH$_4$OH yielded a matrix that was highly enriched in fibronectin, compared to whole cells, and relatively free of actin and myosin contamination, although these components were present in minor amounts in the ECM. This method of ECM preparation was used for all subsequent experiments.

A scanning electron micrograph of the ECM is shown in Figure 5A. An array of fibrillar-like structures covered the entire surface area of the culture dish. Some amorphous material was present on the surface of the fibers; it is not known whether this material was an integral part of the extracellular matrix or represented residual cellular material.

Figure 5B shows an indirect immunofluorescent stain of an ECM preparation using an antibody to fibronectin. The fibrillar arrays of the ECM clearly contain fibronectin, which is consistent with the polyacrylamide gel pattern of ECM shown in Figure 4.

2. Effect of chick ECM on the morphology of transformed chick fibro-blasts. It is well-established that when CEF are transformed by RSV their morphology is dramatically altered (7). The transformed cells are less elongated, more refractile, less adherent and more randomly oriented in culture. Some of these alterations have been ascribed to the diminished production of ECM components by transformed cells (8-10). It has also been shown in studies from this laboratory (2,11,12) that treatment of RSV transformed CEF cultures with the tumor promoter TPA causes pronounced clustering of the transformed cells along with a concomitant loss of the residual ECM substratum (initially reduced upon RSV transformation). It was of interest therefore to determine if ECM produced by normal CEF had an effect on the morphology and behavior of transformed CEF. When transformed CEF and TPA-treated transformed CEF were incubated, in serum-free medium, on the cell-free ECM prepared from normal CEF, pronounced morphological changes were observed. Figure 6 shows a direct comparison of such cells grown on ordinary plastic culture dishes and on dishes containing the fibrillar array of ECM shown in Figure 5. When RSV transformed CEF were grown on normal ECM, the cells appeared more elongated, less refractile and less randomly oriented (compare Figures 6c and 6d). More striking was the effect of normal ECM on the TPA-treated RSVCEF cultures. The cell clustering brought about by TPA treatment (2,11) was completely prevented by the presence of the normal ECM (compare Figures 6e and 6f). The TPA-treated RSVCEF cells remained elongated and appeared completely aligned within or on the underlying normal ECM. However, the inhibitory effect of intact normal ECM on cell clustering was only temporary. If the TPA-treated cultures were incubated for additional periods of time (1-2 da), the cells became disorganized and eventually clustered (Figure 6h). There was little

320

morphological evidence of matrix in these cultures. Parallel cultures of RSVCEF incubated with TPA under identical conditions on plastic exhibited well-advanced morphological changes with tight clusters of cells floating free in the medium (compare Figures 6g and 6h).

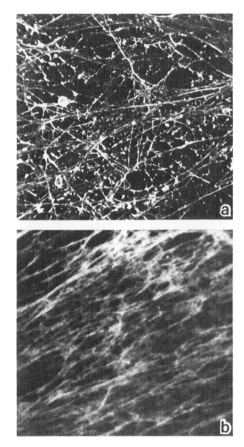

FIGURE 5. Analysis of ECM by Scanning Electron Microscopy and Immuno-fluorescence. ECM was prepared by the NH$_4$OH method and analyzed by (A) scanning electron microscopy and (B) indirect immunofluorescence microscopy using an antibody to chick fibronectin. Separate preparations of ECM were used for each procedure. Magnification: A, 2250 x and B, 720 x.

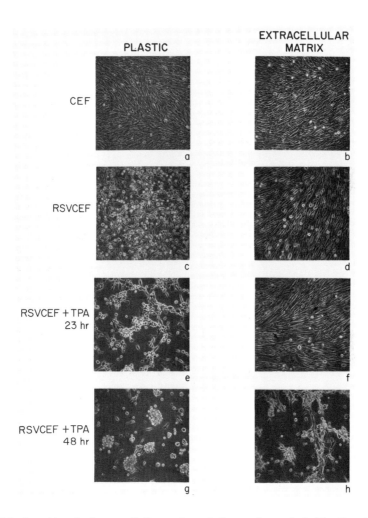

PLASTIC

EXTRACELLULAR
MATRIX

CEF

RSVCEF

RSVCEF + TPA
23 hr

RSVCEF + TPA
48 hr

FIGURE 6. Morphology of Normal and Transformed Cells Incubated on
Tissue Culture Plastic or ECM. Normal CEF and RSV transformed CEF were
seeded (1.5 x 10^6 cells/35 mm dish) in MEM containing 5% plasminogen-
depleted FCS onto ordinary plastic tissue culture dishes which
contained ECM prepared from CEF. After 24 hr the culture dishes were
washed in MEM and the incubation was continued in serum-free MEM. Some
of the RSVCEF cultures were supplemented with TPA (100 ng/ml). Phase
contrast photomicrographs were taken 23 hr (a-f) or 48 hr (g,h) after
the addition of serum-free MEM.

322

3. Alteration and degradation of ECM by transformed and TPA-treated
transformed cells. It appeared from the morphological studies above
that the ECM is altered or lost upon prolonged incubation of
transformed cultures in TPA. In order to biochemically confirm these
observations and quantitate the apparent loss of ECM, radiolabeled
matrices were incubated with different cells in serum-free medium for
varying periods of time in the presence or absence of TPA. The fate of
the matrix was examined by determining the ^{35}S radioactivity released
into the culture supernatant with time. Figure 7 shows that the ECM
was relatively stable when incubated in serum-free medium alone. Less
than 5% of the labeled material was released during a 48 hr incubation.
Normal CEF cultured on the ECM released approximately 5-15% of the
radiolabeled material over the same period of time. RSV transformed CEF
induced a progressive breakdown of ECM components, releasing over 35%
of the protein components in 48 hr. TPA-treated RSVCEF cultures
rapidly destroyed the ECM releasing 40% of the radioactivity in 24 hr
and approximately 70% after 48 hr, coincident with cell migration and
clustering.

4. Plasminogen-dependent and -independent degradation of ECM. The
degradation of ECM by transformed cells in serum-free medium observed
in Figure 7 was enhanced in the presence of purified chicken
plasminogen (Figure 8A). The enhanced rate of degradation (50% release
of radioactivity in 8 hr) could be prevented by Trasylol, an inhibitor
of plasmin. This indicates that plasminogen activator, produced at
elevated levels by the TPA-treated cultures (2,11), catalytically
converted plasminogen to plasmin which in turn rapidly degraded the
ECM. Plasminogen in medium in the absence of cells released less than
10% of the radioactivity. Trasylol had no effect on the cell-mediated
degradation of ECM as 70-80% of the radiolabeled ECM was progressively
released by cells over 48 hr either in the presence or absence of
Trasylol (Figure 8A). Figure 8B shows the cell-mediated polypeptide
loss from ECM over a 6-48 hr time period as well as the rapid loss (6
hr) of polypeptides in the presence of cells plus plasminogen. Trasylol
prevented the plasminogen-dependent loss, again indicating that
degradation occurred via the generated plasmin. The apparent
resistance of specific ECM polypeptides to plasmin degradation (arrows
in lane 5) and their relative susceptibility to cellular degradative
processes (lanes 3 and 4) suggests that cellular enzyme(s) with
somewhat different specificities than plasmin may also be involved in
the cell-mediated ECM degradation. Further evidence that the cell-
mediated degradation of ECM may be distinct from the plasmin-mediated
degradation is shown in Figure 9. The polypeptide pattern of the ECM
supernatant from a 6 hr plasminogen/plasmin incubation (30-40% release
of radioactivity) was distinct from the polypeptide pattern of the ECM
supernatant from a 48 hr incubation of ECM and cells in the absence of
plasminogen (40-50% release of radioactivity). The gel patterns shown
in Figure 9 also demonstrate that most of the ECM proteins were not
released intact from the surface of the culture dish. Little or no
intact fibronectin was present in either supernatant.

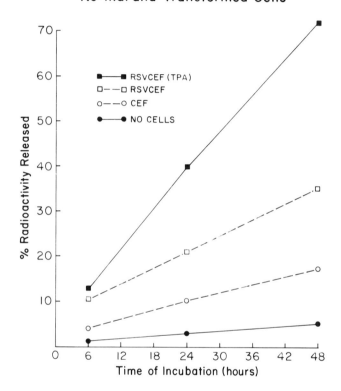

Degradation of CEF Extracellular Matrix by Normal and Transformed Cells

FIGURE 7. Degradation of Radiolabeled ECM by Normal and Transformed Cells. CEF and RSVCEF were seeded (1.5 x 10⁶ cells) onto 35 mm petri dishes containing ³⁵S-labeled ECM. At zero time (18 hr after seeding) the cultures were washed with MEM and incubated in serum-free MEM. Some of the RSVCEF cultures were incubated in serum-free MEM containing TPA (100 ng/ml). As a control, dishes containing ³⁵S-labeled ECM were incubated in MEM without cells. At the indicated times the supernatants were removed from the culture dishes and counted for radioactivity and the percent of total radioactivity was calculated as described in Section III.

5. Effect of serum and serum components on ECM degradation. All of the previously described ECM degradation studies were performed in serum-free medium. Since fetal calf serum (FCS) is often a standard media supplement in transformed cell cultures, the effect of FCS on matrix degradation was examined (Figure 10). The addition of 5% FCS to cultures of TPA-treated RSVCEF incubated on radiolabeled ECM increased the degradation of ECM over that of parallel cultures incubated in serum-free medium. This increase in degradation (approximately 5% to 15% in 6 hr and approximately 40% to 55% in 24 hr) was not as substantial as the increase observed when purified plasminogen was added to serum-free cultures (Figure 8). Since the diminished increase might be due to natural proteinase inhibitors present in serum, FCS was acid-treated and reneutralized to inactivate most of the proteinase-inhibitory capacity of FCS (13) and examined for its effect on ECM degradation. Acid-treated FCS enhanced the degradation of ECM by RSVCEF (25% in 6 hr and 70% in 24 hr) to the levels observed when purified plasminogen was added to serum-free cultures (Figure 8). That the increase in ECM degradation in the presence of FCS (or acid-treated FCS) was dependent on serum plasminogen was further illustrated by the reduction in ECM degradation that occurred when FCS or acid-treated FCS which had been depleted of plasminogen was used as a supplement (Figure 10).

6. The effect of proteinase inhibitors on plasminogen-independent ECM degradation. The nature of the cell-mediated, plasminogen-independent degradation was examined further by the use of selective proteinase inhibitors (Figure 11). Leupeptin and NPGB, inhibitors of arginine-preferring serine proteinases, inhibited ECM degradation by TPA-treated RSVCEF cultures 30-40%, or down to or below the level exhibited by untreated RSVCEF cultures. The combined use of leupeptin and NPGB, however, did not significantly alter the inhibition pattern exhibited by either compound alone. In other experiments inhibitors of serine proteinases (DFP), cysteine proteinases (E64C) and metallo proteinases (1,10 Phenanthroline) were employed. Figure 12 shows that each of these inhibitors reduced ECM degradation by 30-50%. The combined addition of all three inhibitors reduced ECM degradation by 80%. These results suggest that a serine proteinase of arginine specificity and undefined metallo and cysteine proteinases contribute to the degradation of ECM by RSVCEF.

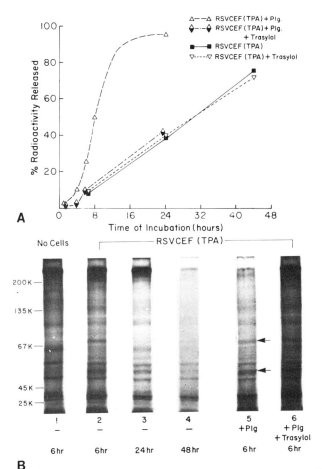

B

FIGURE 8. Plasminogen/Plasmin-Mediated Degradation of ECM: Effect of
a Plasmin Inhibitor and Comparison with Cell-Mediated, Plasminogen
Independent ECM Degradation. Cultures of RSVCEF were incubated in
serum-free medium containing TPA on 35 mm dishes containing ^{35}S-labeled
ECM. Purified chicken plasminogen (2 μg) was added to some of the
cultures at zero time in the presence or absence of Trasylol (20 U/ml),
a plasmin inhibitor. Other cultures were incubated in the absence of
plasminogen but in the presence or absence of Trasylol. At the
indicated times the supernatants were removed from the dishes and the
remaining matrix and cells were dissolved in 1% SDS. Both the supernatants and the dissolved matrices were counted for radioactivity and
analyzed by polyacrylamide gel electrophoresis and autoradiography as
described in Section III. A. The radioactivity released into the
supernatants as a function of incubation time for the different
cultures. B. Autoradiograph of a polyacrylamide gel showing the ECM
proteins remaining on the culture dish at the indicated times for the
indicated culture conditions. The arrows in lane 5 indicate two
polypeptides that were relatively insensitive to plasmin digestion.

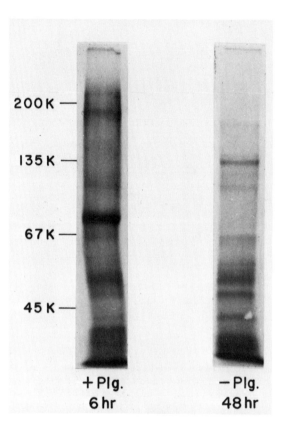

FIGURE 9. Autoradiographic Analysis of Radiolabeled Polypeptides Released into the Culture Supernatant from ^{35}S Labeled ECM. The supernatant polypeptides from cultures of RSVCEF incubated in TPA plus plasminogen for 6 hr are compared to the supernatant polypeptides from parallel cultures of RSVCEF incubated in TPA in the absence of plasminogen for 48 hr. Equal volumes of supernatants were dialyzed, lyophilized and analyzed by polyacrylamide gel electrophoresis and autoradiography. The polypeptide patterns representing released and degraded ECM proteins were distinct for the two culture conditions.

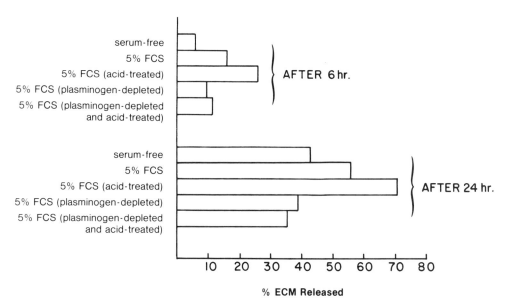

FIGURE 10. The Effect of Serum and Serum Components on ECM Degradation. Parallel cultures of RSVCEF, 18 hr after seeding onto radiolabeled ECM, were incubated in medium supplemented with TPA (100 ng/ml) and 5% FCS treated as indicated. After 6 hr and 24 hr the release of radioactivity into the supernatant from the different cultures was analyzed. The depletion of plasminogen from the serum and the inactivation of acid-sensitive serum proteinase inhibitors are described in Section III.

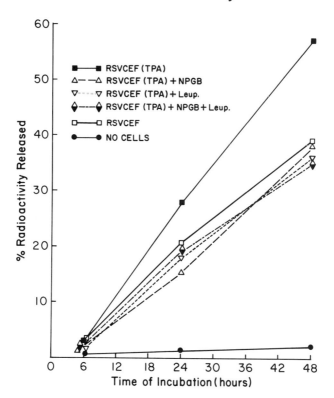

Effects of Protease Inhibitors on the Degradation of Extracellular Matrix by RSVCEF

FIGURE 11. Effect of Proteinase Inhibitors on the Degradation of ECM by Transformed Cells. Cultures of RSVCEF (1.5 x 10^6 cells) were incubated in serum-free medium in 35 mm dishes containing ^{35}S-labeled ECM. TPA was added at a concentration of 100 ng/ml. Parallel cultures contained in addition either NPGB (20 µM), leupeptin (100 µg/ml) or NPGB (20 µM) plus leupeptin (100 µg/ml). Cultures of RSVCEF incubated on radiolabeled ECM in the presence of medium alone were run in parallel as controls. The release of radioactivity into the supernatant from the different cultures was analyzed as described in Section III.

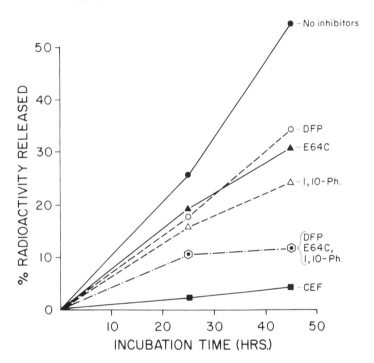

MATRIX DEGRADATION BY RSVCEF:
EFFECT OF INHIBITORS OF SERINE,
THIOL, AND METALLO PROTESSES
IN SINGLET AND IN COMBINATION.

FIGURE 12. Effect of Inhibitors of Serine, Cysteine and Metallo Proteinases in Singlet and in Combination on ECM Degradation. Cultures of RSVCEF (1.5 x 10^6 cells) were incubated in serum-free medium containing TPA (100 ng/ml) on 35 mm dishes containing ^{35}S-labeled ECM. Parallel cultures contained in addition either DFP (250 μM), 1,10 phenanthroline (10 μg/ml), E64C (50 μg/ml) [a reported inhibitor of cysteine proteinases (14)], and all three inhibitors at their respective concentrations. Cultures of normal CEF were incubated in parallel as a control. The release of radioactivity into the supernatant from the different cultures was analyzed as described in Section III.

330

7. Induction of plasminogen activator activity by cultures incubated on ECM. Since RSVCEF cultures and TPA-treated RSVCEF cultures produce elevated levels of PA, an arginine-preferring serine proteinase (2,11) which may be linked to ECM degradation, it was of interest to examine the production of this enzyme when cells were cultured on ECM. Figure 13 shows that the levels of both secreted and cell-associated PA were increased when RSVCEF cells were incubated on ECM compared to

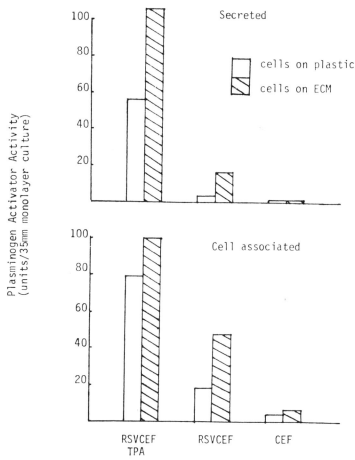

FIGURE 13. Plasminogen Activator Activity of Normal and Transformed Cells Cultured on Plastic or Extracellular Matrix. RSVCEF and CEF (1.5×10^6 cells) were cultured in parallel on ordinary 35 mm tissue culture dishes or dishes coated with ECM in the absence or presence of TPA (100 ng/ml). After 18 hr in serum-free medium, the culture supernatants were removed and assayed for secreted PA. Cell lysates were prepared and assayed for cell-associated PA.

standard cell culture dishes. The levels of PA in TPA-treated RSVCEF were also enhanced on ECM but the percent increase was not as great, possibly because TPA-treated cultures were already producing highly elevated levels of the enzyme. Normal CEF cultures produced low or baseline levels of PA and the effect of ECM on PA production by these cultures was not significant. This induction of PA activity by culturing RSVCEF cells on ECM was similar to the induction of PA activity observed when B16 cells were incubated on fibronectin-coated filters during a migration assay (Table 4).

8. <u>Ultrastructure of ECM degradation</u>. Scanning electron microscopy of RSVCEF cells cultured on ECM demonstrate that the transformed cells were firmly enmeshed in the fibrillar network of ECM. The transformed cells were flattened and elongated within the matrix and strands of ECM material contiguous with the surface of the transformed cells were readily apparent (Figure 14A). After 24 hr in TPA, the RSVCEF cells were still enmeshed in the ECM but early stages of ECM degradation were observed (Figure 14B) as the transformed cells began to clear the immediately surrounding matrix. By 48 hr, the TPA-treated cells had cleared or degraded most of their surrounding ECM although portions of matrix were still present in the spaces devoid of cells (Figure 14C). The cells, free of matrix restrictions, had begun to cluster together. At 67 hr (Figure 14D), the transformed cells had cleared away almost all of the ECM and formed networks of clustered cells. If the serine proteinase inhibitor, NPGB, was present, matrix degradation was diminished (Figure 14E, also see Figure 11). The cells remained relatively flattened in the NPGB-treated cultures and the meshwork of attached matrix appeared to have prevented the cells from forming tight-multicellular clusters (compare Figures 14D and 14E). In contrast to the relatively prolonged time required for cell-mediated matrix alterations to occur, plasmin-mediated matrix clearing was nearly complete by 7 hr (Figure 14F). However, some strands of matrix adjacent to and under the cells were still present and cell clustering had not yet occurred. By 24 hr plasmin cleared the underlying matrix and cell clustering took place (not shown).

III. EXPERIMENTAL METHODS

Cell culture. B16 melanoma cells were cultured under standard conditions as described previously (1). Primary chick embryo fibroblasts (CEF) were prepared from 11 day old embryos and maintained in cultures as described previously (2). CEF secondary cultures were infected and transformed with RSV as described previously (2). All experiments were performed on third, fourth and fifth passage cultures of CEF and RSVCEF.

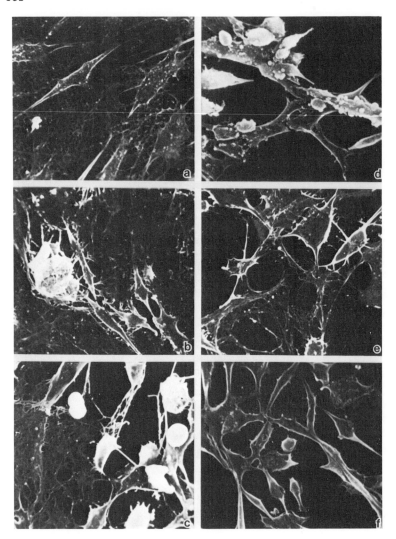

FIGURE 14.   Ultrastructural Analysis of ECM Degradation by Scanning
Electron Microscopy.   Cultures of RSVCEF 18 hr after seeding onto ECM
were incubated in serum-free medium in the presence of TPA for varying
periods of time (A-E).   Some cultures contained 20 μM NPGB (E) or 2 μg
of purified chicken plasminogen (F).   The zero time micrograph (A)
represents the RSVCEF cells 18 hr after seeding before the start of the
incubation in serum-free medium.   Subsequent incubation times were 24
hr (B), 48 hr (C), 67 hr (D), 67 hr in the presence of NPGB (E) and 7
hr in the presence of plasminogen (F).   All micrographs are 2,250 x.

Cell migration assay. A 12 µM pore, 180 µm thick nitrocellulose filter (Schleicher and Schuell, Keane, NH) prewetted with PBS was fitted between the upper and lower compartments of a blindwell chemotactic chamber (Neuroprobe Institute of Biological Research, Bethesda, MD). Human plasma fibronectin or other indicated proteins were added (0.2 ml; 300 µg/ml in medium or PBS) to the lower chamber. A suspension of B16 cells (0.5 ml; 5×10^5 cells/ml) was inoculated into the upper chamber. The chambers were incubated at 37°C in a 10% CO_2 atmosphere for 5 hr unless otherwise indicated. After incubation, filters were removed and fixed with 2.5% glutaraldehyde in 0.1 M potassium phosphate buffer, pH 7.4, for 30 min, rinsed with phosphate buffer, and postfixed with 1% osmium tetroxide in 0.1 M phosphate buffer. The filters were then rinsed with 0.85% NaCl solution (saline) and dehydrated with ethanol, cleared with propylene oxide, and embedded in Epon-812. These blocks were allowed to polymerize in a 60°C oven for at least 24 hr, and transverse sections (1.5 µm thick) were cut with an LKB microtome and stained with 0.1% toluidine blue in sodium borate.

The extent of B16 cell migration into the filter was measured with a 40 x objective and 10 x ocular-micrometer. Five random fields/thick section of filter were studied. In general, a total of approximately 100 cells was counted for each variable in any given experiment. The number of cells migrating into the filter in 10 µm increments of depth was divided by the total number of cells in the filter, and a percentage was calculated. The percentage values were shown to be an accurate representation of the total B16 cell population in control experiments using ^{3}H-thymidine-labeled cells; the number of cells in the filter represented 80 to 100% of the total number of cells inoculated into the upper chamber. All experimental conditions were performed in triplicate, and Student's t test was used to determine the statistical significance of results.

Treatment of fibronectin. Human plasma fibronectin was obtained from Dr. M. Mosesson (Mt. Sinai Medical Center, Milwaukee, WI) and was judged to be pure by polyacrylamide gel electrophoresis. Reduced fibronectin was used following reduction in 10 mM dithiothreitol and treatment with 10 mM iodoacetamide which resulted in a change of a M_r 440,000 species to a M_r 220,000 species as judged by polyacrylamide gel electrophoresis. Fibronectin was also dialyzed in a M_r 10,000 exclusion limit dialysis bag for 24 hr with 3 changes of 1 liter of PBS. Trypsinized fibronectin was used following a 37°C incubation for 60 min of 1 ml of fibronectin (600 µg/ml) containing 10 µg of trypsin. Soybean trypsin inhibitor (30 µg) was added at the end of the incubation to terminate the trypsinization. Fibronectin was radio-labeled with ^{125}I by the iodogen method according to the method described by the manufacturer (Pierce Chemical Co.). The fibronectin was shown to be active in a cell migration assay and the radiolabel was shown to be incorporated into a 220,000 daltons species that co-migrated with standard fibronectin.

Nuclear emulsion autoradiography. Blocks of filters used for time course studies of ^{125}I-labeled fibronectin distribution were used to provide thick sections for autoradiography of the labeled protein. The Ilford Emulsion K5 was prepared by thawing at 43°C and diluting 1:1 with double-distilled water. The slides were held with the long edge on the vertical and dipped into the warm emulsion. Excess emulsion was blotted from the short edge, and the slides were allowed to dry for two hours. Once dry, the slides were placed in slide boxes with a small amount of dessicator. The box was sealed with electrical tape, covered in aluminum foil and stored at 4°C for 9 da. At the end of this exposure time, the slides were developed under safelight conditions by immersion into Kodak Developer D-19 for 4 min, rinsed in distilled water, and immersed in Kodak Fixer for 5 min. All these solutions were kept at 18°C. The slides were then allowed to dry, and examined by bright-field light microscopy.

Preparation of extracellular matrix (ECM). Trial preparations of ECM were carried out according to a number of different methods (3-6). The method of choice used for all preparations, except when noted, was a modification of the procedures described by Jones and DeClerk (3). Petri dishes were seeded with CEF (4 x 10^5 cells in 35 mm dishes) and incubated in MEM supplemented with 10% FCS. When the cultures had reached confluency, they were washed once with phosphate buffered saline (PBS) deficient in calcium and magnesium containing 5 mM EDTA and incubated in the same solution for 10 min at 37°C. The partially-detached cells were lysed away from the underlying ECM by a wash and two ten minute incubations with 0.025 M NH$_4$OH at room temperature. The ECM and remaining material was washed twice with PBS deficient in calcium and magnesium and sterilized with 70% ethanol for 10-15 min. The matrices, still firmly attached to the petri dishes, were stored in PBS at 4°C, and were used for experiments within one week.

Radiolabeling of ECM. One to two days after seeding CEF, when the cultures were 50-75% confluent, ^{35}S methionine (10 μCi/ml) was introduced into the cultures in fresh medium containing 1/20 the normal MEM concentration of methionine. When cultures had reached confluency the matrices were prepared as described above.

ECM degradation assay. Radiolabeled ECM preparations were washed with MEM before cells (CEF or RSVCEF) were seeded onto them at 1.5 x 10^6 cells/35 mm dish in MEM containing 5% plasminogen-depleted FCS prepared as previously described (15). Approximately 18-24 hr later the cultures were washed with MEM and incubated in 2 ml of serum-free MEM in the presence or absence of 100 ng/ml of TPA. ECM-containing dishes were incubated in MEM in the absence of cells as controls. At selected time intervals thereafter triplicate representative dishes were taken for analysis. The supernatant was removed, phenylmethyl-sulfonyl fluoride (PMSF) was added to a final concentration of 2 mM, and a 200 μl aliquot was mixed with 5 ml of Aquasol-2 and counted in a beta-liquid scintillation counter. The remaining supernatant was dialyzed and lyophilized in preparation for polyacrylamide gel electro-phoresis. The remaining ECM and cells were collected from the dishes by scraping with a Teflon policeman in 0.5 ml of 1% sodium dodecyl sulfate (SDS). A 50 µl aliquot was added to 5 ml of Aquasol-2 and counted and the remaining material was prepared for polyacrylamide gel electrophoresis. The total cpm in the supernatant and in the residual matrix was calculated and the % radioactivity released was based on cpm in supernatant/total cpm in supernatant + matrix x 100.

SDS polyacrylamide gel electrophoresis. Analysis on poly-acrylamide gels was carried out according to Laemmli (16). Samples to be analyzed were mixed with appropriate volumes of electrophoresis sample buffer containing β mercaptoethanol, boiled and applied onto 8.5% polyacrylamide slab gels. Unless otherwise noted, equal volumes of supernatant and equal volumes of resuspended matrices corresponding to one culture dish or an equal fraction thereof were applied onto the gels. Autoradiography was performed on gels containing ^{125}I- or ^{35}S-labeled proteins with Kodak R film Ready Pack.

Plasminogen activator (PA) assay. PA activity on cell lysates (cell associated PA) and conditioned medium (secreted PA) was based on the plasmin-mediated hydrolysis of ^{125}I-fibrin employing purified plasminogen and fibrin as previously described (2). Plasminogen free serum was prepared as previously described (2). Acid-treated serum was prepared according to established procedures (13).

IV. CONCLUSIONS

The effect of fibronectin on cellular behavior has been extensively documented. Initial reports published a decade ago by Hynes (17) demonstrated the presence of this molecule on the surface of fibroblasts and its near absence on transformed cells. Subsequently, numerous investigations focused on the role of fibronectin in mediating the social behavior of various cell types and the influence of fibronectin on cell adhesion, cell shape, and cytoskeletal organization (18,19). More recently, fibronectin has been implicated in cell locomotion and morphogenetic movement in embryonic and adult tissues (20-24) suggesting a nearly ubiquitous role for this molecule in tissue and cellular organization. Our studies, in which chemotaxis chambers and thick, porous nitrocellulose filters have been used, have allowed for direct observation of malignant cell migration and of the influence of fibronectin on such migration. The enhancement of directional migration of B16 melanoma cells caused by native fibronectin appears to be specific, since structurally modified fibronectin and other plasma proteins fail to elicit such a response (Table 1). The assay system used permits migratory responses to be observed in a relatively short period of time, from 1 to 5 hr. This eliminates the involvement of cell doubling time and differential cell proliferation and also reduces the potentially deleterious effect of prolonged incubation of cells in serum-free medium.

The use of relatively thick filters (100 to 200 µm) permits the entire population of cells to be observed (Figure 1) as they migrate with time into and along the pores of the nitrocellulose filter. The most distinct advantage of the present assay system, however, is the manipulation of both the removable filters and the separate upper and lower chambers. Results obtained by such manipulations have indicated that: (a) a gradient of fibronectin is the major effector of enhanced B16 cell-directed migration; (b) fibronectin is affecting the actual movement of the cells, and does so in a manner independent of the cell's initial adhesion and attachment to the filter; and (c) the fibronectin molecule appears to be acting as a haptotactic agent in mediating the directed locomotion of the malignant cells as they migrate along a positive gradient of substratum-bound fibronectin.

The exact mechanism and the physiological significance of enhanced B16 cell migration in response to fibronectin are not elucidated by the present study. Nevertheless, it appears that locomotion of many cell types, normal and malignant, is due to the continuous making and breaking of specific cell contacts with the substratum (25). A concentration gradient of specific substratum adhesion molecule(s) may be the driving force for the making and subsequent breaking of the cell contacts resulting in a continuous unidirectional mode of locomotion along a path of preferential adhesion. Such a concept was originally proposed by Carter (26) to explain the directionality of malignant cell movement in tumor invasion. It was hypothesized that movement towards surfaces of greater adhesion is a general phenomenon applicable to cells which are dependent for their motility on contact with a surface (26). In the very simple in vitro model described herein, fibronectin bound to the nitrocellulose filter might provide the adhesion traction necessary for enhanced B16 cell migration as the cells initially attach, then detach and pull themselves along a gradient of bound fibronectin. The detachment process is not well-understood, but evidence presented in this study suggests that selective proteolysis of the fibronectin or a putative fibronectin-cell attachment protein might provide a catalytic driving force for detachment and subsequent migration and then re-attachment. Such a catalytic mechanism repeated over again might add directionality to the cell movement.

In the second experimental system described in this study, directed migration is not involved. Nevertheless, a somewhat similar phenomenon occurs in that RSVCEF cells attach and become enmeshed in a biological substratum. They subsequently degrade that substatum, resulting in an apparent random migration, i.e., cell clustering. The nature of the degradative ability of transformed fibroblasts is complex but some aspects of their catalytic activity toward ECM are illustrated. When a source of plasminogen is present, the degradation of the ECM is rapid and extensive (Figure 8). This is due to the conversion of plasminogen to the active proteinase plasmin which is mediated by the elevated levels of PA produced by the transformed cells (2,11).

The present studies also demonstrate that a plasminogen-independent ECM degradation can occur. This degradation is not as rapid as plasmin-dependent degradation, but is progressive and eventually all or most of the ECM present in a culture dish is solubilized (Figure 8). Such plasminogen-independent degradation has been observed by several laboratories employing a variety of tumor cells (4,27,28); however, the enzymatic nature of the process remains unresolved. In the CEF/RSVCEF culture systems described herein, certain aspects of the process have been resolved. Firstly, the process is mediated by cellular enzymes distinct in specificity from plasmin since it is completely insensitive to Trasylol. The polypeptide patterns of both the solubilized components and residual matrix are different from plasmin-mediated degradation patterns (Figures 8 and 9). Secondly, the cell-mediated degradation of ECM is partially sensitive to inhibitors of arginine-preferring proteinases (Figure 11). The partial sensitivity to these inhibitors and the partial sensitivity to inhibitors of cysteine and metallo proteinases (Figure 12) suggests that a number of cellular enzymes are involved in ECM degradation. The identity of the arginine-specific proteinase(s) remains unknown. Previous studies (11) from this laboratory, however, have indicated that the distinct morphological alterations that occur in TPA-treated RSVCEF cultures are mediated in part by the direct catalytic activty of PA, an arginine-preferring proteinase. The PA activity in this culture system is elevated upon TPA treatment (11), is secreted and associated with a plasma membrane fraction (29) and is sensitive to NPGB and leupeptin and insensitive to Trasylol (11), all results that are consistent with a direct role for the enzyme in ECM degradation.

Two distinct malignant cell culture systems have been discussed. Both systems have limitations as models for invasive and metastatic tumor cell behavior, not the least of which is that they are cell cultures systems and far removed from the complex in vivo interactions that occur in an animal with an invasive and metastatic tumor burden. Nevertheless, results from both systems suggest that when malignant cells encounter a natural substratum or its component parts, an initial attachment occurs possibly through specific cell receptors for adhesive proteins. That attachment can induce the production and secretion of specific proteolytic enzymes which are capable of further activating zymogens resulting in a cascade phenomenon, not unlike the serine proteinase cascades that occur in coagulation and complement. The result is that substratum proteins are selectively degraded, thereby freeing the cells from the restrictions imposed by the adhesive molecules in the substratum. The final result is cell translocation either as a random movement or if a gradient exists a unidirectional translocation of cells in response to that gradient.

ACKNOWLEDGMENTS

The authors acknowledge Mr. Angelo Albano and Ms. Kathy Revesz for their skilled technical assistance and Ms. Roseann Lingeza and Ms. Dorothy Ronayne for the preparation of the manuscript. The work was supported by grants CA 16740 from NIH and BC163 from the American Cancer Society.

338

REFERENCES

1. Lacovara J, Cramer EB, Quigley JP: Fibronectin enhancement of directed migration of B16 melanoma cells. Cancer Res. 44:1657-1663, 1984.
2. Quigley JP: Phorbol ester-induced morphological changes in transformed chick fibroblasts: Evidence for direct catalytic involvement of plasminogen activator. Cell 17:131-141, 1979.
3. Jones PA, DeClerck Y: Destruction of extracellular matrices containing glycoprotiens, elastin, and collagen by metastatic human tumor cells. Cancer Res. 40:3222-3227, 1980.
4. Kramer RH, Vogel KG, Nicolson G: Solubilization and degradation of subendothelial matrix glycoproteins and proteoglycans by metastatic tumor cells. J. Biol. Chem. 257:2678-2686, 1982.
5. Keski-Oja J, Vaheri A: The cellular target for the plasminogen activator, urokinase, in human fibroblasts 66,000-dalton protein. Biochim. Biophys. Acta 720:141-146, 1982.
6. Vlodavsky I, Lui GM, Gospodarowicz D: Morphological appearance, growth behavior and migratory activity of human tumor cells maintained on extracellular matrix versus plastic. Cell 19:607-616, 1980.
7. Hanafusa H: Cell transformation by RNA tumor viruses. Comprehensive Virol. 10:401-483, 1977.
8. Yamada K: Immunological characterization of a major transformation sensitive fibroblast cell surface glycoprotein. J. Cell Biol. 78:520-541, 1978.
9. Vaheri A, Kurkinen M, Lehto V-P, Linder E, Timpl R: Codistribution of pericellular matrix proteins in cultured fibroblasts and loss in transformation: Fibronectin and procollagen. Proc. Natl. Acad. Sci. USA 75:4944-4948, 1978.
10. Hynes RO: Cell surface proteins and malignant transformation. Biochim. Biophys. Acta 458:73-107, 1976.
11. Goldfarb RH, Quigley JP: Production of plasminogen activator by chick embryo fibroblasts: Synergistic effect of Rous sarcoma virus transformation and treatment with the tumor promoter phorbol myristate acetate. Cancer Res. 38:4601-4609, 1978.
12. Quigley JP, Goldfarb RH, Scheiner C, O'Donnell-Tormey J, Yeo TK: Plasminogen activator and the membrane of transformed cells. IN: Hynes RO and Fox CF (eds.) Tumor Cell Surfaces and Malignancy. Alan R. Liss, Inc., New York, pp. 773-796, 1980.
13. Loskutoff D: Effects of acidified fetal bovine serum on the fibrinolytic activity and growth of cells in culture. J. Cell. Physiol. 96:361-370, 1978.
14. Hasida S, Towatari T, Kominami E, Katunuma N: Inhibitions by E-64 derivatives of rat liver cathepsin B and cathepsin L in vitro and in vivo. J. Biochem. 88:1805-1811, 1980.
15. Quigley JP, Ossowski L, Reich E: Plasminogen the serum proenzyme activated by factors from cells transformed on oncogenic viruses. J. Biol. Chem. 249:4306-4311, 1974.
16. Laemmli UK: Cleavage of structural proteins during the assembly of the head of bacteriophage T_4. Nature (London) 277:680-685, 1970.

17. Hynes RO: Alteration of cell surface proteins by viral transformation and proteolysis. Proc. Natl. Acad. Sci. USA 70:3170-3174, 1973.
18. Hynes RO: Fibronectin and its relations to cellular structure and behavior. IN: Hay ED (ed.) Cell Biology of the Extracellular Matrix. Plenum Publishing Corp., New York, pp. 295-334, 1981.
19. Yamada KM, Olden K: Fibronectin-adhesive glycoproteins of cell surface and blood. Nature (London) 275:179-184, 1978.
20. Bowersox JC, Sorgente N: Chemotaxis of aortic endothelial cells in response to fibronectin. Cancer Res. 42:2547-2551, 1982.
21. Gauss-Muller V, Kleinman HK, Martin GR, Schiffman E: Role of attachment factors and attractants in fibroblast chemotaxis. J. Lab. Clin. Med. 96:1071-1080, 1980.
22. Heasman J, Hynes RO, Swan AP, Thomas V, Wylie CC: Primordial germ cells of xenopus embryos: The role of fibronectin in their adhesion during migration. Cell 27:437-447, 1981.
23. Newgreen D, Thiery J-P: Fibronectin in early avian embryos. Synthesis and distribution along the migration pathways of neural crest cells. Cell. Tiss. Res. 211:269-291, 1980.
24. Postlethwaite AE, Keski-Oja J, Balian G, Kang AH: Introduction of fibroblast chemotaxis by fibronectin. J. Exp. Med. 153:494-499, 1981.
25. Harris A: Behavior of cultured cells on substrata of variable adhesiveness. Exp. Cell. Res. 77:285-297, 1973.
26. Carter SB: Principles of cell motility: The direction of cell movement and cancer invasion. Nature (London) 208:1183-1187, 1965.
27. Sheela S, Barrett JC: In vitro degradation of radio-labelled, intact basement membrane mediated by cellular plasminogen activator. Carcinogenesis 4:363-369, 1982.
28. Laug WE, DeClerck Y, Jones PA: Degradation of the subendothelial matrix by tumor cells. Cancer Res. 43:1827-1834, 1983.
29. Quigley JP: Association of a protease (plasminogen activator) with a specific membrane fraction from transformed cells. J. Cell. Biol. 71:472-486, 1976.

CHAPTER 21. PROTEOLYTIC ENZYMES IN TUMOR INVASION AND DEGRADATION OF HOST EXTRACELLULAR MATRICES

RONALD H. GOLDFARB

I. INTRODUCTION

A fact widely recognized by clinical oncologists is that rather than the primary tumor, the secondary metastatic tumor(s) usually leads to the lethality of human malignant disease (1-4). Tumor invasion, the destructive penetration of surrounding normal tissues by malignant cells, is an important feature of the metastatic spread and dissemination of cancer (5-9). Invasive tumor cells must penetrate a number of host extracellular barriers and matrices, including basement membranes, at several stages of tumor metastasis. Investigation of the biochemical mechanisms involved in tumor invasion and degradation of host extracellular matrices have indicated that proteolytic enzymes play a role in these processes (5-13). This chapter will review the role of various proteolytic enzymes in the destruction of several host matrices and their specific components during tumor invasion and metastasis. In addition, the potential significance of matrix degradation by proteolytic enzymes during tumor invasion to the diagnosis and therapy of human metastatic disease will be discussed.

II. TUMOR INVASION

A. Extracellular Matrices

During tumor invasion malignant cells penetrate matrix barriers including basement membranes and interstitial stroma (5,7,8). In order to enter interstitial stroma invasive tumor cells must penetrate the basement membrane. Basement membranes delineate boundaries between organ parenchyma and interstitial stroma, and are composed of molecular components including type IV collagen, laminin, fibronectin, type V collagen, entactin and heparan sulfate proteoglycan (7-8). The basement membrane also forms a scaffolding support for organ parenchymal cells and is usually a stable and resilient structural barrier with a slow turnover rate (8,9). During tumor invasion, however, the basement membrane undergoes a rapid and localized degradation. Intact basement membrane, which excludes the passage of colloidal carbon, does not normally contain pre-existing pores through which tumor cells can migrate passively.

Following penetration of the basement membrane, malignant cells can invade into the underlying interstitial stroma, which separates lymphatics and blood vessels from organ parenchyma. The interstitial connective stroma can be comprised of collagen, elastin, and anchoring fibers and fibrils as well as ground substance; molecular components include type I collagen, type III collagen, type V collagen, fibronectin, elastin and proteoglycans (7). Following stromal invasion, tumor cells can gain entry to the blood vessels and lymphatics and disseminate to distant sites; tumor invasion through small blood vessel walls during intravasation or extravasation requires tumor cell penetration of the subendothelial basement membrane (8). Upon extravasation, tumor cells must invade through the perivascular interstitial stroma prior to metastatic colony formation in the target organ parenchyma (7-8). Therefore, tumor invasion of various extracellular matrices takes place at several stages during the metastatic process and metastasizing tumor cells must invade the vascular basement membrane during both intravasation and extravasation.

B. Tumor Cell Interactions with the Extracellular Matrix

Tumor cells can interact with, or modify, extracellular matrices in a number of distinct ways: degradation of matrix components during tumor invasion (7,14), tumor cell attachment to the matrix by specific plasma membrane receptors (8), desmoplasia, i.e., increased production of matrix components by the host in response to the tumor (7,15) or production of matrix components by tumor cells (7,16,17). The extracellular matrix, composed of a network of collagen and elastin within a ground substance made up of glycoproteins and proteoglycans, has several biological functions: support of tissue compartments, cell attachment, macromolecular filtering and determination of tissue architecture (7). The extracellular matrix also plays a role in mitogenesis, morphogenesis and cytodifferentiation and may play a role in gene expression through changing the association of the cytoskeleton with nuclear components (7,18).

C. Biochemical Steps Involved in Tumor Invasion of the Extracellular Matrix

A hypothesis has been proposed to describe the discrete biochemical steps involved in the invasion of extracellular matrices by malignant cells during tumor invasion (7-9). The first step is tumor cell attachment to the extracellular matrix. The second step is local dissolution of the matrix by tumor cell-derived, or host cell-induced, proteolytic enzymes. The third step is tumor cell locomotion through the localized domains of extracellular matrix which have been modified by proteolytic enzymes in the proximity of invading tumor cells. This biochemical sequence is a useful model for consideration of the diverse factors that appear to play a role in tumor cell invasion of the matrix including cell migration, chemotactic factors, specific tissue matrices and cell-cell interactions (7,19-21).

1. <u>Tumor cell attachment</u>. Attachment appears to be mediated by specific attachment glycoproteins such as laminin or fibronectin (7,8,22). Certain metastatic cells attach more rapidly to type IV collagen than to type I collagen whereas nonmetastatic cells bind preferentially to type I collagen (23). In addition, metastatic and nonmetastatic cells utilize different attachment proteins in their interactions with various collagens (24). For example, laminin has been shown to enhance the attachment of metastatic cells to type IV collagen whereas fibronectin increased the attachment of nonmetastatic cells to both type I and type IV collagen (24). Metastatic PM2 sarcoma and B16-BL6 melanoma cells preferentially utilize laminin over fibronectin in binding to type IV collagen whereas nonmetastatic C3H cells preferentially utilize fibronectin rather than laminin for such attachment (24). Cells selected on the basis of attachment to type IV collagen in the presence of laminin <u>in vitro</u> display enhanced metastatic potential <u>in vivo</u> when compared to either cells that did not attach to type IV collagen or cells selected by fibronectin-mediated attachment (24).

Tumor cell attachment to the extracellular matrix by specific attachment glycoproteins employs receptors on the tumor cell plasma membrane (7,8,25). For example, a specific high affinity receptor has been identified on the surface of human breast carcinoma cells that has a high affinity for laminin (8,25). Experiments with proteinase-derived fragments of laminin have identified domains of the laminin molecule that bind to the cell surface and domains that bind to type IV collagen (7,8,26-28). The biochemical properties of laminin and proteinase-derived fragments of laminin have been directly compared to their molecular structure with rotary shadowing electron microscopy (7,8,27,28). In summary, laminin receptors on tumor cells may facilitate tumor cell interaction with the host matrix during tumor invasion via laminin domains which can mediate binding to both tumor cells and host matrix components.

2. <u>Matrix dissolution</u>. Subsequent to matrix attachment, invasive tumor cells produce degradative enzymes, or induce host cells to produce proteolytic enzymes, that can locally degrade extracellular matrices and components including attachment glycoproteins. Matrix degradation probably takes place in the microenvironment of the cell surface of invasive tumor cells where the local concentration of proteolytic activities titrates proteinase inhibitors and/or excludes them in the contact zone between invasive tumor cells and their substrates. Endogenous proteinase inhibitors can be derived from serum as well as the matrix itself. Degradative enzymes produced by invasive tumor cells can be active in both extracellular, released forms and in cell surface associated forms.

Histological studies have indicated rapid and local breakdown of the basement membrane during tumor invasion (9). Multiple proteolytic enzymes may be directly or indirectly associated with the dissolution of extracellular matrices, as discussed in detail below.

3. Tumor cell locomotion. Following tumor cell attachment and matrix
dissolution, the third step in the penetration of the extracellular
matrix by invasive tumor cells is locomotion through the region of the
matrix which has been locally degraded by proteolytic enzymes. The
direction of invasive tumor cell locomotion may be regulated to some
extent by chemotactic factors derived from host cells, connective
tissue or serum (7,8). Chemotaxis may effect the organ homing of
metastases (19). Detachment of malignant cells from the substrates
through which they migrate contributes to the locomotion of invasive
cells (29). In addition, proteolytic enzymes which play a role in
matrix dissolution may contribute to the locomotion of invasive tumor
cells (8). Tumor cell migration may also be in response to noncollagenous adhesive glycoproteins. Fibronectin and laminin have
recently been shown to enhance specific haptotactic/chemotactic
migration of B16 melanoma cells (30,31). The chemotactic stimulus,
N-formyl-methionyl-leucyl-phenylalanine (FMLP), significantly
stimulates the migration of invasive M5076 cells through amnion
connective tissue at a concentration similar to that found to be
optimal for stimulating the migration of tumor cells and phagocytes
across artificial porous filters (32,33).

III.   PROTEOLYTIC ENZYMES IN TUMOR INVASION AND METASTASIS

   A.   Proteolytic Enzymes and Malignant Cells

      Considerable experimental evidence exists which documents an
association between elevated proteolytic activities and malignant
transformation (8,13,34).   Glycosyl transferases, glycosidases,
peptidases and proteinases of tumor interstitial fluids, various
cathepsins and various neutral serine proteinases have been studied
for their role in malignant transformation (13,34).   Elevated
proteolytic activities, relative to proteinase levels of normal
tissues, have suggested that proteolytic enzymes may play a role in
tumor invasion and metastasis as well as neoplastic transformation and
promotion (8,13,34). Degradative penetration of host extracellular
matrices by invasive malignant cells appears to involve proteolytic
enzymes directly or indirectly associated with tumor cells (5-13).
Since the extracellular matrices of different tissues have distinct
quantitative compositions of collagens, glycoproteins, proteoglycans,
proteins and elastin with equally distinct molecular, adhesive and
structural interactions among matrix components, it is likely that
multiple degradative proteolytic enzymes may be responsible for
degradation of the various extracellular matrices encountered by
metastatic cells (5,8,9).   Cells with metastatic potential produce a
number of proteolytic enzymes that may contribute to matrix degradation
including collagenases, plasminogen activators, cathepsin B, endo-
glucuronidases and procoagulants (8,21).   The role of specific
degradative enzymes in tumor invasion and metastasis is reviewed below.

B.   Role of Type IV Collagenase and Type V Collagenase in Matrix
     Degradation, Tumor Invasion and Metastasis

Evidence has accumulated to indicate that collagenases play an
important role in facilitating tumor cell invasion of the extracellular
matrix (8,9,11).   Type IV collagenase recognizes and degrades type IV
collagen; type IV collagen is uniquely localized to the basement
membrane (8,9,11).   Type IV collagenase, which is distinct from classic
collagenases, has been shown to be elevated in a number of metastatic
cells.   Type IV collagenase produced by cultured metastatic cells is
found in both an active form as well as a plasmin or trypsin
activatable latent form.   Type IV collagenase is a metalloproteinase
which is inhibited by α_2-macroglobulin, EDTA and cartilage-derived
natural collagenase inhibitors.   The enzyme is not inhibited by DFP,
PMSF or N-ethylmaleimide (9,11).   Type IV collagenase purified from
human tumor cells migrates as a doublet on gel electrophoresis with a
M_r of 70,000 (9,11).   At 37°C type IV collagenase cleaves type IV
collagen into several fragments.   Below 35°C, however, specific large
cleavage products are obtained including a specific cleavage within a
pepsin-resistant domain of type IV collagen (9,11).   Degradation of
type IV collagen by the enzyme at 25°C yields a major cleavage product
at a region one third of the way from one end of the intact substrate.
The exact sequence of the cleavage site has not been determined.   Type
IV collagenase does not degrade collagens I, II, III or V, or native
elastin.

A correlation between production of type IV collagenase and the
capacity to give rise to spontaneous murine metastases has been
reported (35).   All highly metastatic tumors tested to date including
carcinomas, fibrosarcomas, hepatomas, melanomas and reticulum cell
sarcomas have consistently shown elevated type IV collagenase activity
when compared to benign control cells (9,11).   Although it is unlikely
that type IV collagenase will correlate with metastatic potential in
all types of tumors it appears that some minimal ability to degrade
type IV collagen would be required for hematogenous metastasis.   In
studies employing three pairs of related tumor variants, each comprised
of a more and less metastatic line in each case, it was found that
whereas imperfect correlations of lytic activity were noted for
purified substrates including laminin and type IV collagen, the more
metastatic tumor line of each pair was always able to solubilize more
iodinated lens capsule basement membrane matrix (36).   Using primary
cell cultures B16-F10 cells did not display more degradative activity
than B16-F1 cells for type IV collagen (36).   Studies indicating that
B16-F10 cells exhibit greater degradation of type IV collagen than
B16-F1 cells have employed tissue-culture passaged cells (35).   Type IV
collagenase production is correlated with metastasis formation for many
malignant tumors (35-38).   Recent studies with tumor cell hybrids
derived from fusions of high metastatic, low metastatic, benign or
normal cells indicate that type IV collagenase activity in the hybrids
correlates with the resulting changes in metastatic potential following
hybridization (39).   In summary, type IV collagenase has an important
function in degradation of basement membrane type IV collagen and also
seems to be correlated with the formation of metastases.

A distinct tumor metalloproteinase produced by metastatic cells which preferentially degrades type V collagen has also been identified (40). Type V collagenase, which is not able to degrade type IV collagen, produces specific large molecular weight cleavage products of type V collagen. The molecular weight of the isolated type V collagenase is 80,000.

Metalloproteinases that degrade type IV and V collagens are not unique to tumor cells. Type V collagen-degrading enzymatic activity has also been found in normal alveolar macrophages (41) and a type IV collagen degrading elastase has been isolated from polymorphonuclear leukocytes (42). Normal involuting epithelial ducts have been shown to contain enzymes that degrade both type IV and type V collagens (43). Type IV and type V collagenases, which contribute to degradation of the host matrix during tumor invasion, also appear to play a role in the selective turnover of the matrix during normal tissue remodeling (11). A recent report has suggested that macrophages and Lewis lung carcinoma cells cooperate in the degradation of basement membrane type IV collagen and that this interaction may be of importance in cancer invasion and metastasis (44). The interaction of matrix-degrading collagenases with the plasminogen activator/plasmin system is considered below (also see Chapter 19).

C.   Role of Plasminogen Activators and Plasmin in Matrix Degradation, Tumor Invasion and Metastasis

1.   Structural, biochemical and enzymatic aspects of PA function. Plasminogen activators (PA) are highly selective, neutral, serine proteinases that proteolytically convert the inactive serum proenzyme plasminogen to the active enzyme plasmin, a neutral proteinase of broad enzymatic specificity (34,45-47). Although PAs are considered to have trypsin-like enzymatic activity, they differ from trypsin and plasmin by having an extremely narrow substrate specificity, confined to very limited cleavage domains. Whereas plasmin, for example, has multiple biological substrates including fibrin, fibronectin, laminin, matrix glycoproteins, plasma membrane components, procollagenases, casein and immunoglobulins, PA has only one well characterized natural, physiological substrate: plasminogen (5,47). This is probably a reflection of the important physiological degradative capacity of PAs in the lysis of fibrin clots and of their role in endogenous thrombolysis. Recent reports have suggested that PA can also function catalytically on a cellular substrate other than plasminogen resulting in a plasminogen-independent modification of the behavior and morphology of malignantly transformed cells (48-51). Colonial morphology resulting from extemely high levels of PA is observed during super-transformation mediated by synergistic inter-action between a tumor virus and a tumor promoter under plasminogen-free conditions; this is blocked by inhibitors of PA but not plasmin. The use of a fluorogenic peptide substrate for the direct determination of PA, independently of plasmin, demonstrated that PA itself, and not plasmin, is involved in mediating these morphological alterations

(48-52). It has also been shown that PA cleaves a 66,000 M_r peri-cellular matrix protein of human lung to a 62,000 M_r product (54). In the studies described below it is therefore worthwhile to keep in mind that PA is a proteinase that may have important biological functions independent of its capacity to generate plasminogen from plasmin.

PAs are classified as being urokinase (UK)-like, or non-urokinase-like (47). Human UK, produced in the kidney and excreted in urine, has several molecular weight forms including a single chain with a M_r value of 56,000, predominantly high molecular weight forms of approximately 54,000 M_r and low molecular weight forms of approximately 32,000 M_r (47). Tissue PAs (TPA) are distinct and immunologically unrelated to UK but identical to the PAs in the vascular wall and to human uterine PA. The M_r of TPAs, which exist in both single and double chain forms, ranges between 60,000 and 75,000 (47). Unlike most forms of UK, TPA efficiently adsorbs to fibrin and fibrin clots, and has recently received considerable attention for potential use in thrombolytic therapy (47). The majority of human PA produced by tumor cells is biochemically and immunologically similar to or identical to UK, whereas some tumors produce TPA (13,47). The primary structure of high molecular weight UK from human urokinase has been reported (55) as has the amino acid sequence of TPA (56). A model for UK was recently described which was constructed on the basis of chymotrypsin structure (57). The high and low molecular weight forms of UK are identical in their B chains which contain the catalytic active site (55); the difference in M_r is due to a cleavage in the A chain leaving an Al chain linked to the B chain by a single disulfide bridge (55). Studies dealing with the sequence of the light, A chain, of high M_r UK have determined three domains within the A chain: a connecting peptide domain, a "kringle" domain and a growth factor domain. The N-terminal region of the A chain may be a growth factor with substantial similarity to the sequence of epidermal growth factor (EGF). The growth factor component of PA may contribute activities to tumor cells in addition to those mediated by the catalytic active site. The kringle domain is also of interest (55,58). Kringles are homologous triple-loop, 3-disulfide-bridge structures which play an important role in molecular interactions in prothrombin-thrombin conversion, plasminogen activation and fibrinolysis (58). Both TPA and UK kringles have recently been reported to be similar to fibronectin kringles suggesting that the homologous kringles of PAs and the gelatin-binding region of fibronectin play important roles in protein-binding behavior (58). With respect to the growth factor domain of UK it is of interest that an enhanced rate of EGF receptor inactivation is closely correlated with increased cellular PA activity. PA-mediated events may initiate the inactivation of the EGF receptor during down-regulation (59). In addition, EGF has been found to stimulate PA activity (60,61).

PAs exist in both cell-surface associated forms as well as extra-cellular, soluble forms (47,52,62). In addition, PAs of many cell types exist in precursor, zymogen forms as well as in active catalytic forms (47,63-66). Cells that produce active or precursor forms of PA have also been shown to produce inhibitors of PA (67-72). The processing of PA, from a cell surface-associated enzyme to a soluble proteinase is not fully understood or characterized, although it has recently been shown that a chymostatin-sensitive enzyme associated with a membrane fraction may play a direct role in the proteolytic release of PA from its membrane association (73). Chymostatin, an inhibitor of chymotryptic enzymes, inhibits the release of PA and leads to the build-up of cell-associated PA levels (74).

In summary, a great deal of information exists dealing with PA at the biochemical, cellular, structural and regulatory levels. In order to fully evaluate the exact role of PAs in malignant transformation, tumor invasion and metastasis, it will be necessary to critically explore issues of PA type (extracellular vs cell-associated; UK-like vs TPA-like), zymogen and/or inhibitor presence, growth factor domain-containing or lacking M_r species, and aspects of the processing of PA in a particular cell type. Following a brief synopsis of the role of PAs in malignant transformation the role of PA in invasion and metastasis is reviewed below.

2. PA/plasmin and malignant transformation. The expression of PA and the proteolytic generation of plasmin from plasminogen play roles in the migration and degradative action of normal cell types involved in tissue remodeling (45). The PA/plasmin enzymatic system has also been associated with several aspects of malignant transformation including tumorigenesis of viral transformants in nude mice, anchorage independent growth of tumor cells in agar, tumorigenesis of bromodeoxy-uridine-regulated murine melanoma cells and hormone-dependent murine mammary carcinoma cells, temperature sensitive expression of the Rous sarcoma virus sarcomagenesis (Src) gene product, tumor promoter treatment of normal and Rous sarcoma virus transformed cells, loss of intracellular actin cables, induction of cellular proliferation and tumorigenicity of carcinogen induced transformed guinea pig fibroblasts (8,34,45-48,75). Recent reports have demonstrated that TPA has a direct role in a morphological aspect of transformation (76). Recent studies have also shown that the production of PA by one cell type can be influenced by additional cell types or by the extracellular matrix (77-79). PA-producing cells might therefore be able to recruit adjacent non-PA producing cells to synthesize PA and thereby contribute to enhanced microenvironmental proteolysis. The induction of PA by u.v. light is correlated with diminished capacity for DNA repair; thus, the expression of PA may play a role in the alteration of gene regulation and contribute to the initiation of malignant transformation (80-84).

Although normal cells involved in invasive, degradative activities also produce PA and generate plasmin, normal cell PA biosynthesis appears to be under developmental, hormonal or temporal regulatory controls that may fail to regulate PA production by tumor cells (45,85). For example, degradation of the Graafian follicle at the time of ovulation and embryonic implantation of trophoblasts are associated with transient production of PA as a function of the invasive phase of these processes (45,47,85).

Exceptions to the correlation between PA production and malignant transformation have been noted (85-87); although most malignant tumors produce more PA than normal tissues the correlation is not exact. Discussions attempting to reconcile conflicting results have been presented previously (47,86,87). Since cell migration, tissue remodeling and malignant transformation may be associated with modifications to host extracellular matrices, PA and plasmin have also been extensively examined for their potential role in degradation of the host extracellular matrix during tumor invasion (see Chapter 20 for more detail on PAs).

3. <u>PA/plasmin in matrix degradation and tumor invasion</u>. A number of studies have demonstrated that matrix glycoproteins are sensitive to proteolytic degradation mediated by plasmin (5,8,88-95). Plasmin, resulting from macrophage plasminogen activation, degrades 50-70 percent of smooth muscle cell matrices composed of glycoproteins, elastin and collagens (88). Matrix glycoproteins inhibit the rate of digestion of other macromolecules including elastin, whereas plasminogen activation with concomitant degradation of glycoproteins allows for more efficient degradation of elastin by macrophage elastase (89). Plasminogen activation by macrophages thereby enhances hydrolysis of elastin and the rate of matrix degradation (90). For alveolar macrophages, PA and plasminogen rather than elastase may be rate limiting in the degradation of elastase (91a). Plasmin generation also appears to contribute significantly to glycoprotein degradation by tumor cells (5,8,9,94).

Four human tumor cell lines were found to digest glycoproteins present in the extracellular matrix produced by cultured rat smooth muscle cells (92). Whereas all four of the metastatic human tumor cells digest matrix glycoproteins, human fibroblasts fail to mediate glycoprotein degradation (92). Jones and DeClerck (92) concluded that tumor cell PA and the generation of plasmin play a key role in the hydrolysis of all matrix components since glycoprotein removal from the matrix is required for the maximal digestion of collagen and elastin. In contrast, Kramer <u>et al</u>. (93) reported that solubilization of vascular subendothelial matrix by metastatic cells is not dependent on serum plasminogen, suggesting that the generation of plasmin by invasive metastatic cells is not necessary for matrix degradation. Nevertheless, Kramer <u>et al</u>. (93) did observe that inactivation of serum proteinase inhibitors by acid treatment increases matrix solubilization in the presence of serum plasminogen. Acid-treated serum also increases tumor cell-mediated digestion of the subendothelial matrix even in the absence of plasminogen (93). The plasminogen independent cleavage of matrix glycoproteins could be due to the direct action of tumor cell PA or to an additional serum inhibitor-sensitive cell-associated or extracellular proteinase (8,49,50,93).

Additional studies probing the role of PA and plasmin in matrix degradation have also been reported. The serine proteinases PA, plasmin, and alpha thrombin have been directly evaluated for their role in the degradation of both components of the basement membrane and intact human amnion basement membrane (94,95). Homogeneously pure enzymes were incubated with whole human amnion basement membrane and with isolated components of basement membrane: acid-extracted type IV collagen, pepsin fragments of collagen type IV, laminin, fibronectin and type V collagen associated with the peri-basement membrane zone (95). Human PA (urokinase) does not significantly degrade fibronectin, or any of the other components of the basement membrane (94,95). Although PA or the inactive zymogen plasminogen are unable to degrade fibronectin or laminin, plasmin and alpha thrombin cleave these substrates into multiple, specific fragments (95,96). Plasmin degrades both the 400,000 and 200,000 M_r chains of laminin to produce specific cleavage products; alpha thrombin degrades only the 400,000 M_r chain of laminin (94-96). Plasmin and alpha thrombin do not yield major cleavages of acid-extracted type IV collagen, pepsinized type IV collagen or type V collagen under native conditions (94-96). At high concentrations plasmin produces a small reduction in the lower of the two chains of type IV collagen suggesting nonspecific removal of a portion of the non-helical telopeptide region of this substrate (95). Type V collagen is cleaved by plasmin and alpha thrombin at 35°C, but such cleavage is not observed at temperatures below 33°C. The biological relevance of laminin degradation was examined by testing extracts from a variety of different cell types for their laminin-degrading capacity employing ^{14}C laminin prepared from cultured EHS cells. Metastatic mouse sarcoma cells, leukocytes and macrophages all exhibit substantial degradation of laminin (95). For the metastatic tumor cells, the major fraction of laminin degradation is plasminogen dependent (95). The majority of the plasminogen-independent laminin-degrading proteolytic activity is removed by inhibitors of metallo-proteinases (95). Since plasmin degrades two noncollagenous components associated with the basement membrane zone, laminin and fibronectin, and has some effect on acid-extracted type IV collagen, plasmin was also studied for its effects on intact isolated human amnion epithelial basement membrane (94,95). Following treatment of the denuded basement membrane with purified plasmin, the basement membrane ultra-structure is not greatly altered (95). Further studies with plasmin have taken advantage of the observation that amnion basement membrane exhibits uniform binding of antibodies to both laminin and type IV collagen, binding which is preserved after epithelial denudation (95). The immunofluorescent localization of anti-type IV collagen and anti-laminin antibodies in denuded basement membrane, following plasmin treatment of the basement membrane, has been examined. Even though electron microscopy indicates that the basement membrane lamina densa is not completely destroyed by plasmin treatment, immunohistology studies have shown that plasmin treatment does lead to loss of immuno-reactivity for anti-laminin antibodies and anti-fibronectin antibodies (95). In contrast, immunoreactivity for anti-type IV collagen antibodies in the basement membrane is retained following plasmin treatment (95). Identical results are noted upon plasmin treatment of human capillary basement membranes (95). It, therefore, appears that plasmin alone is not sufficient for complete degradation of the whole basement membrane. Plasmin may nevertheless play an important role in the proteolytic digestion of the basement membrane by activation of latent tumor cell proteinases which could play a role in degradation of basement membrane collagen, glycoprotein or glycosaminoglycan components (96-100). Plasmin may therefore play a role in both removal of basement membrane glycoproteins from the basement membrane and exposure of type IV collagen to degradation by additional proteolytic enzymes that plasmin can activate from latent forms. A key function of PA in matrix degradation by invasive, metastatic tumor cells might therefore be regulation and control over a cascade of degradative proteolytic activities (8,9,95).

The role of PA, plasmin and plasminogen in matrix degradation have been further defined by additional studies (101-103). Malignant fibrosarcoma cells digest preparations of basement membrane from Syrian hamster lung and the degradation of the basement membrane is correlated with the fibrinolytic activity of the tumor cells (101). Basement membrane degradation is dependent upon the presence of plasminogen in the medium and degradation is not observed when plasminogen-depleted serum is employed; in addition, inhibitors of plasmin inhibit basement membrane degradation (101). The results indicate that degradation of basement membrane by BP6T fibrosarcoma cells is most likely due to PA-mediated degradation of basement membrane glycoproteins (101). Human HT1080 fibrosarcoma cells, which produce large amounts of PA, have been studied for their capacity to degrade bovine subendothelial matrix, which resembles vascular basement membrane (102). The glycoprotein components of this matrix are degraded by plasmin whereas the matrix collagens, including type IV collagen, are insensitive to plasmin. HT1080 cells were found to degrade labeled matrix glycoproteins at maximal rates in the presence of plasminogen (102). Plasminogen-independent glycoprotein digestion was also noted for these cells. Human rhabdomyosarcoma, osteogenic sarcoma and neuroblastoma cells digest mainly the glycoprotein components of the subendothelial matrix with only little collagenolytic activity (102). Clones of HT1080 cells have been isolated from the parental fibrosarcoma line which produce similar levels of cell-associated PA but produce either large or small levels of extracellular PA; each class of PA-producing clones digest the glycoprotein components of the subendothelial matrix at similar rates (102). The results suggest that cell-associated PA plays a predominant role in matrix degradation or that a plasminogen-independent proteolytic activity is also involved in matrix degradation (102). HT1080 clones were also found to differ in collagenolytic activities. HT1080 clones secreting high levels of PA and containing low levels of collagenolytic activity digest more of both collagenase-sensitive and glycoprotein-sensitive components of the matrix than clones secreting low levels of PA with high collagenolytic activity (102). The results therefore suggest that both PA/plasmin and collagenases play significant roles in matrix degradation by invasive metastatic cells. Subsequent studies with HT1080 cells, as well as with B16-F1 cells and human rhabdomyosarcoma cells, have further elucidated the role of plasminogen in matrix degradation by tumor cells (103,104). Each of the cell lines degrade a portion of the smooth muscle cell matrix. Degradation of the matrix by human HT1080 fibro-sarcoma cells and murine B16-F1 melanoma cells shows a plasminogen dependency related to cell density, whereas human rhabdomyosarcoma RD cells digest the matrix at all cell densities only in the presence of plasminogen (103). The results suggest that the generation of plasmin from plasminogen by tumor cell PA is important for matrix digestion at low cell densities for some tumor cell lines which show plasminogen independent matrix degradation with increased cell numbers (103). For other tumor cell lines, degradation of the matrix appears to absolutely require plasmin generation at all cell densities (103). Results with B16-F1 melanoma cells were similar in earlier studies (93). The identity of the proteinase that leads to plasminogen independent glycoprotein degradation remains unidentified, and could include PA itself, a glycosidase, or cathepsin B (49,50,93,105; also see Chapters 18 and 22; and sections below for more detail). To date it has been observed and confirmed that PA (urokinase), plasminogen (94-96) and PA (TPA; 106) fail to cleave laminin. In the presence of plasminogen and either class of PA, or in the presence of plasmin, laminin is efficiently cleaved as discussed above (94-96,106). It is of interest that laminin binds plasminogen and PA (TPA) but not PA (urokinase; 106). Although human PA (urokinase) fails to degrade human plasma fibronectin (94-96), PA from Rous sarcoma virus transformed chick embryo fibroblasts might have a direct role in the degradation of chick cell extracellular matrix highly enriched in fibronectin (107). This PA (RSVCEF) might catalytically remove fibronectin from cells and substratum or cleave a protein responsible for the attachment of fibronectin to the cell surface and substratum (52). Recent studies with Rous sarcoma virus transformed cells have indicated that a proteinase(s) can degrade fibronectin at extracellular matrix contact sites; although inhibitors of PA can block the observed effects, it is not clear whether the fibronectin degrading activity is PA or a distinct enzymatic activity (108). In studies dealing with human umbilical vein endothelial cells, human kidney PA (urokinase)-treatment of human fibronectin in plastic cell culture dishes leads to enhanced morphological organizational behavior of the endothelial cells, i.e., when added to the PA-treated fibronectin-containing dishes (109). Endothelial cells can inhibit matrix glycoprotein degradation mediated by HT1080 PA and plasminogen activation, yet the unidentified proteolytic activity that plays a role in glycoprotein degradation by HT1080 cells at high cell density is not affected by the endothelial cell factor (104).

In summary, the generation of plasmin by tumor cell PA can contribute to tumor invasion by degradation of the glycoprotein components of the extracellular matrix and exposure of other substrates, including type IV collagen, to additional tumor-associated proteinases. In addition, plasmin can activate the latent forms of collagenases which degrade basement membrane type IV collagen and associated type V collagen (97-102). Both the PA/plasmin and collagenolytic system may play important roles in degradation of the subendothelial matrix and the secretion of PA, concomitantly with that of basement membrane collagenase, may be a prerequisite for metastasis (100,102). In addition, the direct enzymatic activity of PA may play a role in plasminogen independent degradation of glycoprotein components of the extracellular matrix (49,50,54,93,102,103).

4. PA in tumor growth and metastasis. A number of studies have examined the potential role of PA in tumor growth, progression, and metastasis and several reviews on the subject have recently appeared (21,47,110-112).

Homogeneously purified PAs (high and low molecular weight urokinase) are angiogenic in the rabbit cornea, suggesting that PA might contribute to tumor neovascularization during tumor invasion and metastasis (8,13,113). In contrast, DFP-inhibited PA, for which ^{3}H-DFP has been incorporated into both the high and low molecular weight forms of PA (urokinase), failed to mediate neovascularization in the rabbit cornea (R.H. Goldfarb, L.A. Liotta, G.M. Murano and M. Ziche, unpublished observations). In addition to a direct role for PA in angiogenesis, PA/plasmin can play additional roles in neovascularization. Upon stimulation by angiogenic factors, endothelial cells may produce active PA and latent collagenase which is activated upon generation of plasmin from plasminogen by the active PA (114). Extracts of adult bovine retina, which contain a potent stimulator of neovascularization, trigger the dose-dependent release of PA by fetal bovine aortic endothelial cells grown in culture (115). The retinal extracts do not contain PA in either latent or active forms but stimulate the release of PA by vascular endothelial cells (114). In addition, the retinal extract also stimulates degradation of basement membrane type IV collagen by vascular endothelial cells (115). PA, and the generation of plasmin from plasminogen, may play important roles in early steps in the formation of new blood vessels by tumor cells and these roles might be related to degradation of the basement membrane (8,13,113-115).

A recent study examined the levels of PA in normal and tumor-bearing mice (116). B16, colon 26, Lewis lung and M5076 tumors have high to intermediate levels of PA. The specific activities of PA in extracts of B16 and colon 26 tumors are three to four times higher than those in normal organs with PA activity (kidney, lung, brain and intestine). High PA levels in the B16 tumor correlate with substantial elevations in the levels of fibrin degradation products (four to thirty fold higher) in the serum of B16 tumor-bearing mice (116). Breusch et al. (116) suggest that the observed tumor-associated PA activity is less subject to in vivo inhibitory control than the PA of normal tissues studied since the majority of fibrin degradation products are caused by the tumor even though the tumor mass is far less than the mass of normal organs yielding fibrinolytic activity.

A number of studies have examined the issue of whether a quantitative correlation exists between the production of PA by malignant cells and their capacity to metastasize. Some of these studies, with conflicting conclusions, will be reviewed here. One report has shown that low metastatic B16-F1 and variants of increasing metastatic potential (B16-F5, B16-F10 and B16-F13) display similar levels of high PA activity (117). Studies with UV2237 fibrosarcoma cells have demonstrated that some cloned tumor cell lines with high in vivo metastatic potential produce low levels of PA when compared to cells with lower metastatic potential (118). Studies with metastatic variants from cloned cell lines of hepatic origin have also found no correlation between metastatic capacity and fibrinolytic activity (119). Studies with Lewis lung carcinoma cells have also been reported in which no consistent differences are detectable in PA levels between primary and metastatic cultures (120). Recent studies have also examined the PA activity of metastatic variants from a murine fibrosarcoma and have failed to show any significant correlation between tumor cell metastatic potential and cellular PA activity (121). A number of studies have recently examined a variety of proteolytic activities for possible correlations with metastatic activities, including PA, cathepsin D, cathepsin B, cathepsin G, elastase-like activities, and collagenases and have found no differences between proteinase activities in: homogenates of normal and Lewis lung carcinoma cells (122); clones derived from a methylcholanthrene-induced fibrosarcoma (123); and sublines of rat prostatic adenocarcinomas (124). In the studies with rat prostatic adenocarcinomas only the levels of elastase and chymotrypsin-like activities are consistently elevated in highly metastatic prostatic cancers when compared to those in either normal prostate or prostatic cancers with low metastatic potential (124). With regard to some of the studies described above the following should be noted. The studies with UV2237 cells are not considered to be a conclusive test of the role of PA in metastasis for a variety of reasons including: questions concerning the hormonal regulation of these lines in vivo; lack of determination of PA production by subpopulations of cultured cells that form metastases; comparatively low levels of PA produced by clones of high metastatic activity may provide sufficient PA to contribute to metastasis; and the observation that when immunosuppressed animals were employed, clones with normally low metastatic potential are highly metastatic (118). The studies with Lewis lung carcinoma employed cultures atypical of parental tumors which grow slowly upon reinjection at primary tumor sites and which have impaired metastatic potential (120) or described methodological problems with the assay of proteolytic activities in cellular homogenates (122).

In contrast, a number of reports have indicated a good correlation between PA production and metastatic potential. Quantitative differences in PA production between low metastatic B16-F1 and high metastatic B16-F10 sublines have been reported (125). B16-F10 cells consistently produce more PA than B16-F1 cells when $10^5 - 10^7$ cells are cultured for at least twenty-four hours (125); in contrast, there is no significant difference in PA production between B16-F10 and B16-F1 cells when 10^4 cells, or less, are tested. The studies with B16-F1-F13 sublines which failed to show a positive correlation between PA levels and metastasis employed 10^4 cells (117). B16 cells harvested from pulmonary metastatic nodules of host mice show higher PA activity than do B16 cells from primary tumors in the same mice (125). PA has also been associated with the metastatic spread of rat prostatic adenocarcinoma cells and it has been suggested that the high level of PA in these cancer cells is involved in metastasis (126). Studies with rat mammary adenocarcinoma have also suggested that PA activity is an indicator of metastatic tumor colonization and may play a role in the mechanisms of tumor nidation and colonization (127). Cell populations derived from metastatic foci have high PA levels whereas lectin resistant variants, which have lost their capacity to nidate in the lung, have the lowest PA activity (127). Studies with highly metastatic rat mammary adenocarcinomas,and their fusion with non-metastatic cells, have indicated that PA is involved in the formation of metastatic lung foci (128). Highly metastatic parental cells produce large quantities of PA, whereas none can be detected in the non-metastatic lines; although hybrid clones have decreased metastatic potential and decreased PA activity, one clone reverted to a more metastatic line without an increase in PA activity (128). Additional studies with this rat mammary adenocarcinoma have indicated that this cell line is heterogenous with respect to PA production (129). A strong correlation has been reported for PA activity and metastatic potential for this system and it has been suggested that PA production may play an important role in tumor metastasis (129). This study is of significance since it employed cells selected for differing levels of PA activity among heterogenous cells with metastatic potential rather than employing cells selected only for differences in metastatic potential; the latter selection process, used in most studies examining the role of PA in metastasis, does not select for PA levels alone, but rather selects for multiple cellular changes that could contribute to metastasis. Recent immunohistological studies have also suggested that PA plays a role in tumor invasion and metastasis (130). Invasive and metastasizing Lewis lung carcinoma cells were examined immunocyto-chemically with antibodies directed against PA (urokinase-like); different portions of individual tumors show heterogeneity in the intensity of staining. Strong staining with antibodies directed against PA are found in areas with invasive growth and degradation of surrounding normal tissue whereas other areas do not stain (130). Immunoreactivity is observed with both a perinuclear cytoplasmic localization in tumor cells and also in association with extracellular material (130). The results suggest that PA in the Lewis lung carcinoma plays a role in invasive growth and tissue degradation. Interestingly, the administration of PA (urokinase) to mice has been reported to significantly increase hematogenous pulmonary metastases of Lewis lung (130a).

A number of studies with human tumor cells have also indicated a role for PA in tumor progression and metastasis. Human epidermoid HEp-3 cells, which have been used in a quantitative model of metastasis in chick embryos, express human PA in chick tissues (131). The human PA can be distinguished from chick PA since each enzyme has a preference for homologous plasminogen. Human PA in chick tissues and body fluids has therefore been used as a quantitative marker for HEp-3 metastasis in both chick embryos and newly hatched chicks (131). Anti-PA (human urokinase) which inhibits HEp-3 but not chick PA prevents or strongly inhibits the metastasis of HEp-3 cells to the chick embryo lung upon intravenous administration (132). The results suggest that PA is required in the early stages of human HEp-3 cell metastasis in chick embryos (132).

The induction of PA production in response to the tumor promoter 12-0-tetradecanoylphorbol-13-acetate, TPA, has been used to rank distinct histological classes of human colonic adenomas in primary culture from the most benign to an advanced premalignant state (133,134). Benign tubular adenomas in culture do not respond to TPA by PA secretion since they are not at a sufficiently preneoplastic state to respond (134). During tumor evolution, villous subpopulations of adenomas are the first preneoplastic cells to express responsiveness to TPA by secretion of PA and this phenotypic property is maintained as the cells evolve through more advanced premalignant stages to carcinomas (134). TPA treatment yields multicellular clusters concomitant with PA secretion that are similar to areas of carcinoma found within adenomas and also similar to the morphology observed in cells supertransformed by Rous sarcoma virus and TPA (48-50). The cytoskeletons of PA-secreting "late stage" preneoplastic cells from adenomas demonstrate disorganized actin filaments in response to TPA, whereas non PA-secreting "early stage" preneoplastic cells retain actin organization following TPA treatment (135). Loss of actin organization may be a marker for the transition of noninvasive benign colonic tumors to human invasive, malignant colonic tumors; this transition seems to be reflected in vitro by induction of PA secretion by "late stage" preneoplastic cells in response to TPA (135).

Systematic studies to evaluate the PA content of human tumors and corresponding normal tissues have recently been reviewed (110). In studies dealing with tumors of the lung, colon, prostate and breast the mean enzyme content of tumors was found to be higher than in the normal tissues presumed to be the tissue of origin (110). In studies dealing with PA content of human colon tumors and normal mucosae the PA content of tumors that showed invasive or metastatic spread is higher than primary colon tumors that lack this phenotype (136). Recent studies have demonstrated that the measurement of PA secretion rates results in better distinction between normal and malignant tissue than the amount of extractable PA (137). The secretion rate of PA by metastatic tumors of the colon is lower than the secretion rate of primary tumors, suggesting an important role for cell-associated PA, perhaps related to the responsiveness of metastatic cells to growth factors in vivo (137). Immunohistochemical studies have shown that PA (urokinase) is present within the neoplastic component of human colon tumors (137). Studies with human prostatic cancer explants have indicated that the mean PA activity of prostatic carcinomas is significantly higher than that of benign prostatic hyperplasia (138). In contrast to studies indicating that human melanomas produce PA (TPA), it was recently reported that human malignant melanoma PA is predominantly of the urokinase type. Immunoperoxidase reaction for the detection of PA (urokinase) has shown that PA is localized predominantly within the cell membrane of human melanoma cells (139). One study with human breast tumors has indicated that PA activity in tumor bearing patients is very high in malignant tissue but decreasd in plasma as a correlate of metastases in the axillary lymph nodes (140). In contrast, another study with human breast tumor has indicated no quantitative correlation between proteinases, including PA, cathepsin B and collagenases, and invasive properties of breast cancer (141).

In summary, many studies indicate that PA can contribute to various aspects of tumor progression and metastasis in a number of cell types and in a number of species. A full description of the role of PA in tumor metastasis will require careful analysis of a large number of experimental variables. For example, careful experimental design will have to take into account: clonal subpopulations of metastatic variants; heterogeneity of PA production among metastatic variants; consideration of cell surface-associated PA as well as extracellular; soluble PA; the role of zymogen precursor forms of PA and zymogen activation by PA or plasmin; the role of tumor cell or host cell derived inhibitors of PA and/or plasmin; immunologic and biophysical forms of PA: urokinase and/or TPA-like forms of PA; strengths and pitfalls of assays for PA activity: assay of PA vs plasmin; evaluation of TPA-like activity of fibrin or non-fibrin substrates, etc.; modulation of PA activity by direct tumor cell or host cell interaction with adjacent cells by direct cell-cell contact or by the release of soluble mediators; the direct role of PA vs plasminogen activation vs activation of additional proteolytic activities; presence or absence of hormonal modulation; immune status of the host; contribution to tumor cell PA activity by host endothelial cells and cells of the immune response including macrophages and large granular lymphocytes that account for natural killer cell activity (47,52,63-72,77,78,85,87, 97-100,110,113-115,129,142,143).

D. Role of Heparan Sulfate Endoglycosidase in Matrix Degradation, Tumor Invasion and Metastasis

Invasive, metastatic tumor cells have the capacity to digest proteoglycans from the subendothelial matrix (93,144). Metastatic B16 melanoma cells produce a glycosidase that specifically cleaves glyco-saminoglycans and releases heparan sulfate-rich fragments (93). Upon comparison of metastatic sublines for their abilities to degrade basal lamina, invasive metastatic variants, such as B16-BL6 melanoma sublines, are found to solubilize matrix glycosaminoglycans and purified heparan sulfate faster than do B16 cells with poor potential for metastatic lung colonization (145-148). Analysis of the degradation products of heparan sulfate and other purified glycosamino-glycans and determination of their reducing terminal saccharides has determined that a B16 melanoma cell specific endoglucuronidase (heparanase) is responsible for the degradation of matrix sulfated glycosaminoglycans and purified heparan sulfate (93,145-149). Kramer and Vogel (148) suggest that metastatic cells may degrade matrix proteoglycans more readily than other matrix-containing proteins.

Cloned lines of a methylcholanthrene-induced DBA/2 low metastatic T lymphoma Eb line and its highly metastatic variant line, ESb, show differential abilities in degradation of subendothelial matrix proteo-glycans (150). The highly metastatic ESb cells digest the subendothelial proteoglycans to low M_r fragments to a greater extent than the low metastatic Eb cells. Radiolabeled low M_r degradation

358

products are also found upon incubation of radiolabeled extracellular
matrix with a cell-free medium from high metastatic but not low
metastatic lymphoma cells (150).

Since heparan sulfate is an important scaffolding glycosaminoglycan of extracellular matrices, including the basement membrane, its
preferential degradation by high metastatic tumor cells may contribute
to tumor invasion through tissues and blood vessels during hematogenous
metastasis (146-150). The endoglucuronidase most likely works in
concert with proteolytic enzymes that also play a role in tumor
invasion by degradation of additional matrix components (5,8,9,92,95).
Both macrophages and T lymphocytes, upon stimulation, produce an
endoglycosidase with the capacity to cleave glycosaminoglycans and
release heparan-sulfate rich fragments from the matrix (151). Thus
activated cells that play a role in cell-mediated immunity, as well as
high metastatic cells, may degrade sulfated proteoglycans in a similar
manner (144,151). Heparan sulfate proteoglycan isolated from basement
membrane can bind to type IV collagen and laminin and the interaction
of laminin, type IV collagen and heparan sulfate proteoglycan probably
contributes to the structure of extracellular matrices such as the
basement membrane which must be degraded by invasive, metastatic cells
(152). Interestingly, studies with a bacterial heparanase which has a
potent sulfated-glycosaminoglycan-degrading capacity have shown that
upon heparanase digestion of human fibroblast matrix > 95% of sulfated
glycosaminoglycans are degraded in the matrix without the release of
biochemically or immunochemically detectable fibronectin or other major
pericellular matrix glycoproteins (153). The possibility that the
glucuronidase (heparanase) of metastatic cells has a direct catalytic
role in the degradation of matrix fibonectin or laminin has not been
determined (93,95).

The interrelationships among the production of heparan sulfate
proteoglycan by invasive, metastatic cells, the influence of matrix
components on heparan sulfate production, the role of heparan sulfate
proteoglycans in adhesion phenomena with fibronectin, laminin and
collagen, and the elaboration by metastatic cells of endoglucuronidase
(heparanase) degradative activity may be of interest (93,144,148-150,
154-157).

In summary, a number of recent studies have demonstrated that
metastatic cells produce an endoglucuronidase (heparanase) which has
the capacity to degrade basal lamina proteoglycans in addition to their
capacity to digest glycoproteins and proteins of the basal lamina
(93,144-151). The correlation of this enzymatic activity with the high
metastatic potential of murine B16 melanoma sublines and the ESb
T-lymphoma variant suggests a role for this enzyme in matrix
degradation by metastatic cells during tumor invasion (147,150; see
Chapter 18 for further discussion).

E. Role of Cathepsin B in Tumor Invasion and Metastasis

Recent studies have indicated that a cathepsin B-like activity in the high metastatic B16-F10 melanoma cell variant is elevated in comparison to the low metastatic B16-F1 variant (158). It is therefore likely that cathepsin B can contribute to tumor metastasis by playing either a direct or a regulatory role (158,159). In addition, it has been reported that cathepsin B is released from malignant human breast tumors to a greater extent than from normal breast tissue or non-malignant tumors (160,161). An elevation of cathepsin B levels has also been noted in the serum of patients with vaginal clear-cell adenocarcinoma (162). A 39,000 M_r cathepsin B has also been found to be released from cultured spontaneous murine mammary tumors; this enzyme is similar in enzymatic properties to lysosomal cathepsin B (163).

The cathepsin B activity of the high metastatic B16-F10 melanoma cells has been localized to the light mitochondrial fraction of this cell type (159). In the case of human neoplastic cervical epithelial cells, it has been reported that cathepsin B-like activity can also be found in the plasma membrane and nuclear fraction of this cell type (164). Approximately 70% of cathepsin B-like activity occurs in the mitochondrial-lysosomal fraction of control cell homogenates, yet only 33-52% of such activity is found in the corresponding fraction in neoplastic cells; approximately 14% of the total cellular cathepsin B-like activity is found in association with plasma membrane-enriched cellular subfractions (164).

A recent report has shown that a latent cysteine proteinase within ascitic fluid of patients with ovarian carcinoma is a high molecular weight form of cathepsin B. The latent form of the enzyme was found to be a single chain with a M_r of 40,000 while upon pepsin activation the M_r was 33,000. The 33,000 M_r form is similar to the 25,000 M_r form of lysosomal cathepsin B (165). It has been suggested that the latent enzyme is a high molecular weight precursor form of cathepsin B which is released extracellularly as opposed to being processed and directed to the lysosome (163,165).

A number of reports have indicated potential roles for cathepsin B in tumor invasion and metastasis. It has been suggested that cathepsin B could play a role in the induction of platelet aggregation by tumor cells; inhibitors of cysteine proteinases were found to inhibit both B16 amelanotic melanoma cell-induced aggregation of platelets and cathepsin B activity (166). Prostacyclin, which has been shown to exhibit antimetastatic activity, inhibits both tumor cell-induced and cathepsin B-like papain-induced platelet aggregation (166). Inhibitors of cysteine proteinases have also been employed to inhibit platelet aggregation mediated by murine mammary adenocarcinoma cells and membrane vesicles shed from these tumor cells in culture; it was suggested that a correlation exists between a cathepsin B-like proteinase in the mammary adenocarcinoma cells and shed vesicles and their ability to induce platelet aggregation (167). Cathepsin B might play some role in matrix degradation; the enzyme has been reported to

cleave proteoglycans and native collagen and to activate a procollagenase (reviewed in 158,159). Cathepsin B may also have some
laminin-degrading capacity (8 and Chapter 22).

Some studies have shown that tumor cathepsin B is a property of
viable tumor cells and not macrophages and that murine resident
peritoneal macrophages have negligible cathepsin B activity, however,
some reports have indicated cathepsin B activity in subpopulations of
rodent macrophages (158,168). Rat peritoneal and pulmonary macrophages
contain high levels of cathepsin B activity and it has been suggested
that cathepsin B is also found in human bronchoalveolar lavage fluids,
derived mostly from human macrophages (168).

In summary, cathepsin B has been shown to be correlated with
metastatic tumor cells as well as a number of other tumor cells and
this enzymatic activity has been related to tumor-associated platelet
aggregation. Although cathepsin B may cleave laminin, the full
matrix-degrading potential of this proteinase has not yet been fully
explored. Studies to determine whether this proteinase plays a
critical role in degradation of laminin, fibronectin, type IV collagen,
type V collagen and heparan sulfated glycosaminoglycans and to
elucidate the role, if any, of cathepsin B in activation or regulation
of latent forms of PA, type IV collagenase, and type V collagenase will
be of interest. (See Chapter 22 for a complete discussion of cathepsin
B in tumor invasion and metastasis).

F. Role of Tumor Cell Procoagulants in Tumor Invasion and
   Metastasis

A number of reports have shown that a variety of transformed cells
and tumors produce procoagulants (169-172). The procoagulants have
been described as tissue-factor like; a procoagulant associated with
plasma membrane vesicles; and a procoagulant with the capacity to
directly activate factor X. The factor X activating procoagulant has
been shown to be a cysteine proteinase. The latter class of procoagulant activity has been identified in Lewis lung carcinoma,
extracts of malignant human tissue and transformed fibroblast cell
lines (169 and Chapter 11).

A strong correlation exists between procoagulant activity levels
and the number of B16-F1 and B16-F10 melanoma pulmonary metastases
formed, suggesting a role for tumor cell procoagulants and fibrin
formation during metastatic spread (169). Studies with sarcoma
sublines with varying metastatic potential have indicated that cells
with the lowest metastatic capacity display the highest level of
procoagulant activity (172); it is of interest that in studies with the
same murine fibrosarcoma sublines it has been noted that thrombin can
modulate cellular PA activity (121). Direct correlations with
metastatic behavior have also been noted for malignant cells of hepatic
origin and procoagulant activities of cellular lysates (119).

In summary, procoagulants appear to play a role in aspects of tumor metastasis dealing with fibrin formation. The role of these activities in invasive, degradative aspects of matrix degradation remain undefined.

IV. SIGNIFICANCE OF MATRIX DEGRADATION BY PROTEOLYTIC ENZYMES

A. Diagnosis of Metastasis

An understanding of the biochemical mechanism of tumor cell penetration of the extracellular matrix may yield important insights into the diagnosis of human malignant disease. For example, micrometastases of breast carcinoma can be detected by the presence of basement membrane type IV collagen (173). Immunoperoxidase staining with antibodies to specific components of the basement membrane may be of diagnostic use in the distinction of intraductal carcinoma from true microinvasive carcinoma of the breast, as well as the identification of micrometastases in secondary sites. In intraductal carcinoma, intact basement membrane surrounds the lobules and ducts; antibodies to type IV collagen and laminin yield linear, extracellular staining patterns. In contrast, in intraductal carcinoma with microinvasion, fragmentation or absence of the basement membrane within areas of microinvasion has been noted (174). Antibodies to laminin and type IV collagen have also been employed in the study of fresh-frozen as well as formalin-fixed sections of several types of invasive carcinomas in situ, as well as benign counterparts (14). By immunofluorescent and immunoperoxidase techniques, benign lesions demonstrated linear staining of type IV collagen and laminin whereas the majority of invasive carcinomas lack immunoreactivity for these basement membrane components (14). For in situ carcinoma with microinvasion, thinning, fragmentation and disruption of the basement membrane is observed within the locus of microinvasion but not at other sites (14). Antibodies to type IV collagen seem to be of value in confirming conventional diagnosis of vascular invasion in breast cancer and also increase the accuracy and rate of detection (175). Antibodies to basement membrane components have also been found to be of use in helping to differentiate between tubular carcinoma and sclerosing adenosis of the breast (176). The demonstration of type IV collagenase immunoreactivity in human breast carcinoma has also been employed in the identification of tumor invasion in tissue sections (177). Anti-type IV collagen and anti-laminin rarely stain the basement membrane of metastatic human colorectal carcinomas and draining lymph nodes from breast carcinomas (178); in contrast anti-type IV collagen is noted in the peritumoral stroma. Recent studies with immunohistology of PAs also suggest that detection of PA might be of potential use in the diagnosis of tumor invasion (130,137,139). An independent diagnostic application for PA is related to the type of PA released by the leukemic cells of patients with acute myeloid leukemia; it has been observed that the patients whose cells released only TPA do not respond to combination chemotherapy (179).

362

B. Therapy of Established Micrometastatic Disease

Although considerable evidence indicates that a variety of
proteolytic enzymes contribute to matrix degradation during metastatic
tumor invasion, the potential therapeutic significance of this evidence
remains undefined. Criticial resolution of the issue of whether
inhibitors of invasive proteolytic enzymes can play a role in the
therapy of metastatic disease will likely depend upon the development
of specific and efficient, non-toxic, bioavailable inhibitors (180). It
remains unclear whether inhibitors of specific enzymatic activities
involved in matrix degradation and metastasis could contribute to
maintenance of micrometastatic dormancy and overcome issues related to
drug resistance and tumor heterogeneity by a non-toxic mode of action.
Reviews summarizing studies with proteinase inhibitors in metastasis
have recently appeared (180-182). Prodrugs that are substrates for
tumor associated proteinases have been described which are designed to
be locally activated by the conversion of plasminogen to plasmin by PA
in the tumor microenvironment (183,184). In addition, studies with the
plasminogen-plasmin inhibitor, tranexamic acid, demonstrated
suppression of the growth of human tumors in nude mice or potentiation
of the effects of anticancer drugs; decreased number of pulmonary
metastases of Lewis lung carcinoma; decreased tumor vascularization;
and arrested growth of human ovarian tumors (130a, 185-187). As highly
potent, selective, non-toxic, pharmacokinetically suitable inhibitors
against collagenases; PAs; glycosidases; cathepsins; and procoagulants
of metastatic tumor cells are derived, the exact role and scope of
potential therapy against these degradative enzymes can be elucidated.

V. CONCLUSION

This chapter has reviewed the evidence linking a variety of
degradative enzymes with the invasive, metastatic spread of cancer. A
battery of enzymes from metastatic cells have the capacity to
contribute to the destruction of a variety of host extracellular
matrices which must be degraded during tumor invasion and metastasis.
Multiple matrices exist with molecular components which vary
qualitatively and quantitatively. Therefore, matrix degradation by
metastatic cells requires a variety of enzymatic activities with
selectivities for different matrix substrates. It is likely that the
degradative enzymes of metastatic cells contribute to an enzymatic
cascade for matrix degradation under the selective and regulatory
specificity of irreversible, limited proteolytic action. The
degradation of the host matrix by metastatic cells is of importance to
our understanding of the pathophysiology of metastatic spread, the
development of early diagnosis of micrometastatic disease and the
potential development of antimetastatic agents for the prevention or
treatment of human metastatic disease.

REFERENCES

1. Fidler IJ, Gersten DM, Hart IR: The biology of cancer invasion
    and metastasis. Adv. Cancer Res. 28:149-250, 1978.
2. Sugarbaker EV, Weingard DN, Roseman JM: Observations on cancer
    metastasis in man. IN: Liotta LA and Hart IR (eds.) Tumor
    Invasion and Metastasis. Martinus Nijhoff, The Hague, pp.
    427-465, 1982.
3. Poste G, Fidler IJ: The pathogenesis of cancer metastasis. Nature
    (London) 283:139-146, 1980.
4. Hart IR, Fidler IJ: Cancer invasion and metastasis. Quart. Rev.
    Biol. 55:121-142, 1980.
5. Jones PA, DeClerck YA: Extracellular matrix destruction by
    invasive tumor cells. Cancer Metastasis Rev. 1:289-317, 1982.
6. Pauli BU, Schwartz DE, Thonar EJ-M, Keuttner K: Tumor invasion
    and host extracellular matrix. Cancer Metastasis Rev. 2:129-152,
    1983.
7. Liotta LA, Rao CN, Barsky SH: Tumor invasion and the extra-
    cellular matrix. Lab. Invest. 49:636-649, 1983.
8. Liotta LA, Goldfarb RH: Interactions of tumor cells with the
    basement membrane of endothelium. IN: Honn KV and Sloane BF
    (eds.) Hemostatic Mechanisms and Metastasis. Martinus Nijhoff,
    The Hague, pp. 319-336, 1984.
9. Liotta LA, Garbisa S, Tryggvason K: Biochemical mechanisms
    involved in tumor cell penetration of the basement membrane. IN:
    Liotta LA and Hart IR (eds.) Tumor Invasion and Metastasis.
    Martinus Nijhoff, The Hague, pp. 318-333, 1982.
10. Strauli P, Barrett AJ, Baici A (eds.): Proteinases and Tumor
    Invasion. Raven Press, New York, 1980.
11. Liotta LA, Thorgeirsson UP, Garbisa S: Role of collagenases in
    tumor cell invasion. Cancer Metastasis Rev. 1:277-288, 1982.
12. Recklies AD, Poole AR: Proteolytic mechanisms of tissue
    destruction in tumor growth and metastasis. IN: Weiss L and
    Gilbert HA (eds.) Liver Metastasis. GK Hall, Boston, pp. 77-95,
    1982.
13. Goldfarb RH: Proteases in tumor invasion and metastasis. IN:
    Liotta and Hart IR (eds.) Tumor Invasion and Metastasis. Martinus
    Nijhoff, The Hague, pp. 375-390, 1982.
14. Barsky SH, Siegal GP, Jannotta F, Liotta LA: Loss of basement
    membrane components by invasive tumors but not by their benign
    counterparts. Lab. Invest. 49:140-147, 1983.
15. Barsky SH, Rao CN, Grotendorst GR, Liotta LA: Increased content
    of type V collagen in desmoplasia of human breast carcinoma. Am.
    J. Pathol. 108:276-282, 1982.
16. Alitalo K, Vaheri A: Pericellular matrix in malignant trans-
    formation. Adv. Cancer Res. 37:111-158, 1982.
17. Auersperg N, Erber H, Worth A: Histologic variation among poorly
    differentiated invasive carcinomas of the human uterine cervix. J.
    Natl. Cancer Inst. 51:1461-1477, 1973.
18. Bissell MJ, Hall HG, Parry G: How does the extracellular matrix
    direct gene expression? J. Theor. Biol. 99:31-64, 1982.

19. Nicolson GL: Cancer metastasis organ colonization and the cell-surface properties of malignant cells. Biochim. Biophys. Acta 695:113-176, 1982.

20. Nicolson GL, Poste G: Tumor cell diversity and host responses in cancer metastasis - part 1, properties of metastatic cells. Curr. Prob. Cancer 7:1-83, 1982.

21. Nicolson GL: Tumor implantation and invasion at metastatic sites. Int. Rev. Exp. Pathol. 25:77-181, 1983.

22. Yamada KM: Cell surface interactions with extracellular materials. Ann. Rev. Biochem. 52:761-799, 1983.

23. Murray JC, Liotta LA, Rennard SI, Martin GR: Adhesion characteristics of murine metastatic and nonmetastatic tumor cells in vitro. Cancer Res. 40:347-351, 1980.

24. Terranova VP, Liotta LA, Russo RG, Martin GR: Role of laminin in the attachment and metastasis of murine tumor cells. Cancer Res. 42:2265-2269, 1982.

25. Terranova VP, Rao CN, Kalebic T, Margulies IM, Liotta LA: Laminin receptor on human breast carcinoma cells. Proc. Natl. Acad. Sci. USA 80:444-448, 1983.

26. Liotta LA, Goldfarb RH, Terranova VP: Cleavage of laminin by thrombin and plasmin: Alpha thrombin selectively cleaves the beta chain of laminin. Thromb. Res. 21:663-673, 1981.

27. Rao CN, Margulies IMK, Tralka TS, Terranova VP, Madri JA, Liotta LA: Isolation of a subunit of laminin and its role in molecular structure and tumor cell attachment. J. Biol. Chem. 257:9740-9744, 1982.

28. Rao CN, Margulies IMK, Goldfarb RH, Madri JA, Woodley DT, Liotta LA: Differential proteolytic susceptibility of laminin alpha and beta subunits. Arch. Biochem. Biophys. 219:65-70, 1982.

29. Weiss L, Ward PM: Cell detachment and metastasis. Cancer Metastasis Rev. 2:111-127, 1983.

30. Lacovara J, Cramer EB, Quigley JP: Fibronectin enhancement of directed migration of B16 melanoma cells. Cancer Res. 44:1657-1663, 1984.

31. McCarthy JB, Furcht LT: Laminin and fibronectin promote the haptotactic migration of B16 melanoma cells in vitro. J. Cell Biol. 98:1474-1480, 1984.

32. Thorgeirsson UP, Liotta LA, Kalebic T, Margulies IM, Thomas K, Rios-Candelore M, Russo RG: Effect of natural protease inhibitors and a chemoattractant on tumor cell invasion in vitro. J. Natl. Cancer Inst. 69:1049-1054, 1982.

33. Russo RG, Thorgeirsson U, Liotta LA: In vitro quantitative assay of invasion using human amnion. IN: Liotta LA and Hart IR (eds.) Tumor Invasion and Metastasis. Martinus Nijhoff, The Hague, pp. 173-187, 1982.

34. Quigley JP: Proteolytic enzymes of normal and malignant cells. IN: Hynes RO (ed.) Surfaces of Normal and Malignant Cells. John Wiley and Sons, Chichester, pp. 247-285, 1979.

35. Liotta LA, Tryggvason K, Garbisa S, Hart I, Foltz CM, Schafie S: Metastatic potential correlates with enzymatic degradation of basement membrane collagen. Nature (London) 284:67-68, 1980.

36. Starkey JR, Hosick H, Stanford DR, Liggitt HD: Interaction of metastatic tumor cells with bovine lens capsule basement membrane. Cancer Res. 44:1585-1594, 1984.

37. Nakajima M, Custead SE, Welch DR, Nicolson GL: Type IV collagenase: Relation to metastatic properties of rat 13762 mammary adenocarcinoma metastatic clones. Proc. Am. Assoc. Cancer Res. 24:62, 1984.

38. Shields SE, Ogilvie DJ, McKinnell RG, Tarin D: Degradation of basement membrane collagens by metalloproteases released by human, murine, and amphibian tumors. J. Pathol. 143:193-197, 1984.

39. Turpeenniemi-Hujanen T, Thorgeirsson UP, Hart I, Liotta LA: Expression of basement membrane collagen degrading metalloprotease activity in tumor cell hybrids which differ in metastatic potential. Proc. Am. Assoc. Cancer Res. 24:62, 1984.

40. Liotta LA, Lanzer WL, Garbisa S: Identification of a type V collagenolytic enzyme. Biochem. Biophys. Res. Commun. 98:184-190, 1981.

41. Mainardi LL, Seyer JM, Kang AH: Specific collagenolysis: Identification of a type V degrading activity in alveolar macrophages. Biochem. Biophys. Res. Commun. 97:1108-1115, 1980.

42. Mainardi C, Dixit SN, Kang AH: Degradation of type IV (basement membrane) collagen by a proteinase isolated from polymorphonuclear leukocyte granules. J. Biol. Chem. 225:5435-5441, 1980.

43. Liotta LA, Wicha MS, Foidart JM, Rennard SI, Garbisa S, Kidwell WR: Hormonal requirements for basement membrane collagen deposition by cultured rat mammary epithelium. Lab. Invest. 41:511-518, 1979.

44. Henry N, Eeckhout Y, van Lamsweerde A-L, Vaes G: Cooperation between metastatic tumor cells and macrophages in the degradation of basement membrane (type IV) collagen. FEBS Lett. 161:243-246, 1983.

45. Reich E: Activation of plasminogen: A general mechanism for producing localized extracellular proteolysis. IN: Berlin RD, Herrmann M, Lepow IH and Tanzer JM (eds.) Molecular Basis of Biological Degradative Processes. Academic Press, New York, pp. 155-169, 1978.

46. Christman JK, Silverstein SC, Acs G: Plasminogen activators. IN: Barrett AJ (ed.) Proteinases in Mammalian Cells and Tissues. Elsevier/North Holland, Amsterdam, pp. 91-148, 1977.

47. Goldfarb RH: Plasminogen activators. Ann. Rep. Med. Chem. 18:257-264, 1983.

48. Goldfarb RH, Quigley JP: Production of plasminogen activator by chick embryo fibroblasts: Synergistic effect of Rous sarcoma virus transformation and treatment with the tumor promoter phorbol myristate acetate. Cancer Res. 38:4601-4608, 1978.

49. Quigley JP, Goldfarb RH: Morphological changes induced by endogenous protease activity in cultures of phorbol ester treated RSV-transformed chick fibroblasts: Evidence for direct proteolytic activity of plasminogen activator. J. Cell Biol. 79:73a, 1978.

50. Quigley JP: Phorbol ester-induced morphological changes in transformed chick fibroblasts: Evidence for direct catalytic involvement of plasminogen activator. Cell 17:131-141, 1979.

366

51. Quigley JP, Martin BM, Goldfarb RH, Scheiner CJ, Muller WD: Involvement of serine proteases in growth control and malignant transformation. Cold Spring Harbor Conf. Cell Proliferation 6:219-238, 1979.
52. Quigley JP, Goldfarb RH, Scheiner CJ, O'Donnell-Tormey J, Yeo T: Transformed cell membranes and plasminogen activator. Prog. Clin. Biol. Res. 42:773-795, 1980.
53. Zimmerman M, Quigley JP, Ashe B, Dorn C. Goldfarb RH, Troll W: A direct fluorescent assay for urokinase and normal and malignant tissue plasminogen activator: Kinetics and inhibitor profile. Proc. Natl. Acad. Sci. USA 75:750-753, 1978.
54. Keski-Oja J, Vaheri A: The cellular target for the plasminogen activator, urokinase, in human fibroblasts-66,000 dalton protein. Biochim. Biophys. Acta 720:141-148, 1982.
55. Gunzler WA, Steffens GJ, Otting F, Kim S-MA, Frankus E, Flohe L: The primary structure of high molecular weight urokinase from human urine: The complete amino acid sequence of the A chain. Hoppe-Seyler's Z. Physiol. Chem. 363:1155-1165, 1982.
56. Pohl G, Kallstrom M, Bergsdorf N, Wallen P, Jornvall H: Tissue plasminogen activator: Peptide analyses confirm an indirectly derived amino acid sequence, identify the active site serine residue, establish glycosylation sites, and localize variant differences. Biochemistry 23:3701-3707, 1984.
57. Strassburger W, Wollmer A, Pitts JE, Glover ID, Tickle IJ, Blundell TL, Steffens GJ, Gunzler WA, Otting F, Flohe L: Adaptation of plasminogen activator sequences to known protease structures. FEBS Lett. 157:219-223, 1983.
58. Patthy L, Trexler M, Vali Z, Banyai L, Varadi A: Kringles: Modules specialized for protein binding. Homology of the gelatin-binding region of fibronectin with the kringle structures of proteases. FEBS Lett. 171:131-136, 1984.
59. Gross JL, Krupp MN, Rifkin DB, Lane MD: Down-regulation of epidermal growth factor receptor correlates with plasminogen activator activity in A431 epidermoid carcinoma cells. Proc. Natl. Acad. Sci. USA 80:2276-2280, 1983.
60. Lee L, Weinstein IB: Epidermal growth factor, like phorbol esters, induces plasminogen activator in HeLa cells. Nature (London) 274:696-697, 1978.
61. Jetten AM, Goldfarb RH: Action of epidermal growth factor and retinoids on anchorage-dependent and -independent growth of nontransformed rat kidney cells. Cancer Res. 43:2094-2099, 1983.
62. Quigley JP: Association of a protease (plasminogen activator) with a specific membrane fraction isolated from transformed cells. J. Cell Biol. 71:472-486, 1976.
63. Wun T-C, Ossowski L, Reich E: A proenzyme form of human urokinase. J. Biol. Chem. 257:7262-7268, 1982.
64. Skriver L, Nielsen LS, Stephens R, Danø K: Plasminogen activator released as inactive proenzyme from murine cells transformed by sarcoma virus. Eur. J. Biochem. 124:409-414, 1982.

65. Nielsen LS, Hansen JG, Skriver L, Wilson EL, Kaltoft K, Zeuther J, Danø K: Purification of zymogen to plasminogen activator from human glioblastoma cells by affinity chromatography with monoclonal antibody. Biochemistry 21:6410-6415, 1982.

66. Andreasen PA, Nielsen LS, Grøndahl-Hansen J, Skriver L, Zeuthen J, Stephens RW, Danø K: Inactive proenzyme to tissue type plasminogen activator from human melanoma cells, identified after affinity purification with a monoclonal antibody. EMBO J. 3:51-56, 1984.

67. Levin E: Latent tissue plasminogen activator produced by human endothelial cells in culture: Evidence for an enzyme-inhibitor complex. Proc. Natl. Acad. Sci. USA 80:6804-6808, 1983.

68. Vassalli J-D, Dayer J-M, Wohlwend A, Belin D: Concomitant secretion of pro-urokinase and of a plasminogen activator-specific inhibitor by cultured human monocytes-macrophages. J. Exp. Med. 159:1653-1668, 1984.

69. Hoal EG, Wilson EL, Dowdle DB: The regulation of tissue plasminogen activator activity by human fibroblasts. Cell 34:273-279, 1983.

70. Cwikel BJ, Barouski-Miller PA, Coleman PL, Gelehrter TD: Dexamethasone induction of an inhibitor of plasminogen activator in HTC hepatoma cells. J. Biol. Chem. 259:6847-6851, 1984.

71. Eaton DL, Scott RW, Baker JB: Purification of human fibroblast urokinase proenzyme and analysis of its regulation by proteases and protease nexin. J. Biol. Chem. 259:6241-6247, 1984.

72. Saksela O, Vaheri A, Schleuning W-D, Mignatti P, Barlati S: Plasminogen activators, activation inhibitors and alpha$_2$-macroglobulin produced by cultured normal and malignant human cells. Int. J. Cancer 33:609-616, 1984.

73. O'Donnell-Tormey J, Quigley JP: Detection and partial characterization of a chymostatin sensitive endopeptidase in transformed fibroblasts. Proc. Natl. Acad. Sci. USA 80:344-348, 1983.

74. O'Donnell-Tormey J, Quigley JP: Inhibition of plasminogen activator release from transformed chicken fibroblasts by a protease inhibitor. Cell 27:85-95, 1981.

75. Goldfarb RH, Quigley JP: Purification of plasminogen activator from Rous sarcoma virus transformed chick embryo fibroblasts treated with the tumor promoter phorbol-12-myristate-13-acetate. Biochemistry 19:5463-5471, 1980.

76. DePetro G, Vartio T, Salonen EM, Vaheri A, Barlati S: Tissue type plasminogen activator, but not urokinase, exerts transformation-enhancing activity. Int. J. Cancer 33:563-567, 1984.

77. Davies RL, Rifkin DB, Tepper R, Miller A, Kucherlapati R: A polypeptide secreted by transformed cells that modulates human plasminogen activator production. Science 221:171-173, 1983.

78. Liu H-Y, Yang PP, Toledo DL, Mangel WF: Modulation of cell-associated plasminogen activator activity by cocultivation of a stem cell and its tumorigenic descendant. Mol. Cell. Biol. 4:160-165, 1984.

368

79. Yang N-S, Park C, Longley C, Furmanski P: Effect of the extra-cellular matrix of plasminogen activator isozyme activities of human mammary epithelial cells in culture. Mol. Cell. Biol. 3:982-990, 1983.

80. Miskin R, Reich E: Plasminogen activator: Induction of synthesis by DNA damage. Cell 19:217-224, 1980.

81. Miskin R, Ben-Ishai R: Induction of plasminogen activator by UV light in normal and xeroderma pigmentosum fibroblasts. Proc. Natl. Acad. Sci. USA 78:6236-6240, 1981.

82. Ben-Ishai R, Sharon R, Rothman M, Miskin R: DNA repair and induction of plasminogen activator in human fetal cells treated with ultraviolet light. Carcinogenesis 5:357-362, 1984.

83. Meyn MS, Rossman T, Troll W: A protease inhibitor blocks SOS-functions in Escherichia coli: Antipain prevents lambda-repressor inactivation, ultraviolet mutagenesis, and filamentous growth. Proc. Natl. Acad. Sci. USA 74:1152-1156, 1977.

84. Radman M, Villani G, Boiteux S, Defais M, Caillet-Fauquest P, Spadari S: On the mechanism and genetic control of mutagenesis induced by carcinogenic mutagens. IN: Hiatt HH, Watson JD and Winsten JA (eds.) Origins of Human Cancer. Cold Spring Harbor Laboratory Press, Cold Spring Harbor, pp. 903-922, 1977.

85. Rohrlich ST, Rifkin DB: Proteases and cell invasion. Ann. Rep. Med. Chem. 14:229-239, 1979.

86. Skehan P, Friedman SJ: Malignant transformation: In vivo methods and in vitro correlates. IN: Cameron IL and Pool TB (eds.) The Transformed Cell. Academic Press, New York, pp. 8-65, 1981.

87. Mullins DE, Rohrlich ST: The role of proteinases in cellular invasiveness. Biochim. Biophys. Acta 695:177-214, 1983.

88. Werb A, Banda MJ, Jones PA: Degradation of connective tissue matrices by macrophages. I. Proteolysis of elastin, glyco-proteins, and collagen by proteinases isolated from macrophages. J. Exp. Med. 152:1340-1357, 1980.

89. Jones PA, Werb Z: Degradation of connective tissue matrices by macrophages. II. Influence of matrix composition on proteolysis of glycoproteins, elastin, and collagen by macrophages in culture. J. Exp. Med. 152:1527-1536, 1980.

90. Werb Z, Bainton DF, Jones PA: Degradation of connective tissue matrices by macrophages. III. Morphological and biochemical studies on extracellular, pericellular and intracellular events in matrix degradation by macrophages in culture. J. Exp. Med. 152:1537-1553, 1980.

91. Jones PA, Scott-Burden T: Activated macrophages digest the extracellular matrix proteins produced by cultured cells. Biochem. Biophys. Res. Commun. 86:71-77, 1979.

91a. Chapman HA, Stone DL, Vavrin Z: Degradation of fibrin and elastin by intact human alveolar macrophages in vitro. Characterization of a plasminogen activator and its role in matrix degradation. J. Clin. Invest. 73:806-815, 1984.

92. Jones PA, DeClerck YA: Destruction of extracellular matrices containing glycoproteins, elastin and collagen by metastatic human tumor cells. Cancer Res. 40:3222-3227, 1980.

93. Kramer RH, Vogel KG, Nicolson GL: Solubilization and degradation of subendothelial matrix glycoproteins and proteoglycans by metastatic tumor cells. J. Biol. Chem. 257:2678-2686, 1982.

94. Goldfarb RH, Liotta LA, Garbisa S: Degradation of basement membrane components: Effects of plasminogen activator, plasmin, and alpha thrombin. Proc. Am. Assoc. Cancer Res. 22:59, 1981.

95. Liotta LA, Goldfarb RH, Brundage RG, Siegal GP, Terranova VP, Garbisa S: Effect of plasminogen activator (urokinase), plasmin, and thrombin on glycoprotein and collagenous components of basement membrane. Cancer Res. 41:4629-4636, 1981.

96. Liotta LA, Goldfarb RH, Terranova VP: Cleavage of laminin by thrombin and plasmin: Alpha thrombin selectively cleaves the beta chain of laminin. Thromb. Res. 21:663-673, 1981.

97. Werb Z, Mainardi C, Vater C, Harris ED: Endogenous activation of latent collagenase by rheumatoid synovial cells. Evidence for a role of plasminogen activator. N. Eng. J. Med. 296:1017-1023, 1977.

98. Paranjpe M, Engel L, Young N, Liotta LA: Activation of human breast carcinoma collagenase through plasminogen activator. Life Sci. 26:1223-1231, 1980.

99. O'Grady R, Upfold LI, Stephens RW: Rat mammary carcinoma cells secrete active collagenase and activate latent enzyme in the stroma via plasminogen activator. Int. J. Cancer 28:509-515, 1981.

100. Salo T, Liotta LA, Keski-Oja J, Turpeenniemi-Hujanen T, Tryggvason K: Secretion of basement membrane collagen degrading enzyme and plasminogen activator by transformed cells - role in metastasis. Int. J. Cancer 30:669-673, 1982.

101. Sheela S, Barrett JC: In vitro degradation of radiolabeled, intact basement membrane mediated by cellular plasminogen activator. Carcinogenesis 3:363-369, 1982.

102. Laug WE, DeClerck YA, Jones PA: Degradation of the subendothelial matrix by tumor cells. Cancer Res. 43:1827-1834, 1983.

103. Bogenmann E, Jones PA: Role of plasminogen in matrix breakdown by neoplastic cells. J. Natl. Cancer Inst. 71:1177-1182, 1983.

104. Heisel M, Laug WE, Jones PA: Inhibition by bovine endothelial cells of degradation by HT-1080 fibrosarcoma cells of extra-cellular matrix proteins. J. Natl. Cancer Inst. 71:1183-1187, 1983.

105. Sloane BF, Honn KV, Sadler JG, Turner WA, Kimpson JJ, Taylor JD: Cathepsin B activity in B16 melanoma cells: A possible marker for metastatic potential. Cancer Res. 42:980-986, 1982.

106. Salonen E-M, Zitting A, Vaheri A: Laminin interacts with plasminogen and its tissue-type activator. FEBS Lett. 172:29-32, 1984.

107. Quigley JP: Morphological alterations and degradative ability of RSV-transformed chick fibroblasts when cultured on the extra-cellular matrix produced by normal chick fibroblasts. Proc. Am. Assoc. Cancer Res. 24:29, 1983.

108. Chen W-T, Olden K, Bernard BA, Chu F-F: Expression of transformation-associated protease(s) that degrade fibronectin at cell contact sites. J. Cell Biol. 98:1546-1555, 1984.

109. Maciag T, Kadish J, Wilkins L, Stemerman MB, Weinstein R: Organizational behavior of human umbilical vein endothelial cells. J. Cell Biol. 94:511-520, 1982.

110. Markus G: Plasminogen activators in malignant growth. IN: Davidson JF (ed.) Progress in Fibrinolysis, Churchill-Livingstone, Edinburgh, pp. 587-600, 1983.

111. Markus G: The role of hemostasis and fibrinolysis in the metastatic spread of cancer. Semin. Thromb. Hemostasis 10:61-79, 1984.

112. Duffy MJ, O'Grady P: Plasminogen activator and cancer. Eur. J. Cancer Clin. Oncol. 20:577-582, 1984.

113. Berman M, Winthrop S, Ausprunk D, Rose J, Langer R, Gage J: Plasminogen activator (urokinase) causes vascularization of the cornea. Invest. Opthalmol. Vis. Sci. 22:191-199, 1982.

114. Rifkin DB, Moscatelli D, Cross J, Jaffe E: Proteases, angiogenesis, and invasion. IN: Nicolson G and Milas L (eds.) Cancer Invasion and Metastasis: Biologic and Therapeutic Aspects Raven Press, New York, pp. 187-200, 1984.

115. Glaser BM, Kalebic T, Garbisa S, Connor TB, Liotta LA: Degradation of basement membrane components by vascular endothelial cells: Role in neovascularization. IN: Wolpert L (ed.) Development of the Vascular System (Ciba Foundation Symposium 100), Pitman Books Ltd., London, pp. 150-162, 1983.

116. Bruesch MR, Johnson GL, Palackdharry CS, Weber MJ, Carl PL: Plasminogen activator in normal and tumor-bearing mice. Int. J. Cancer 32:121-126, 1983.

117. Nicolson GL, Winkelhake JL, Nussey AC: An approach to studying the cellular properties associated with metastasis: Some in vitro properties of tumor variants selected in vivo for enhanced metastasis. IN: Weiss L (ed.) Fundamental Aspects of Metastasis North Holland Publishing Co., Amsterdam, pp. 291-303, 1976.

118. Roblin R: Contributions of secreted tumor cell products to metastasis. Cancer Biol. Rev. 2:59-94, 1981.

119. Talmadge JE, Starkey JR, Stanford DR: In vitro characteristics of metastatic variant subclones of restricted genetic origin. J. Supramol. Struc. Cell. Biochem. 15:139-151, 1981.

120. Whur P, Magudia M, Boston J, Lockwood J, Williams DC: Plasminogen activator in cultured Lewis lung carcinoma cells measured by chromogenic aubstrate assay. Br. J. Cancer 42:305-313, 1980.

121. Coen D, Bottazzi B, Bini A, Conforti MG, Mantovani A, Mussoni L, Donati MB: Plasminogen activator activity of metastatic variants from a murine fibrosarcoma: Effect of thrombin in vitro. Int. J. Cancer 32:67-70, 1983.

122. Giraldi T, Sava G, Kopitar M, Suhar A, Turk V, Baici A: Methodologic problems encountered in the assay of proteinases in Lewis lung carcinoma, a mouse metastasizing tumor. Tumori 68:381-387, 1982.

123. McLaughlin MEH, Liener IE, Wang N: Proteolytic and metastatic activities of clones derived from a methylcholanthrene induced murine fibrosarcoma. Clin. Exp. Metastasis 1:359-371, 1983.

124. Lowe FC, Isaacs JT: Biochemical methods for predicting metastatic ability of prostatic cancer utilizing the Dunning R-3327 rat prostatic adenocarcinoma system as a model. Cancer Res. 44:744-752, 1984.

125. Wang BS, McLoughlin GA, Richie JP, Mannick JA: Correlation of the production of plasminogen activator with tumor metastasis in B16 melanoma cell lines. Cancer Res. 40:288-292, 1980.

126. Pollard M, Luckert PH, Bruckner-Kardoss E: The association of plasminogen activator (PLA) with metastatic spread of rat prostate adenocarcinoma. Fed. Proc. Fed. Am. Soc. Exp. Biol. 42:773, 1983.

127. Ng R, Kellen JA, Wong ACH: Plasminogen activators as markers of tumor colonization potential. Invasion Metastasis 3:243-248, 1983.

128. Ramshaw IA, Carlsen S, Wang HC, Badenoch-Jones P: The use of cell fusion to analyze factors involved in tumor cell metastasis. Int. J. Cancer 32:471-478, 1983.

129. Carlsen SA, Ramshaw IA, Warrington RC: Involvement of plasminogen activator production with tumor metastasis in a rat model. Cancer Res. 44:3012-3016, 1984.

130. Skriver L, Larsson L-I, Kielberg V, Nielsen LS, Andresen PB, Kristensen P, Danø K: Immunocytochemical localization of urokinase-type plasminogen activator in Lewis lung carcinoma. J. Cell Biol. 99:752-757, 1984.

130a. Tanaka N, Ogawa H, Tanaka K, Kinjo M, Kohga S: Effects of tranexamic acid and urokinase on hematogenous metastases of Lewis lung carcinoma in mice. Invasion Metastasis 1:149-157, 1981.

131. Ossowski L, Reich E: Experimental model for quantitative study of metastasis. Cancer Res. 40:2300-2309, 1980.

132. Ossowski L, Reich E: Antibodies to plasminogen activator inhibit tumor metastasis. Cell 35:611-619, 1983.

133. Friedman EA: Differential response of premalignant epithelial cell classes to phorbol ester tumor promoters and to deoxycholic acid. Cancer Res. 41:4588-4599, 1981.

134. Friedman E, Urmacher C, Winawer S: A model for human colon carcinoma evolution based on the differential response of cultured preneoplastic, premalignant, and malignant cells to 12-0-tetradecanoylphorbol-13-acetate. Cancer Res. 44:1568-1578, 1984.

135. Friedman E, Verderame M, Winawer S, Pollack R: Actin cytoskeletal organization loss in the benign-to-malignant tumor transition in cultured human colonic epithelial cells. Cancer Res. 44:3040-3050, 1984.

136. Corasanti JG, Celik C, Camiolo SM, Mittelman A, Evers JL, Barbasch A, Hobika GH, Markus G: Plasminogen activator content of human colon tumors and normal mucosae: Separation of enzymes and partial purification. J. Natl. Cancer Inst. 65:345-351, 1980.

137. Markus G, Camiolo SM, Kohga S, Madeja JM, Mittelman A: Plasminogen activator secretion of human tumors in short-term organ culture, including a comparison of primary and metastatic tumors. Cancer Res. 43:5517-5525, 1983.

138. Camiolo SM, Markus G, Englander LS, Siuta M, Hobika GH, Kohga S: Plasminogen activator content and secretion in explants of neoplastic and benign human prostate tissues. Cancer Res. 44:311-318, 1984.

139. Markus G, Kohga S, Camiolo SM, Madeja JM, Ambrus JL, Karakousis C: Plasminogen activators in human malignant melanoma. J. Natl. Cancer Inst. 72:1213-1222, 1984.

140. Colombi M, Barlati S, Magdelenat H, Fiszer-Szafarz B: Relationship between multiple forms of plasminogen activator in human breast tumors and plasma and the presence of metastases in lymph nodes. Cancer Res. 44:2971-2975, 1984.

141. Abecassis J, Collard R, Eber M, Pusel J, Fricker JP, Methlin G: Proteinases and sialyltransferase in human breast tumors. Int. J. Cancer 33:821-824, 1984.

142. Stephens RW, Golder JP: Novel properties of human monocyte plasminogen activator. Eur. J. Biochem. 139:253-258, 1984.

143. Goldfarb RH, Timonen T, Herberman RB: Production of plasminogen activator by human natural killer cells: Large granular lymphocytes. J. Exp. Med. 159:935-951, 1984.

144. Nicolson GL, Irimura T, Nakajima N, Estrada J: Metastatic cell attachment to and invasion of vascular endothelium and its underlying basal lamina using endothelial cell monolayers. IN: Nicolson GL and Milas (eds.) Cancer Invasion and Metastasis: Biologic and Therapeutic Aspects Raven Press, New York, pp. 145-167, 1984.

145. Nicolson GL: Metastatic tumor cell attachment and invasion assay utilizing vascular endothelial cell monolayers. J. Histochem. Cytochem. 30:214-220, 1982.

146. Vlodavsky I, Ariav Y, Atzmon R, Fuks Z: Tumor cell attachment to the vascular endothelium and subsequent degradation of the subendothelial extracellular matrix. Exp. Cell Res. 140:149-159, 1982.

147. Nakajima M, Irimura T, DiFerrante D, DiFerrante N, Nicolson GL: Heparan sulfate degradation: Relation to tumor invasive and metastatic properties of mouse B16 melanoma sublines. Science 220:611-613, 1983.

148. Kramer RH, Vogel KG: Selective degradation of basement membrane macromolecules by metastatic melanoma cells. J. Natl. Cancer Inst. 72:889-899, 1984.

149. Nakajima M, Irimura T, DiFerrante N, Nicolson GL: Metastatic melanoma cell heparanase. Characterization of heparan sulfate degradation fragments produced by B16 melanoma endoglucuronidase. J. Biol. Chem. 259:2283-2290, 1984.

150. Vlodavsky I, Fuks Z, Bar-Ner M, Ariav Y, Schirrmacher V: Lymphoma cell-mediated degradation of sulfated proteoglycans in the subendothelial extracellular matrix: Relationship to tumor cell metastasis. Cancer Res. 43:2704-2711, 1983.

151. Savion N, Vlodavsky I, Fuks Z: Interaction of T lymphocytes and macrophages with cultured vascular endothelial cells: Attachment, invasion and subsequent degradation of the subendothelial matrix. J. Cell. Physiol. 118:169-178, 1984.

152. Woodley DT, Rao CN, Hassell JR, Liotta LA, Martin GR, Kleinman HK: Interactions of basement membrane components. Biochim. Biophys. Acta 761:278-283, 1983.
153. Hedman K, Vartio T, Johansson S, Kjellen L, Hook M, Linker A, Salonen M, Vaheri A: Integrity of the pericellular fibronectin matrix of fibroblasts is independent of sulfated glycosaminoglycans. EMBO J. 3:581-584, 1984.
154. Iozzo RV: Biosynthesis of heparan sulfate proteoglycan by human colon carcinoma cells and its localization at the cell surface. J. Cell Biol. 99:403-417, 1984.
155. Luikart SD, Maniglia CA, Sartorelli AC: Influence of collagen substrata on glycosaminoglycan production by B16 melanoma cells. Proc. Natl. Acad. Sci. USA 80:3738-3742, 1983.
156. Lark MW, Culp LA: Multiple classes of heparan sulfate proteoglycans from fibroblast substratum adhesion sites. Affinity fractionation on columns of platelet factor 4, plasma fibronectin, and octyl-Sepharose. J. Biol. Chem. 259:6773-6782, 1984.
157. Gallagher JT, Hampson IN: Proteoglycans in cellular differentiation and neoplasia. Biochem. Soc. Trans. 12:541-543, 1984.
158. Sloane BF, Honn KV, Sadler JG, Turner WA, Kimpson JJ, Taylor JD: Cathepsin B activity in B16 melanoma cells: A possible marker for metastatic potential. Cancer Res. 42:980-986, 1982.
159. Sloane BF, Dunn JR, Honn KV: Lysosomal cathepsin B: Correlation with metastatic potential. Science 212:1151-1153, 1981.
160. Poole AR, Tiltman KJ, Recklies AD, Stoker TAM: Differences in secretion of the proteinase cathepsin B at the edges of human breast carcinomas and fibroadenomas. Nature (London) 273:545-547, 1978.
161. Recklies AD, Tiltman KJ, Stoker TAM, Poole AR: Secretion of proteinases from malignant and nonmalignant human breast tissue. Cancer Res. 40:550-556, 1980.
162. Pietras RJ, Szego CM, Mangan CE, Seeler BJ, Burtnett MM: Elevated serum cathepsin B1-like activity in women with neoplastic disease. Gynecol. Oncol. 7:1-17, 1979.
163. Recklies AD, Mort JS, Poole AR: Secretion of a thiol proteinase from mouse mammary carcinomas and its characterization. Cancer Res. 42:1026-1032, 1982.
164. Pietras RJ, Roberts JA: Cathepsin B-like enzymes: Subcellular distribution and properties in neoplastic and control cells from human ectocervix. J. Biol. Chem. 256:8536-8544, 1981.
165. Mort JS, Leduc MS, Recklies AD: Characterization of a latent cysteine proteinase from ascitic fluid as a high molecular weight form of cathepsin B. Biochim. Biophys. Acta 755:369-375, 1983.
166. Honn KV, Cavanaugh P, Evens C, Taylor JD, Sloane BF: Tumor cell-platelet aggregation: Induced by cathepsin B-like proteinase and inhibited by prostacyclin. Science 217:540-542, 1982.
167. Cavanaugh PG, Sloane BF, Bajkowski AS, Gasic GJ, Gasic TB, Honn KV: Involvement of a cathepsin B-like cysteine proteinase in platelet aggregation induced by tumor cells and their shed membrane vesicles. Clin. Exp. Metastasis 1:297-307, 1983.

374

168. Lesser M, Chang JC, Orlowski J, Kilburn K, Orlowski M: Cathepsin B and prolyl endopeptidase activity in peritoneal and alveolar macrophages. J. Lab. Clin. Med. 101:327-334, 1983.

169. Gilbert LC, Gordon SG: Relationship between cellular procoagulant activity and metastatic activity of B16 melanoma variants. Cancer Res. 43:536-540, 1983.

170. Dvorak HF, Van DeWater L, Bitzer AM, Dvorak AM, Anderson D, Harvey VS, Bach R, Davis GL, DeWolf W, Carvalho CA: Procoagulant activity associated with plasma membrane vesicles shed by cultured tumor cells. Cancer Res. 43:4334-4342, 1983.

171. Gordon SG, Franks JJ, Lewis B: Cancer procoagulant A: A factor X activating procoagulant from malignant tissue. Thromb. Res. 6:127-137, 1975.

172. Colucci M, Giavazzi M, Allesandri G, Semeraro N, Mantovani A, Donati MB: Procoagulant activity of sarcoma sublines with different metastatic potential. Blood 57:733-735, 1981.

173. Liotta LA, Foidart JM, Gehon Robey P, Martin GR, Gullino PM: Identification of micrometastasis of breast carcinomas by presence of basement membrane collagen. Lancet 2:146-147, 1979.

174. Siegal GP, Barsky SH, Terranova VP, Liotta LA: Stages of neoplastic transformation of human breast tissue as monitored by dissolution of basement membrane components. Invasion Metastasis 1:54-70, 1981.

175. Bettelheim R, Mitchell D, Gusterson BA: Immunocytochemistry in the identification of vascular invasion in breast cancer. J. Clin. Pathol. 37:364-366, 1984.

176. Ekblom P, Miettinen M, Forsman L, Andersson L: Basement membrane and apocrine epithelial antigens in differential diagnosis between tubular carcinoma and sclerosing adenosis of the breast. J. Clin. Pathol. 37:357-363, 1984.

177. Burtin P, Chavanel G, Foidart JM, Andre J: Alterations of the basement membrane and connective tissue antigens in human metastatic lymph nodes. Int. J. Cancer 31:719-726, 1983.

178. Barsky SH, Togo S, Garbisa S, Liotta LA: Type IV collagenase immunoreactivity in invasive breast carcinoma. Lancet 1:296-297, 1983.

179. Wilson EL, Jacobs P, Dowdle EB: The secretion of plasminogen activators by human myeloid leukemic cells in vitro. Blood 61:568-574, 1983.

180. Nelles LP, Schnebli HP: Are proteinase inhibitors potentially useful in tumor therapy? Invasion Metastasis 2:113-124, 1982.

181. Giraldi T, Sava G: Selective antimetastatic drugs (review). Anticancer Res. 1:163-174, 1981.

182. Weiss L, Ward PM: Cell detachment and metastasis. Cancer Metastasis Rev. 2:111-127, 1983.

183. Carl PL, Chakravarty PK, Katzenellenbogen JA, Weber MJ: Protease-activated "prodrugs" for cancer chemotherapy. Proc. Natl. Acad. Sci. USA 77:2224-2228, 1980.

184. Chakravarty PK, Carl PL, Weber MJ, Katzenellenbogen JA: Plasmin-activated prodrugs for cancer chemotherapy. 2. Synthesis and biological activity of peptidyl derivatives of doxorubicin. J. Med. Chem. 26:638-644, 1983.

185. Iwakawa A, Tanaka K: Effect of fibrinolysis inhibitor and chemotherapeutics on the growth of human cancers transplanted into nude mice and in tissue culture.   Invasion Metastasis 2:232-248, 1982.
186. Sundbeck A, Myrhage R, Peterson H-I: Influence of tranexamic acid on tumor vascularization.   An experimental microangiographic study.   Anticancer Res.   1:295-298, 1981.
187. Astedt B, Glifberg I, Mattsson W, Trope T: Arrest of growth of ovarian tumor by tranexamic acid.   J. Am. Med. Assoc.   238:154-155, 1977.

CHAPTER 22. CATHEPSIN B-LIKE CYSTEINE PROTEINASES AND METASTASIS

BONNIE F. SLOANE, JURIJ ROZHIN, RANDALL E. RYAN, TAMARA T. LAH, NANCY A. DAY, JOHN D. CRISSMAN AND KENNETH V. HONN

I. INTRODUCTION

During the process of metastasis tumor cells traverse several extracellular matrix barriers in order to gain entry to the vascular space at the site of the primary tumor and to the perivascular space at the sites of metastatic tumors. A number of in vitro model systems have been designed to study tumor cell invasion through extracellular matrices. Several of these model systems including systems to study the concomitant digestion of these matrices by tumor cells are discussed elsewhere in this volume (see Chapters 18-21). A focus of much recent research is the basement membrane which underlies endothelial cells. The physical location of the basement membrane suggests that it must be traversed for tumor cells to form hematogenous metastases. Since the basement membrane in contrast to other extra-cellular matrix barriers contains type IV collagen a number of investigators have hypothesized that tumor cells must be able to degrade type IV collagen in order to invade through the basement membrane (see also Chapter 19). Metastatic variants of the B16 melanoma have been shown to secrete a type IV collagenase (1). However, type IV collagenase is secreted by tumor cells in a latent form which requires activation (2) suggesting that type IV collagenase is not by itself sufficient for basement membrane invasion by tumor cells and that additional proteinases or a proteolytic cascade may participate in basement membrane invasion. Three additional factors which need to be addressed are the following: 1) Tumor cells may be able to penetrate through the type IV collagen lattice found in the basement membrane in the absence of tumor cell or host cell collagenolytic activity. The type IV collagen lattice has holes whose sides are ~ 800 nm (3), i.e., a latticework through which a tumor cell could move. 2) Penetration of the basement membrane may only require limited digestion of the nonhelical regions of type IV collagen or degradation of the proteo-glycans which form the ground substance of the basement membrane. This limited degradation of type IV collagen could be accomplished by proteinases such as plasmin formed by the action of plasminogen activator (see Chapters 20 and 21) or cathepsin B. In addition, heparanase (see Chapter 18) or cathepsin B could singly or in concert induce degradation of basement membrane proteoglycans. 3) Tumor cells may not require proteolytic or hydrolytic enzymes to pass through the basement membrane. However, we (4) and others (5) have observed local dissolution of endothelial basement membrane in regions of contact between tumor cells and basement membrane which would seem to negate this.

II. CATHEPSIN B

        We have hypothesized that the cysteine proteinase cathepsin B
facilitates tumor cell metastasis.   Cysteine proteinases are one of the
four classes of endopeptidases or proteinases (see 6-8 for discussion).
Cysteine proteinases include lysosomal cysteine proteinases like
cathepsins B, H and L, the cytosolic calcium-activated neutral
proteinases and plant proteinases like papain.   Cathepsin B has a pH
optimum of 6.0 - 6.5 against synthetic and some protein substrates
(7,9).   Although this enzyme was believed to be irreversibly inactivated
by exposure to weakly alkaline pH (9), in recent work by Willenbrock
and Brocklehurst (10,11) they suggest that the pH dependent changes
[cathepsin B] in this   pH range [7 - 8] are not due to denaturation.
Barrett and co-workers (12) have reported significant activities for
both cathepsin L and cathepsin B at pH 8.0 when activity is recorded
"continuously over the first 30 s of hydrolysis."   Cathepsin B has
broad specificity as an endopeptidase against protein substrates such
as hemoglobin (9), myosin (13,14), actin (13), troponin (14), tropo-
myosin (14), insulin (15), proteoglycans (16), fibronectin (17) and the
nonhelical portion of types I-IV collagen (18,19) as well as peptidyldi-
eptidase activity against glucagon (20) and aldolase (21).   Thus as an
endopeptidase of broad specificity cathepsin B could degrade the
nonhelical regions of basement membrane type IV collagen (18,19), the
glycoproteins fibronectin (17) and laminin (see below) and the proteoglycans (16) in the basement membrane.   As a peptidyldipeptidase
cathepsin B could activate latent enzymes found in the basement
membrane   including type IV collagenase (22). These properties would
seem to make cathepsin B an ideal proteinase for degradation of the
basement membrane - both directly and indirectly via a proteolytic
cascade.   However, cathepsin B is a lysosomal acid hydrolase whose
activity is regulated in vivo by the acid pH of the lysosome, compart-
mentalization in lysosomes, cytosolic and extracellular inhibitors and
a requirement for thiol activation (6,9).   In the following sections
we will evaluate the current evidence that cathepsin B may play a
role(s) in tumor invasion and metastasis.

III.   SUBCELLULAR LOCALIZATION OF TUMOR CATHEPSIN B

    A.   Release of Cathepsin B

        During the synthesis, processing and packaging of a lysosomal
enzyme a proportion of the enzyme is released extracellularly (23,24).
Under certain pathological conditions like lysosomal storage diseases,
e.g., I-cell disease, the proportion of lysosomal enzymes released is
enhanced; these high extracellular activities led to the secretion-
recapture hypothesis for the packaging of lysosomal enzymes (25).   In
normal cells lysosomal enzymes are packaged intracellularly and extracellular activities may be the result of lysosomal enzyme release
during fusion between plasma membrane, endocytotic or exocytotic
vesicles and lysosomes.   In cells such as macrophages or neutrophils
lysosomes seem to function like secretory granules whose contents are

released in response to given stimuli (26). Thus the proportion of lysosomal enzymes released from macrophages or neutrophils can be quite high.

The synthesis, processing and packaging of cathepsin B has not been studied in normal cells nor in tumor cells. Cathepsin B activity has been measured extracellularly in culture medium of tumor cells (27-33), ascites fluid of women with ovarian carcinomas (33,34) and serum and urine of patients with a diverse variety of malignancies (35-40). Poole and co-workers (41-43) have reported that release of cathepsin B is positively correlated with the malignancy of human and murine mammary carcinoma explants. The cathepsin B appears to be released from viable tumor cells because 1) the cathepsin B activity in media of explants from the invasive and growing edge of the tumor is higher than that in media from explants of the central necrotic core (42), 2) the release of cathepsin B activity requires protein synthesis (42,43) and 3) cathepsin B activity is also present in culture media of tumor cells (33). Pietras et al. (28) reported that release of cathepsin B from human cervical epithelial cells correlates with the malignancy of the cells in vivo and their rate of cell proliferation in vitro. We have demonstrated cathepsin B activity in the culture media of a number of murine tumor lines: B16-F1 and B16-F10 (27), B16 amelanotic melanoma (B16a; 29,31,32) and 15091A mammary adenocarcinoma (30,31). The most suggestive evidence that cathepsin B is also released from tumor cells in vivo is that provided by Mort et al. (33): cathepsin B activity is present in ascites fluid from women with ovarian carcinoma. The ascites cells are believed to be the source of the cathepsin B activity since the ascites cells grown in culture release cathepsin B whereas sera from the same patients has no cathepsin B activity. Host cells might account in part for cathepsin B release in vivo or from tumor explants in vitro. However, macrophages are not believed to be the source of the cathepsin B activity since Recklies et al. (43) did not find cathepsin B activity in culture media of resident or stimulated murine macrophages. Baici et al. (44) recently reported that cathepsin B is released both from explants of rabbit V2 carcinoma and from explants of normal sub-cutaneous tissue from tumor-bearing rabbits. This release, like that from human and murine mammary carcinoma explants, requires protein synthesis. Cathepsin B release from the V2 carcinoma, normal tissue and co-cultures of the two can be stimulated by a diffusible factor present in tumor explant-conditioned culture medium.

Arachidonic acid metabolites may play a role in release of cathepsin B from tumor cells. Release of lysosomal glycosidases from neutrophils has been shown to be stimulated by lipoxygenase products (principally leukotriene B_4) of arachidonic acid metabolism (45,46) and inhibited by inhibitors of the lipoxygenase pathway (47,48). Pre-liminary evidence indicates that cathepsin B release from B16a cells can be stimulated by lipoxygenase products and inhibited by inhibitors of the lipoxygenase pathway (32,49). The cellular source in a solid tumor of lipoxygenase products which could stimulate cathepsin B release and account for the enhanced levels of cathepsin B measured extracellularly has not been identified. Tumor cell release of cathepsin B in response to the stimulus of lipoxygenase products is not associated with release of lysosomal glycosidases (32,49), thus suggesting that tumor cells do not release their entire lysosomal contents as do neutrophils in response to lipoxygenase products (45,46). Interactions among tumor cells, host cells, diffusible factors, lipoxygenase products, etc. which might result in enhanced release of cathepsin B in vivo clearly require further study.

We have demonstrated that several lines of tumor cells in culture release cathepsin B activity into the culture medium. Cathepsin B activity released from B16-F1 and B16-F10 cells in culture varies with the length of time the tumor cells have been in culture as well as with the number of passages in culture. We found that cathepsin B activity could not be measured in the culture medium of primary cultures, i.e., in tumor cells isolated from a subcutaneous tumor (27). However, cathepsin B activity is present in the media of 3rd passage and 6th passage cells (27). The amount of cathepsin B activity released by 3rd passage cells correlates with the metastatic potential of the B16-F1 and B16-F10 cell lines, whereas that released by 6th passage cells is reduced and does not correlate (24). Recklies et al. (43) reported that release of cathepsin B activity from explants of murine breast tumors decreases after culture periods of 9-11 da. This decrease may be due to loss of viability of the explants, however, loss of viability does not account for the decreased release from B16-F1 and B16-F10 variants in monolayer culture which we observed (27). The decreased release of cathepsin B may be due to the lack of host cell-tumor cell interactions. We have also found that cathepsin B activity released into the culture medium of B16a cells decreased with the number of passages in vivo as a subcutaneous tumor (before establishment in culture) as well as with the number of passages in vivo; the metastatic potential of the B16a tumor decreased in parallel (unpublished observations). Similarly, Recklies et al. (43) found that cathepsin B secretion rates from explants of the first transplant generation of a spontaneous tumor are significantly less than from explants of the original spontaneous tumor.

Mort et al. (33) have established that the cathepsin B released from tumor explants into culture media and present in ascites fluid is primarily in a latent form activatable by pepsin. Mort et al. (34) demonstrated by SDS-PAGE under reducing conditions that pepsin activation of latent ascites cathepsin B results in a change in M_r from 40,000 to 32,000, cathepsin B running as a single band in both cases. Based on this, they feel that latent cathepsin B is an inactive precursor rather than an enzyme-inhibitor complex. Recently we have established that five variants of the B16 melanoma released latent cathepsin B into their culture medium (Table 1). The cathepsin B activity released from B16 variants did not exhibit any correlation with the lung colonization potential of these variants. The rank order of lung colonization potential in Table 1 is B16a > B16-BL6 > B16-B15b > B16-F10 > B16-O13.

Table 1.   Cathepsin B Activity in Culture Media of B16 Variants.

Cell Line	Activity[*]	
	Latent	Total
B16a	100.0	116.3
B16-O13	54.3	56.1
B16-F10	28.8	31.7
B16-BL6	16.7	18.8
B16-B15b	13.7	15.8

B16 variants were cultured and the media harvested after 48 hr in the presence of heat and acid inactivated fetal calf serum, centrifuged at 120,000 x g and concentrated 10-23x using an Amicon YM10 membrane. Latent activity was measured after pepsin (0.5 - 2.0 mg/ml) activation at pH 4.2.

[*]pmoles 4-methoxy-β-napthylamine formed per ml medium per min.

A number of laboratories including our own have established that cathepsin B activity released from tumor cells has enhanced stability to elevated temperature and to mildly alkaline pH. Pietras et al. (28) reported that cathepsin B activity released from neoplastic cervical cells retains 90-96% of its activity after 5 min exposure to 65°C. We have found that cathepsin B activity in the culture media of B16a and 15091A tumor cells retains 62 ± 5% and 67 ± 5% of its activity, respectively, after exposure to pH 8.0 for 60 min (50). Baici et al. (44) reported that the cathepsin B activity released from the inter-action between host cells and tumor cells has stability above pH 7.0; the cellular source of this cathepsin B activity may be either tumor cells or host cells. Dufek et al. (39) found an alkaline stable form of cathepsin B in human serum; this form represents 40% of the total activity in serum and is present in all patients with primary liver carcinoma.

B.   Plasma Membrane Cathepsin B

Release of cathepsin B from tumor cells in culture suggests that cathepsin B may at some point in time be associated with the tumor cell plasma membrane. When normal and neoplastic human cervical cells were subjected to sucrose density gradient centrifugation, cathepsin B activity was found in association with a plasma membrane fraction of the neoplastic cells, but not of the normal cells (51).   Zucker et al.

(52) have recently reported elevated levels of cathepsin B in plasma membrane fractions isolated from human pancreatic adenocarcinoma cells. Although Koppel et al. (53) found cathepsin B activity in rat sarcoma plasma membranes, the cathepsin B activity in the plasma membrane of the metastatic variant was less than that in the nonmetastatic variant. Bohmer et al. (54), on the other hand, found that the activity of an unidentified acid cysteine proteinase is similar in plasma membranes purified from normal bovine lymphoid cells and from bovine lympho-

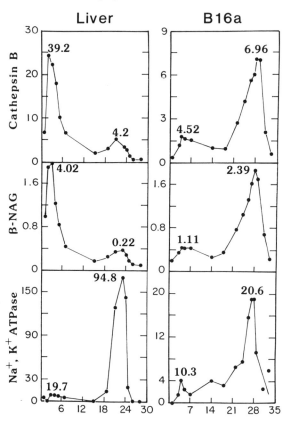

FIGURE 1. Elution Profile of Marker Enzymes Separated from Murine Liver and B16 Amelanotic Melanoma by Percoll Density Gradient Centrifugation. Values on y axes represent enzyme activities per ml; values within graphs represent specific activity of the enzyme in the peak fraction.

sarcoma cells. Kozlowski et al. (55) have provided morphological evidence, using a fluorescent transition-state analog, that a cysteine proteinase is associated with the cell surface of $HSDM_1C_1$ fibrosarcoma cells.

Tumor cells grown in vitro have been shown to shed plasma membrane-derived vesicles (56-58). Poste and Nicolson (58) found that by fusing shed vesicles from B16-F10 melanoma cells (high potential) with B16-F1 cells (low potential) the lung colonization potential of the B16-F1 melanoma can be increased. We had previously established that cathepsin B activity is higher in B16-F10 cells than B16-F1 (27,59) and that both variants release cathepsin B in vitro (27). Therefore we assayed membrane vesicles, from a cell line (15091A) which has been shown to shed vesicles in quantity (56,57), for cathepsin B activity and established that the vesicles do possess cathepsin B activity (30).

We have established that the cathepsin B activity in three melanomas shifts in correspondence with the metastatic potential to the plasma membrane of the tumors (60,61). Differential centrifugation of murine liver and three melanomas of increasing metastatic potential (Cloudman < B16-F1 < B16a) indicates that cathepsin B activity shifts to the light mitochondrial fraction in correspondence with metastatic potential (Table 2). Percoll density gradient centifugation of the light mitochondrial fraction indicates that the shift of cathepsin B activity is to the plasma membrane fraction of the metastatic B16 melanomas (Figure 1). Activity of β-N-acetyl-glucosaminidase (β-NAG) exhibits a similar shift (Figure 1), but activities of two additional lysosomal hydrolases, cathepsin H and β-glucuronidase, do not shift to the plasma membrane fraction of the metastatic B16 melanomas.

Table 2. Ratio of Specific Activity in Light Mitochondrial Fraction (L) to that in Heavy Mitochondrial Fraction (H) for Lysosomal Enzymes in Murine Liver and Melanomas.

Enzyme	L/H			
	Liver	Cloudman	B16-F1	B16a
Cathepsin B	0.44	1.04	1.50	1.82
β-NAG[*]	0.34	0.99	1.52	0.94
Cathepsin H	0.77	1.14	1.33	0.96
β-glucuronidase	0.62	1.15	1.41	0.94

[*]β-N-acetyl-glucosaminidase

Establishing that cathepsin B in tumors is membrane-associated could be of importance as membrane-associated cathepsin B might possess proteolytic activity when free cathepsin B, presumably due to the lesser ability of proteinase inhibitors to bind to a membrane-associated enzyme. In this regard, we have found that cathepsin B activity in 15091A vesicles is less susceptible to inhibition by a cysteine proteinase inhibitor than is cathepsin B activity in 15091A tumor cells (31). Cathepsin B activity in 15091A tumor cells is inhibited ≥ 99% by 5 μM Z-Phe-Ala-CHN$_2$ whereas the cathepsin B activity released into the culture medium is inhibited 87 ± 2% (31). Steven et al. (62) have reported that the activity of a trypsin-like proteinase present on the surface of Ehrlich ascites cells against casein and BANA cannot be inhibited by high M_r proteinase inhibitors such as SBTI but can be inhibited by low M_r inhibitors such as TLCK. In a more detailed study by Steven and co-workers (63), they showed that proteinase inhibitors have a significantly reduced ability to inactivate proteinases which are bound to "artificial membranes" when compared to the same proteinases in solution even when the inhibitors are present in excess.

Cathepsin B released from tumor cells which are in contact with the extracellular matrix such as the basement membrane of the blood vessel wall also might not be accessible to extracellular proteinase inhibitors and thereby not be inhibitable. One example of this was reported by Campbell et al. (64); their studies indicate that proteolysis by elastase released from neutrophils cannot be prevented by proteinase inhibitors when the neutrophils are in contact with their connective tissue substrate (in this case fibronectin). Similarly Johnson and Varani (64a) reported that when inhibitors and substrate are surface bound neutrophils cannot hydrolyze the substrate. In contrast, when the inhibitors are present in the fluid phase neutrophils retain hydrolytic activity.

In addition to reduced binding to inhibitors, cathepsin B associated with the plasma membrane may have enhanced stability. For example, the cathepsin B in membrane vesicles spontaneously shed from 15091A murine mammary adenocarcinoma cells in culture retains a significant proportion (85%) of activity at alkaline pH (pH 8.0; 50) as well as after exposure to 56°C for 30 min. Sixty-eight percent of cathepsin B activity in the vesicles is heat-stable (30). By contrast only 5 - 16% of cathepsin B activity in 15091A cells is alkaline stable and 14% heat stable (30,50). There have been other reports that tumor-associated cathepsin B may be more stable than liver cathepsin B (see A above). Cathepsin B activity in plasma membrane fractions of neoplastic human cervical cells also has been found to have enhanced stability to both alkaline pH and heat (51).

IV. TUMOR CATHEPSIN B

We have partially purified cathepsin B from six human tumors (melanoma, mammary adenocarcinoma, malignant fibrous histiocytoma, renal cell carcinoma, stomach adenocarcinoma and colon adenocarcinoma) and two normal tissues (liver and spleen) from non-tumor-bearing patients (65). Tumor cathepsin B has a greater stability above a pH of 7 then does either liver or spleen cathepsin B (Figure 2). Our studies thus suggest that tumor cathepsin B may have properties which enable it to act extracellularly. However, when Olstein and Liener (66) purified cathepsin B from murine liver and a murine fibrosarcoma induced by methylcholanthrene they found that the enzymes from both tissues are irreversibly denatured above pH 7.0. The recent studies by Willenbrock and Brocklehurst (10,11), however, indicate that the pH-dependent changes in cathepsin B activity from pH 7.0 - 8.0 may not be due to irreversible denaturation. Thus, cathepsin B released from tumor cells or present in the plasma membrane of tumor cells may be able to participate in the proteolytic degradation that seems to accompany tumor cell invasion.

V. DOES CATHEPSIN B PLAY A ROLE IN TUMOR METASTASIS?

No definitive proof exists to indicate that cathepsin B plays a role in tumor invasion and metastasis. There is, however, an increasing body of correlative evidence relating cathepsin B activity to the malignancy of human tumors and the metastatic capabilities of animal tumors.

386

Activity of cathepsin B in homogenates of murine solid tumors correlates with the lung colonization potential of six B16 melanoma variants (27,59,67) and with the potential to spontaneously metastasize to the lungs of B16a and 3LL metastatic variants (31). Cathepsin B activity in homogenates of human mammary tumors that are estrogen and progesterone receptor positive exhibited a positive correlation with tumor malignancy as determined clinically by increased ^{3}H-thymidine incorporation (Figure 3). In contrast, cathepsin B activity in estrogen and progesterone receptor negative mammary tumors exhibited either an inverse or no correlation with malignancy (Figure 3). Although Recklies et al. (42) did not find a correlation between cathepsin B activity and malignancy of human breast tumors, Vashishta et al. (40) did find a correlation. Cathepsin B activity in human mammary tumors may depend on several factors, e.g., rates of synthesis of cathepsin B, rates of processing of inactive precursor to active enzyme, rates of synthesis of cysteine proteinase inhibitors.

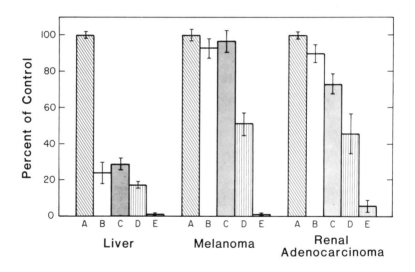

FIGURE 2. pH Stability of Partially Purified Cathepsin B from Human Liver, Melanoma and Renal Adenocarcinoma. A = 50 mM acetate buffer, pH 5.2; B = 50 mM phosphate buffer, pH 7.4; C = 50 mM Tris buffer, pH 7.4; D = 50 mM HEPES buffer, pH 7.4; E = 50 mM Tris buffer, pH 8.0. Exposure was for 30 min at 37°C.

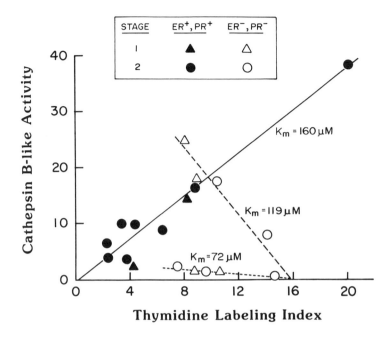

FIGURE 3. Cathepsin B Activity in Human Mammary Tumors versus their
Malignancy (Thymidine Labeling Index). Each symbol represents a single
tumor. The correlation coefficients for the three apparent subpopulations of tumors (represented by differing Km's) were ≥ 0.93. The
activity was determined as V_{max} and expressed as nmol/min/mg protein.

Cathepsin B activity in homogenates of some tumors does not
exhibit any correlation with metastatic potential or malignancy. For
example, McLaughlin et al. (68) did not find any correlation between
cathepsin B activity and the metastatic potential of a methylcholanthrene induced (murine fibrosarcoma) and its 18 clones. McLaughlin et
al. (68) suggested that correlates of proteolytic activity and
metastatic potential "based on a comparison of only two cell variants
[as in our initial study of B16-F1 and B16-F10 tumors; 27,59] may in
fact be fortuitous." However, cathepsin B activity in four additional
B16 variants (B16a, B16-BL6, B16-013, B16-B5b) also correlated with
lung colonization potential (67), thus confirming and extending our
earlier observations (27,59). Takenaga (69) reported that treatment of
Lewis lung carcinoma cells with dimethylsulfoxide increases both their
lung colonization potential and their activity of degradative enzymes
including cathepsin B. In contrast, Lowe and Isaacs (70) did not find
any correlation between cathepsin B activity and the metastatic ability

of rat prostatic adenocarcinoma variants. Cathepsin B activity like
that of other proteolytic enzymes appears to correlate with malignancy
in some tumor lines but not in others.

The inability to establish a correlation between cathepsin B
activity in homogenates of solid tumors and malignancy may be due to
one of many factors (see also Chapter 4). Solid tumors contain a
multiplicity of cell types (macrophages, lymphocytes and stromal cells
as well as tumor cells), any of which could account for enzyme activity
or for activity of cysteine proteinase inhibitors. Centrifugal
elutriation has been used successfully to separate as well as
synchronize tumor cell subpopulations from solid tumors (71,72) and
from multicellular tumor spheroids (73). We have separated rodent
solid tumors into two subpopulations of viable tumor cells (β fraction)
and nonviable tumor cells and host cells (α fraction) using sequential
collagenase digestion followed by centrifugal elutriation (59,67).
These studies definitively demonstrate that 95% of cathepsin B activity
is associated with the viable tumor cells in rodent solid tumors
(59,67). Eight rodent tumors of five histologic types were analyzed in
these studies. The four variants of the B16 melanoma (rank order of
lung colonization potential B16a > B16-BL6 > B16-B15b > B16-013)
exhibit a positive correlation between cathepsin B activity in homogenates of the isolated tumor cells and lung colonization potential
(67). This correlation is not found for homogenates of solid tumors;
the presence of endogenous cysteine proteinase inhibitors in the host
cells of solid tumors might account for this lack of correlation (67).

Studies of lysosomal proteinase activity or of cathepsin B
activity in cultured tumor cells have demonstrated both a correlation
with malignancy or metastatic potential as well as no correlation
(27,35,68,74-78). In our laboratory when the B16-F1 and B16-F10
variants are grown in vivo as subcutaneous tumors, there is either a
positive correlation or no correlation between lung colonization
potential and cathepsin B activity depending on the length of time in
culture (27). Nicolson and co-workers (79,80) recently reported that
the phenotype of malignant cells can change in culture in either the
direction of increased or decreased malignancy. In some in vitro
studies, cathepsin B activity has been shown to correlate negatively
with transformation (76,77) and positively with differentiation (77).
In contrast, we have demonstrated that cathepsin B activity in
chemically-transformed C3H10T½ fibroblasts (clones 15 and 16) was
elevated over that in the parent clone 8 (unpublished observations).
Clones 15 and 16, but not clone 8, have been shown to be tumorigenic
in vivo (81) and also tumorigenic in our hands. Poste (82) questions
the tumorigenicity of some cell lines which have been transformed in
vitro. Apparently several such cell lines, including the Nil hamster
cells used in one of the studies exhibiting a negative correlation
between cathepsin B activity and malignancy (77), are tumorigenic prior
to transformation by tumor viruses (82). Positive correlations between
cathepsin B activity in cultured chick embryo fibroblasts and transformation by Rous sarcoma virus have been reported by Chu and Olden
(83), between cathepsin B activity in cultured rat anaplastic sarcoma
cells and their potential for spontaneous metastasis to the lymphatics

and the lung by Koppel et al. (53) and between cathepsin B activity in cultured human ectocervix cells and malignancy by Pietras et al. (35) and Pietras and Roberts (51).

Further evidence that cathepsin B may play a role in tumor cell invasion during the metastatic cascade may be derived from the studies of cathepsin B activity in the plasma membrane of tumor cells. Our laboratories have demonstrated a quantitative relationship between cathepsin B activity in plasma membrane fractions (purified by Percoll density gradient centrifugation) and lung colonization potential (60,61). Cathepsin B activity in the plasma membrane is enhanced 18 fold when expressed as a percentage of ouabain sensitive Na^+,K^+-ATPase activity in the same fraction (61). Similarly Pietras and Roberts (51) have observed an increase in cathepsin B activity in plasma fractions (purified by sucrose density gradient centrifugation) in correspondence with both malignancy and rate of proliferation in vitro. Koppel et al. (53) on the other hand reported an inverse correlation between cathepsin B activity in the plasma membrane and metastatic potential of two rat anaplastic sarcomas. Such conflicting results between malignancy and/or metastatic potential and amounts of cathepsin B released from tumors also occur in the literature. Although Poole and co-workers (41-43) have demonstrated a correlation between cathepsin B activity released from breast explants and malignancy, we have not been able to demonstrate a correlation between latent, native or total cathepsin B activity released from six B16 metastatic variants and their lung colonization potentials (see Table 1).

Is a quantitative relationship between cathepsin B activity and metastatic potential needed to indicate that cathepsin B plays a role(s) in metastasis? Obviously the answer is no. Several factors may be more important, e.g., 1) the localization of cathepsin B at the site of tumor cell dissolution of the basement membrane, 2) enhanced activity and/or stability of tumor cathepsin B, and 3) ability to degrade components of the extracellular matrix.

1) We recently studied (at the light and electron microscopic levels) the arrest and extravasation of B16a cells injected intravenously (4 and Chapter 9). Figure 4 is a diagrammatic representation of the process(es) by which a B16a tumor cell extravasates into the perivascular space at metastatic sites. The upper figure illustrates a tumor cell arrested in a pulmonary capillary. The middle figure illustrates the retraction of the underlying endothelial cell resulting in exposure of the basement membrane. The lower figure illustrates the dissolution of the basement membrane at the site of contact with the tumor cell plasma membrane. Such focal sites of dissolution would suggest that a proteolytic enzyme (such as cathepsin B) or a glycolytic enzyme localized in the tumor cell plasma membrane or released locally could be an effective mediator of B16a extravasation (see above). With the B16a line there was not any evidence of diapedesis or active invasion by the tumor cells.

2) Cathepsin B released from tumors or in the plasma membrane fractions has previously been shown to exhibit enhanced stabilities to both pH and heat (see above). Recent work in our laboratories on the endogenous inhibitors of cysteine proteinases indicates that tumor cathepsin B could have enhanced activity unrelated to its own intrinsic properties. We have recently purified cysteine proteinase inhibitors of $\sim$ 13,000 M_r and isoelectric points from 4.7 - 7.7 from human liver and human malignant fibrous histiocytoma (84). Two classes of cysteine proteinase inhibitors have been isolated from normal human spleen (85), one with acidic isoelectric points and one with neutral to basic isoelectric points. Of these two classes the acidic are more effective against cathepsin B (85). We found that the sarcoma and liver extracts containing both forms exhibited similar affinities for papain but the sarcoma exhibited less affinity for cathepsin B than did the liver extract (84). Since the isolated sarcoma inhibitors with isoelectric points greater than 6.0 exhibited similar affinities for papain and cathepsin B we hypothesize that the acidic type of cysteine proteinase inhibitors differ in sarcomas.

3) As discussed in section II, cathepsin B has broad substrate specificity. Cathepsin B from normal tissues has been shown to degrade several components of the basement membrane, i.e., proteoglycans (16), fibronectin (17) and the nonhelical regions of type IV collagen (18,19). In preliminary studies we have compared the abilities of cathepsin B isolated from human liver and human colon carcinoma to degrade laminin. These studies were performed for time periods from 4 to 24 hr at pH 6.5 and 25°C. Under these conditions tumor cathepsin B degraded laminin at lower enzyme to substrate ratios than did liver cathepsin B; the digestion products also differed (unpublished observations). Studies of the digestion of other basement membrane components are in progress.

Present evidence supports a link between cathepsin B and tumor cell invasion and metastasis but does not yet support a causal role for cathepsin B in these processes. The recent work in our laboratories demonstrating a correlation between cathepsin B activity in the plasma membrane and metastatic potential, a reduced affinity of tumor endogenous inhibitors for cathepsin B and the ability of tumor cathepsin B to degrade extracellular matrix components all further support this link. However, continuing work in our own and other laboratories will be required to define a causal role for cathepsin B in tumor invasion and metastasis.

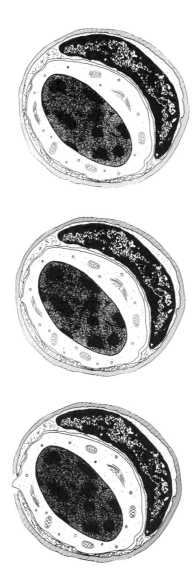

FIGURE 4. Arrest and Extravasation of B16 Amelanotic Melanoma Cell in Pulmonary Microvasculature. Top, arrest and attachment to endothelial cell. Middle, retraction of endothelial cell-cell junctions exposing basement membrane. Bottom, focal dissolution of basement membrane at site of contact with tumor cell plasma membrane.

ACKNOWLEDGMENTS

This work was supported in part by CA36481 awarded by the National Cancer Institute (BFS) and a grant from Harper-Grace Hospitals (KVH and BFS). BFS is the recipient of a Research Career Development Award (CA00921) from the National Cancer Institute.

REFERENCES

1. Liotta LA, Tryggvason K, Garbisa S, Hart I, Foltz CM, Shafie S: Metastatic potential correlates with enzymatic degradation of basement membrane collagen. Nature (London) 284:61-62, 1980.
2. Salo T, Liotta LA, Tryggvason K: Purification and characterization of a murine basement membrane collagen-degrading enzyme secreted by metastatic tumor cells. J. Biol. Chem. 257:3058-3063, 1983.
3. Kuhn K: Collagen family-variations in the molecular and supermolecular structures. In: Tschesche H (ed.) Proteinases in Inflammation and Tumor Invasion. Walter de Gruyter & Co., Berlin, in press.
4. Crissman JD, Hatfield J, Schaldenbrand M, Sloane BF, Honn KV: Arrest and extravasation of B16 amelanotic melanoma in murine lungs. Lab. Invest., in press.
5. Jones PA, DeClerck YA: Extracellular matrix destruction by invasive tumor cells. Cancer Metastasis Rev. 1:289-317, 1982.
6. Barrett AJ: The many forms and functions of cellular proteinases. Fed. Proc. Fed. Am. Soc. Exp. Biol. 39:9-14, 1980.
7. Barrett AJ, McDonald JK: Mammalian Proteases. Academic Press, New York, Vol. 1, 1980.
8. Neurath H: Evolution of proteolytic enzymes. Science 224:350-357, 1984.
9. Barrett AJ: Human cathepsin Bl. Purification and some properties of the enzyme. Biochem. J. 131:809-822, 1973.
10. Willenbrock F, Brocklehurst K: Preparation of cathepsins B and H by covalent chromatography and characterization of their catalytic sites by reaction with a thiol-specific two-protonic-state reactivity probe. Biochem. J. 227:511-519, 1985.
11. Willenbrock F, Brocklehurst K: A general framework of cysteine-proteinase mechanism deduced from studies on enzymes with structurally different analogous catalytic-site residues Asp-158 and -161 (papain and actinidin), Gly-196 (cathepsin B) and Asn-165 (cathepsin H). Biochem. J. 227:521-528, 1985.
12. Mason RW, Green GDJ, Barrett AJ: Human liver cathepsin L. Biochem. J. 226:233-241, 1985.
13. Schwartz WN, Bird JWC: Degradation of myofibrillar proteins by cathepsins B and D. Biochem. J. 167:811-820, 1977.
14. Noda T, Isogai K, Hayashi H, Katunuma N: Susceptibilities of various myofibrillar proteins to cathepsin B and morphological alteration of isolated myofibrils by this enzyme. J. Biochem. (Tokyo) 90:371-379, 1981.

15. McKay MJ, Offermann MK, Barrett AJ, Bond JS: Action of human liver cathepsin B on oxidized insulin B chain. Biochem. J. 213:467-471, 1983.
16. Morrison RIG, Barrett AJ, Dingle JT: Cathepsins Bl and D action on human cartilage proteoglycans. Biochim. Biophys. Acta 302:411-419, 1973.
17. Recklies AD, Poole AR: Proteolytic mechanisms of tissue destruction in tumor growth and metastasis. In: Weiss L, Gilbert HA (eds.) Liver Metastasis. GK Hall, Boston, pp. 77-95, 1982.
18. Burleigh MC, Barrett AJ, Lazarus GS: Cathepsin Bl. A lysosomal enzyme that degrades native collagen. Biochem. J. 137:387-398, 1974.
19. Etherington DJ: The dissolution of insoluble bovine collagens by cathepsin Bl, collagenolytic cathepsin and pepsin. Conn. Tiss. Res. 5:135-145, 1977.
20. Aronson NN, Barrett AJ: The specificity of cathepsin B. Hydrolysis of glucagon at the C-terminus by a peptidyldipeptidase mechanism. Biochem. J. 171:759-765, 1978.
21. Bond JS, Barrett AJ: Degradation of fructose-1-6-biphosphate aldolase by cathepsin B. A further example of peptidyldipeptidase activity of this proteinase. Biochem. J. 189:17-25, 1980.
22. Eeckhout Y, Vaes G: Further studies on the activation of procollagenase, the latent precursor of bone collagenase. Effects of lysosomal cathepsin B, plasmin and kallikrein, and spontaneous activation. Biochem. J. 166:21-31, 1977.
23. Rosenfeld MG, Kreibich G, Popov D, Kato K, Sabatini DD: Biosynthesis of lysosomal hydrolases: Their synthesis in bound polysomes and the role of co- and post-translational processing in determining their subcellular distribution. J. Cell Biol. 93:135-143, 1982.
24. Sly WS, Fischer HD: The phosphomannosyl recognition system for intracellular and intercellular transport of lysosomal enzymes. J. Cell. Biochem. 18:67-85, 1982.
25. Neufeld EF, Lim TW, Shapiro LJ: Inherited disorders of lysosomal metabolism. Annu. Rev. Biochem. 44:357-376, 1975.
26. Skudlarek MD, Swank RT: Turnover of two lysosomal enzymes in macrophages. J. Biol. Chem. 256:10137-10144, 1981.
27. Sloane BF, Honn KV, Sadler JG, Turner WA, Kimpson JJ, Taylor JD: Cathepsin B activity in B16 melanoma cells: A possible marker for metastatic potential. Cancer Res. 42:980-986, 1982.
28. Pietras RJ, Szego CM, Roberts JA, Seeler BJ: Lysosomal cathepsin B-like activity: Mobilization in prereplicative and neoplastic epithelial cells. J. Histochem. Cytochem. 29:440-450, 1981.
29. Honn KV, Cavanaugh P, Evens C, Taylor JD, Sloane BF: Tumor cell-platelet aggregation: Induced by cathepsin B-like proteinase and inhibited by prostacyclin. Science 217:540-542, 1982.
30. Cavanaugh PG, Sloane BF, Bajkowski A, Gasic GJ, Gasic TB, Honn KV: Involvement of a cathepsin B-like cysteine proteinase in platelet aggregation induced by tumor cells and their shed membrane vesicles. Clin. Exp. Metastasis 1:297-308, 1983.
31. Sloane BF, Sadler JG, Evens C, Ryan R, Bajkowski AS, Crissman JD, Honn KV: Cathepsin B-like cysteine proteinases and tumor metastasis. Cancer Bull. 36:196-200, 1984.

32. Sloane BF, Makim S, Dunn JR, Lacoste R, Theodorou M, Battista J, Alex R, Honn KV: In: Bockman RS, Powles T, Honn KV, Ramwell P (eds.) Prostaglandins and Cancer. Alan Liss, New York, pp. 789-792, 1982.

33. Mort JS, Leduc M, Recklies AD: A latent thiol proteinase from ascitic fluid of patients with neoplasia. Biochim. Biophys. Acta 662:173-180, 1981.

34. Mort JS, Leduc M, Recklies AD: Characterization of a latent cysteine proteinase from ascitic fluid as a high molecular weight form of cathepsin B. Biochim. Biophys. Acta 755:369-375, 1983.

35. Pietras RJ, Szego CM, Mangan CE, Seeler BJ, Burtnett MM, Orevi M: Elevated serum cathepsin B1 and vaginal pathology after prenatal DES exposure. Obstet. Gynecol. 52:321-327, 1978.

36. Pietras RJ, Szego CM, Mangan CE, Seeler BJ, Burtnett MM: Elevated serum cathepsin B1-like activity in women with neoplastic disease. Gynecol. Oncol. 7:1-17, 1979.

37. Perras RJ, Cramer J, Bishop R, Averette H, Sevin BU: Detection of increased levels of cysteinyl proteinase activity in urine of gynecological cancer patients. Proc. Am. Assoc. Cancer Res. 24:130, 1983.

38. Perras JP, Sevin BU: Production of monoclonal antibodies against cathepsin B-like enzyme derived from urine of gynecologic cancer patients. Proc. Am. Assoc. Cancer Res. 25:250, 1984.

39. Dufek V, Matous B, Kral V: Serum alkaline-stable acid thiol proteinase - a possible marker for primary liver carcinoma. Neoplasma 31:99-107, 1984.

40. Vasishta A, Baker PR, Preece PE, Wood RAB, Cuschieri A: Serum and tissue proteinase-like peptidase activities in women undergoing total mastectomy for breast cancer. Eur. J. Clin. Oncol. 20:203-208, 1984.

41. Poole AR, Tiltman KJ, Recklies AD, Stoker TAM: Differences in secretion of the proteinase cathepsin B at the edges of human breast carcinomas and fibroadenomas. Nature (London) 273:545-547, 1980.

42. Recklies AD, Tiltman KJ, Stoker TAM, Poole AR: Secretion of proteinases from malignant and nonmalignant human breast tissue. Cancer Res. 40:550-556, 1980.

43. Recklies AD, Mort JS, Poole AR: Secretion of a thiol proteinase from mouse mammary carcinomas and its characterization. Cancer Res. 42:1026-1032, 1982.

44. Baici A, Gyger-Marazzi M, Strauli P: Extracellular cysteine proteinase and collagenase activities as a consequence of tumor-host interaction in the rabbit V2 carcinoma. Invasion Metastasis 4:13-27, 1984.

45. Bokoch GM, Reed PW: Effect of various lipoxygenase metabolites of arachidonic acid on degranulation of polymorphonuclear leukocytes. J. Biol. Chem. 256:5317-5320, 1981.

46. Hafstrom I, Pamblad J, Malsten CL, Radmark O, Samuelsson B: Leukotriene B_4 - a stereospecific stimulator for release of lysosomal enzymes from neutrophils. FEBS Lett. 130:146-148, 1981.

47. Walenga RW, Showell HJ, Feinstein MB, Becker EL: Parallel inhibition of neutrophil arachidonic acid metabolism and lysosomal enzyme secretion by nordihydroguaiaretic acid. Life Sci. 27:1047-1053, 1980.

48. Smith RJ, Sun FF, Bowman BJ, Iden SS, Smith HW, McGuire JC: Effect of 6,9-diepoxy-6,9-(phenylimino)-Δ6,8-prostaglandin I_1 (U-60-257) an inhibitor of leukotriene synthesis on human neutrophil function. Biochem. Biophys. Res. Commun. 109:943-949, 1982.

49. Sloane BF, Honn KV: Proteolytic enzymes and arachidonic acid metabolites. In: Lands WEM (ed.) Biochemistry of Arachidonic Acid Metabolism. Martinus Nihhoff, Boston, pp. 311-321, 1985.

50. Sloane BF, Honn KV: Cysteine proteinases and metastasis. Cancer Metastasis Rev. 3:249-263, 1984.

51. Pietras RJ, Roberts JA: Cathepsin B-like enzymes. Subcellular distribution and properties in neoplastic and control cells from human ectocervix. J. Biol. Chem. 256:8536-8544, 1981.

52. Zucker S, Lysik RM, Wieman J, Wilkie D, Lane B: Tumor cell membrane metalloproteinases are responsible for collagenolysis and cell destruction during cancer invasion. Proc. Am. Assoc. Cancer Res. 26:56, 1985.

53. Koppel P, Baici A, Keist R, Matzku S, Keller R: Cathepsin B-like proteinase as a marker for metastatic tumor cell variants. Exp. Cell Biol. 52:293-299, 1984.

54. Bohmer FD, Schmidt HE, Schon R: Proteolytic activities associated with plasma membrane preparations from tumour cells in enzootic bovine leukosis and from normal bovine lymphoid cells. Acta Biol. Med. Germ. 41:883-890, 1982.

55. Kozlowski KA, Wezeman FH, Schultz RM: Tumor cell proteinase visualization and quantification using a fluorescent transition-state analog probe. Proc. Natl. Acad. Sci. USA 81:1135-1139, 1984.

56. Gasic GJ, Catalfamo JL, Gasic TB, Avdalovic N. In vitro mechanisms of platelet aggregation by purified plasma membrane vesicles shed by mouse 15091A tumor cells. In: Donati MB, Davidson JF, Garattini S (eds.) Malignancy and the Hemostatic System. Raven Press, New York, pp. 27-35, 1981.

57. Gasic GJ, Boettiger D, Catalfamo JL, Gasic TB, Stewart GJ: Aggregation of platelets and cell membrane vesiculation by rat cells transformed in vitro by Rous sarcoma virus. Cancer Res. 38:2950-2955, 1978.

58. Poste G, Nicolson GL: Arrest and metastasis of blood-borne tumor cells are modified by fusion of plasma membrane vesicles from highly metastatic cells. Proc. Natl. Acad. Sci USA 77:399-403, 1980.

59. Sloane BF, Dunn JR, Honn KV: Lysosomal cathepsin B: Correlation with metastatic potential. Science 212:1151-1153, 1981.

60. Sloane BF, Rozhin J, Crissman JD, Bajkowski AS, Honn KV: Association of a cathepsin B-like cysteine proteinase with tumor cell plasma membranes. In: Hellmann K and Eccles SA (eds.) Treatment of Metastasis: Problems and Prospects. Taylor and Francis, London, pp. 377-380, 1985.

61. Sloane BF, Rozhin J, Johnson K, Taylor H, Crissman JD, Honn KV: Cathepsin B: A plasma membrane enzyme in metastatic tumors. Submitted.

62. Steven FS, Griffin MM, Itzhaki S, Al-Habib A: A trypsin-like neutral protease on Ehrlich ascites cell surfaces: Its role in the activation of tumour-cell zymogen of collagenase. Br. J. Cancer 42:712-721, 1980.

63. Steven FS, Griffin MM, Itzhaki S: Inhibition of free and bound trypsin-like enzymes. Eur. J. Biochem. 126:311-318, 1982.

64. Campbell EJ, Senior RM, McDonald JA, Cox DL: Proteolysis by neutrophils. Relative importance of cell-substrate contacts and oxidative inactivation of proteinase inhibitors in vitro. J. Clin. Invest. 70:845-852, 1982.

64a. Johnson KJ, Varani J: Substrate hydrolysis by immune complex-activated neutrophils: Effect of physical presentation of complexes and protease inhibitors. J. Immunol. 127:1875-1879, 1981.

65. Sloane BF, Bajkowski AS, Day NA, Honn KV, Crissman JD: Purification and properties of a cathepsin B-like enzyme from human tumors: Comparison with cathepsin B isolated from human liver and spleen. Proc. Am. Assoc. Cancer Res. 25:4, 1984.

66. Olstein AD, Liener IE: Comparative studies of mouse liver cathepsin B and an analogous tumor thiol proteinase. J. Biol. Chem. 258:11049-11056, 1983.

67. Ryan RE, Crissman JD, Honn KV, Sloane BF: Cathepsin B-like activity in viable tumor cells isolated from rodent tumors. Cancer Res., in press.

68. McLaughlin MEH, Liener IE, Wang N: Proteolytic and metastatic activities of clones derived from a methylcholanthrene-induced murine fibrosarcoma. Clin. Exp. Metastasis 1:359-372, 1983.

69. Takenaga K: Enhanced metastatic potential of cloned low-metastatic Lewis lung carcinoma cells treated in vitro with dimethyl sulfoxide. Cancer Res. 44:1122-1127, 1984.

70. Lowe FC, Isaacs JT: Biochemical methods for predicting metastatic ability of prostatic cancer utilizing the Dunning R-3327 rat prostatic adenocarcinoma system as a model. Cancer Res. 44:744-752, 1984.

71. Meistrich ML, Grdina DJ, Meyn RE, Barlogie B: Separation of cells from mouse solid tumors by centrifugal elutriation. Cancer Res. 37:4291-4296, 1977.

72. Meistrich ML, Meyn RE, Barlogie B: Synchronization of mouse L-P59 cells by centrifugal elutriation separation. Exp. Cell Res. 105:169-177, 1977.

73. Bauer KD, Keng PC, Sutherland RM: Isolation of quiescent cells from multicellular tumor spheroids using centrifugal elutriation. Cancer Res. 42:72-78, 1982.

74. Bosmann HB, Bieber GF, Brown AE, Case KR, Gersten DM, Kimmerer TW, Lione A: Biochemical parameters correlated with tumor cell implantation. Nature (London) 246:487-489, 1973.

75. Nicolson GL, Brunson KL, Fidler IJ: Tumor cell surfaces: Some characteristics of neoplastic cells that determine states of transformation and malignancy. Acta Histochem. Cytochem. 10:114-133, 1977.

76. Dolbeare F, Vanderlaan M, Phares W: Alkaline phosphatase and acid arylamidase as marker enzymes for normal and transformed WI-38 cells. J. Histochem. Cytochem. 28:419-426, 1980.

77. Morgan RA, Inge KL, Christopher CW: Localization and characterization of N-ethylmaleimide sensitive inhibitor(s) of thiol cathepsin activity from cultured Nil and polyoma virus-transformed Nil hamster cells. J. Cell. Physiol. 108:55-66, 1981.

78. Burnett D, Crocker J, Vaughn ATM: Synthesis of cathepsin B by cells derived from the HL60 promyelocytic leukemia cell line. J. Cell. Physiol. 115:249-254, 1983.

79. Miner KM, Kawaguchi T, Uba GW, Nicolson GL: Clonal drift of cell surface, melanogenic, and experimental metastatic properties of in vivo selected, brain meninges-colonizing muring B16 melanoma. Cancer Res. 42:4631-4638, 1982.

80. Welch DR, Nicolson GL: Phenotypic drift and heterogeneity in response of metastatic mammary adenocarcinoma cell clones to Adriamycin, 5-fluoro-2'-deoxyuridine and methotrexate treatment in vitro. Clin. Exp. Metastasis 1:317-325, 1983.

81. Reznikoff CA, Bertram JS, Brankow DW, Heidelberger C: Quantitative and qualitative studies of chemical transformation of cloned C3H mouse embryo cells sensitive to postconfluence inhibition of cell division. Cancer Res. 33:3239-3249, 1973.

82. Poste G: Methods and models for studying tumor invasion. In: Liotta LA and Hart IR (eds.) Tumor Invasion and Metastasis. Martinus Nijhoff, The Hague, pp. 147-171, 1982.

83. Chu FF, Olden K: Distribution of acid hydrolases in subcellular fractions of proliferating versus non-proliferating fibroblasts. Exp. Cell Res. 154:606-612, 1984.

84. Lah TT, Rozhin J, Honn KV, Crissman JD, Sloane BF: Human tumor cysteine proteinase inhibitors: Reduced affinity against cathepsin B. J. Cell Biol., in press.

85. Jarvinen M, Rinne A: Human spleen cysteineproteinase inhibitor. Purification, fractionation into isoelectric variants and some properties of the variants. Biochim. Biophys. Acta 708:210-217, 1982.

CHAPTER 23. APPLICATIONS FOR ANTIMETASTATIC THERAPIES

JOHN D. CRISSMAN AND KENNETH V. HONN

I. INTRODUCTION

The development of therapies directed toward either interrupting the metastatic cascade or decreasing its efficiency is an intriguing concept. For the most part, clinicians and scientists have concentrated their efforts on achieving a cure of malignant neoplasms. Therapies which decrease the efficiency of the metastatic cascade have been viewed as palliative. Surgery and/or radiation therapy are the traditional and most effective methods to excise or sterilize primary and regional disease. However, cure is unlikely if successful metastatic foci have been established prior to or during initial treatment. Small metastases are not often identifiable at the time of initial diagnosis and treatment. Careful clinical staging will usually uncover large metastatic deposits in organs accessible to non-invasive maneuvers. Newer technologies (i.e., CT scans) have resulted in an increased identification of smaller metastases. Cytotoxic chemotherapy was originally reserved for palliative therapy of patients with documented disseminated cancer. Nevertheless, in selected cancers, patients with a high probability of microscopic tumor spread are commonly treated systemically with single or combination cytotoxic chemotherapy. The major exception to this is the use of hormonal therapy for neoplasms arising in the accessory sex organs. In the last decade cytotoxic chemotherapy has improved dramatically resulting in the successful treatment of many types of leukemia, lymphoma and germ cell tumors. Remarkable cytoreduction has occurred in these tumors with a significant number of patients surviving for $\geq$ 5 years. Unfortunately, similar success has not been evident with the more common carcinomas.

Current therapies achieve local tumor control in most patients. However, major improvements in local and regional control will probably not translate to increased survival (1) since local recurrences may remain a problem in selected advanced cancers. The major emphasis in cancer treatment is starting to shift to the early recognition, localization and treatment of clinical micrometastases. A large proportion of previously undiagnosed cancer patients have already developed either regional lymph node or distant metastases. With the advent of more efficacious therapies for treating the primary tumor, considerable effort has been expended on early identification and localization of small metastatic deposits. Monoclonal antibodies to tissue (tumor) antigens are being investigated, both for identification of small metastatic foci with radiolabeled antibodies and as a possible mechanism for delivering therapeutic agents to the micrometastases (see also Chapter 16). Stimulation of host tumoricidal cell populations (e.g., NK cells, activated macrophages) also represents a new area of development which may eventually result in an effective therapy for disseminated malignancies (see also Chapters 14 and 15).

In this chapter we will discuss observations which have the potential for clinical application as "non-toxic" therapies. Because the majority of human tumors are epithelial in origin, emphasis will be placed on the more common carcinomas.

II. CLINICOPATHOLOGIC OBSERVATIONS RELATED TO METASTASES

A. Tumor Size

Larger tumors have a higher incidence of both regional lymph node and systemic metastases. In the National Surgical Adjuvant Breast Project (NSABP) over 2,500 patients were evaluated and increasing primary tumor size was found to be clearly associated with an increased incidence of axillary lymph node metastases (2). However, this relationship is variable and up to 23% of patients with "minimal breast tumors" (defined as invasive cancers of < 5 mm) have axillary lymph node metastases (3). Conversely, a minority of breast cancers reach large proportions without evidence of regional or systemic metastases. These observations reinforce the concept that parameters other than primary tumor size are important for the establishment of successful metastases. Similar observations are available for other common epithelial neoplasms, including colon (4), lung (5) and upper aero-digestive tract squamous cell carcinomas (6). Other common neoplasms such as basal cell carcinoma of the skin undergo extensive local invasion without developing systemic metastases. Rare tumors such as mesotheliomas and adenoid cystic carcinomas also extensively invade host tissues and metastasize by lymphatic or blood channels only late in their clinical course.

B. Growth Rate and Tumor Differentiation

Cancers with short doubling times or a large proliferating fraction have a more rapid clinical course. In studies using tritiated thymidine labeling indices, the probability of relapse has been found to correlate significantly with the fraction of tumor cells incorporating thymidine (8). Cancers with large proliferating fractions usually have an aneuploid chromosome population and tend to be high grade (little evidence of histologic differentiation) cancers (7). All of these factors appear to be interrelated. Rapidly growing tumors appear to have a higher capacity for metastasis than slow growing tumors of equivalent size. The relationship among tumor grade (degree of differentiation), growth rate and propensity to metastasize is highly variable. In general, poorly differentiated "anaplastic" tumors have a short doubling time and metastasize rapidly, whereas differentiated tumors have a more orderly growth rate. Traditionally, histologic assessment of tumor grade includes the evaluation of nuclear pleomorphism, frequency of mitoses, cytoplasmic differentiation, intercellular relationships, etc. The degree of differentiation is often helpful in assessing prognosis, however, this correlation is extremely variable and has resulted in a deemphasis of its role in planning patient therapy. The histologic parameters that are not commonly included in the determination of tumor grade include the relationship between the neoplasm and host stroma.

C. Patterns of Invasion

The pattern by which a neoplasm infiltrates host tissue is extremely valuable in predicting vascular invasion and whether metastases will occur. For many years pathologists have recognized that tumors with well defined, expanding or pushing borders (i.e., verrucous carcinomas) seldom metastasize and accordingly are associated with a good prognosis. For the most part, large neoplasms which do not metastasize have a well demarcated border with the host stroma. In contrast, malignant tumors that invade in a non-cohesive pattern of single cells or small cellular aggregates have a higher frequency of regional lymph node and distant metastases. This observation has been confirmed for numerous human tumors including breast (12), colon (13), stomach (14), urinary bladder (15), uterine cervix (16), larynx (17) and tonsil (18). The pattern of invasion has been studied occasionally in human tumors; only rarely has its correlation with tumor aggressiveness been studied in animal tumors (19).

The correlation between tumor invasion of host stroma by small aggregates or single tumor cells and vascular invasion might be predicted. Large cohesive sheets of tumor cells "pushing" or expanding into the adjacent host connective tissue are unlikely to gain access to either postcapillary venules or lymphatic vessels (Figure 1), whereas single cells infiltrating the host stroma may be more capable of penetrating lymphatic and blood vessels (Figure 2). The possibility that vascular invasion occurs from the main body of the tumor has been suggested. Some investigators believe that infiltration of tumor cells into the peritumoral host stroma is not a requirement for vascular invasion. Since lymphatic vessels are not present within tumors but only in the adjacent host stroma, infiltration of tumor cells into the peritumoral host stroma represents the only access the tumor has for lymphatic invasion. The capacity for distant metastases by several human tumors is best correlated with the identification of vascular (capillary or venule) invasion outside the main mass of the neoplasm. This association reflects the propensity for tumor invasion of blood vessels both within and around the tumor.

The type and origin of the neoplasm and its anatomical location are also important in the development of vascular invasion and dissemination. The latter observations are supported by both clinical data (6) and observations in animal models (7) in which similar tumors arising in different anatomical locations have significant variations in frequency of metastases. These observations may reflect not only differences within histologically similar neoplasms but also the effects of host responses at different anatomic sites.

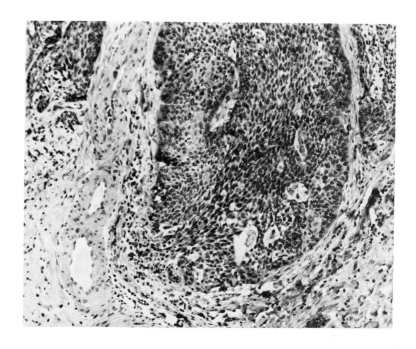

FIGURE 1. Squamous Cell Carcinoma Infiltrating the Host Stroma as a Cohesive Sheet of Cells. Note adjacent blood vessels without evidence of vascular invasion. Carcinomas with similar broad pushing borders of invasion seldom infiltrate blood or lymphatic channels. (Hematoxylin and eosin stain, magnification X 203).

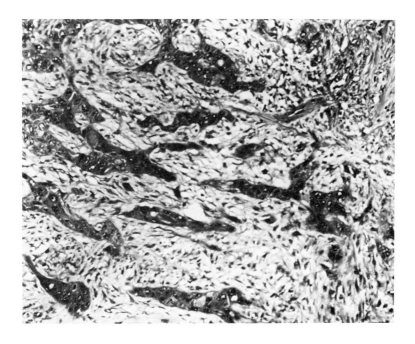

FIGURE 2. Squamous Cell Carcinoma Invading the Host Stroma in Small Irregular Cords of Cells and Single Cells. The neoplasm impinges on an open space in the center that is consistent with a small dilated lymphatic channel. This pattern of invasion is commonly associated with vascular and/or lymphatic penetration. (Hematoxylin and eosin stain, magnification X 203).

D. Vascular/Lymphatic Invasion

Histological evidence of vascular invasion by human carcinomas is consistent with a poor prognosis (Figure 3). The presence of vascular invasion is associated with an increase in regional and distant metastases and with decreased survival. This has been demonstrated in carcinomas of the breast (12,21,22), stomach (23), tonsil (18), uterine cervix (10,24,25), urinary bladder (26) and colon (13,27,28). The majority of clinicopathologic studies have identified vascular invasion by tumor cells to be closely correlated with the presence of regional lymph node and/or systemic metastases, however, not all studies have confirmed this observation. In carcinoma of the colon, two limited studies failed to associate intramural invasion of small vessels with poor prognosis in cancers of equivalent stage (29,30). Other studies evaluating the prognostic value of vascular invasion by colon carcinomas demonstrated an association with metastases (27,28). This association was even more significant when larger extramural vessels are invaded by tumors. Invasion of small venous structures by single cells (Figure 3) does not seem to carry the same ominous prognosis as does invasion of larger muscular veins. The latter may allow the release of large tumor emboli into the blood or lymphatic circulation (Figure 4).

Tumor cell entry into the lymphatics most likely occurs as the tumor invades into the host stroma. As previously described, tumors which invade in small groups of cells or as single cells are associated with a higher frequency of metastases, presumably by gaining easier access to lymphatics and small blood vessels. Venous invasion by cancer cells seems to occur more commonly at the region of the tumor-host interface. This region has a rich supply of blood vessels and the tumor cells are better oxygenated and presumably more metabolically active (31). Sugarbaker (1) hypothesized that areas of tumor necrosis and formation of "vascular lakes" are a potential source of tumor emboli. This is an interesting hypothesis but cannot account for regional lymph node metastasis and hematogenous spread in smaller neoplasms which lack necrotic regions.

Animal (32) and clinical (33) studies have demonstrated that tumor cells are constantly released into the bloodstream. In animal studies up to 10% of a tumor was found to be shed into the bloodstream over a 24 hr period (32). In addition, the number of cells shed per gram of tumor tissue is fairly constant over a wide range of experimental tumor sizes. This observation could explain why more metastases occur in larger tumors as more cells per gram of tumor tissue are released into the circulation. In addition, another study of animal tumors demonstrated that not only did the total number of tumor cells released into circulation increase in growing tumors, but that the metastatic efficiency is proportional to the number and size of tumor clumps found in the tumor effluent (34). This observation is also associated with the density and size of the vessels found within the tumor; larger tumors have larger vessels.

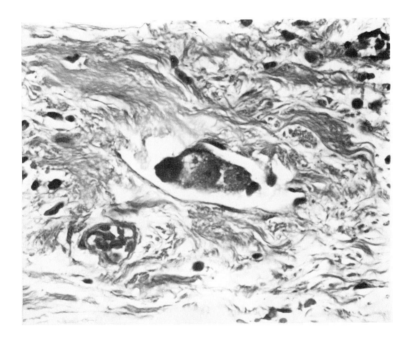

FIGURE 3. Lymphatic Invasion by an Adenocarcinoma of the Breast. Two
cells are present which appear to be attached to each other. The space
is lined by identifiable endothelial cells. (Hematoxylin and eosin,
magnification X 811).

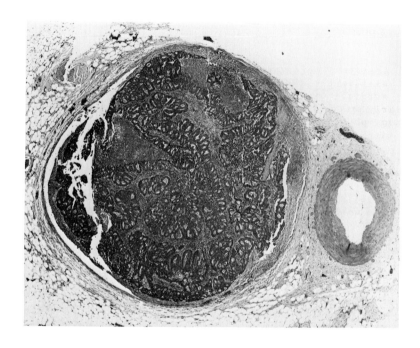

FIGURE 4. Venous Invasion by an Adenocarcinoma of the Colon. Note the adjacent muscular artery in the mesentery. The colon carcinoma has invaded and appears to be proliferating within the muscular vein. The amorphous material surrounding the glandular neoplasm is a thrombus. (Hematoxylin and eosin, magnification X 22).

III. TRAUMA AND INTRAVASCULAR RELEASE OF TUMOR CELLS

Surgical manipulation could theoretically result in the release of tumor cells. Engell (35) demonstrated that up to 10% of cancer patients have circulating tumor cells. This observation created considerable controversy as the prevailing attitudes equated circulating tumor cells with successful development of metastases. However, many of the patients with tumor cells identified in their blood failed to develop metastases, raising a question about the significance of this observation (36). Subsequently, we have learned that very few circulating tumor cells achieve the successful arrest, implantation and growth necessary to form successful metastatic foci (20).

Numerous studies have established that physical manipulation of animal tumors increases the number of circulating tumor cells (34) as well as the number of tumor cell clumps (37). This in turn results in an increase in the number of observed metastases (37,38). Experimental studies have demonstrated an increase in metastases after surgical biopsy (39,40). Cancer cells have been identified in the venous blood of the mesentery in patients with colon cancer. Increased numbers of tumor cells in the venous blood from the colonic neoplasm are noted during surgical manipulation of the tumor (33). The illustrations in this early study all demonstrate multi-cellular tumor emboli (33). In addition, physical examinations, biopsies and scrubbing the patient's skin prior to surgery have been shown to increase the number of circulating tumor cells found in the peripheral circulation.

Poorly differentiated malignant neoplasms have a shorter tumor doubling time, are less cohesive, possess irregular borders and invade as small cellular aggregates or as individual tumor cells. Advanced tumors are associated with large blood vessels and subsequently with a greater blood supply. Vascular invasion is more common in this situation and may extend into the larger veins by intravascular extension. These intravascular tumor proliferations have the potential of releasing tumor cell aggregates into the venous circulation. These tumors have been demonstrated to be associated with a higher efficiency of metastasis formation. Unfortunately, this combination of poor prognostic parameters is not uncommon and is generally associated with a high risk of existing metastases at the time of diagnosis. Controlled trauma such as that which occurs during surgical resection (and less vigorous forms of manipulation) results in an increase of shed tumor cells, especially clumps of tumor cells which in turn may lead to successful establishment of metastases.

The only surgical study addressing this problem is, unfortunately, uncontrolled (41). In a series of bowel resections for colon cancers, the "no touch" technique, defined as ligation of the most proximal mesenteric vascular and lymphatic vessels prior to resection of the primary tumor, resulted in improved five year survivals. However, the observed increase in survival is related to a comparable number of historical controls from the same institution. This technique, which is sound in theory, has evoked considerable controversy. Subsequent uncontrolled studies of patients treated with "radical" surgical resection have resulted in equivalent survivals (42). The explanation is that the "high" ligation of the vascular (and lymphatic) pedicle results in a more extensive and radical resection with greater lymph node removal. Unfortunately, neither concept has ever been tested in a well designed randomized surgical trial, thus leaving the controversy unresolved. Nevertheless, the logic of ligating vessels draining a cancer is recognized and this approach has been adopted by many surgeons. Unfortunately, not all primary neoplasms have an accessible efferent vascular/lymphatic bundle such as found in the colon. The role of surgical manipulation in the release of increased numbers of homotypic tumor emboli has been repeatedly demonstrated in both clinical situations and in animal models. If the homotypic tumor cell emboli released during this apparent critical period of therapy can be blocked from forming metastases, the effect on patient survival could be significant. The possibility of improving survival by decreasing the efficiency of metastases formation during surgery is real and needs to be addressed in a carefully controlled study.

IV. THE METASTATIC CASCADE

Intravasation is the process by which tumor cells gain access to the circulatory or lymphatic systems. Many factors which control tumor growth and invasion contribute to the process of intravasation (42). The continued growth of a malignant neoplasm and associated tumor angiogenesis all contribute to the increase in vascular/lymphatic intravasation. Once a metastatic foci is established it can grow and contribute additional circulating tumor cells to the metastatic cascade, resulting in the development of secondary metastases or metastasis from metastases. This becomes of practical importance in clinical therapies which can successfully control the primary tumor but not the continued invasion of the vascular compartment by tumor cells from existing metastatic foci. Unfortunately, many patients with "cure" of their primary neoplasm still develop lethal body burdens of neoplasms, most likely from secondary metastases. An alternate but unproved source of multiple metastases may include pre-existing micro-metastases originating from the primary tumor (tumor dormancy; 43). Although this mechanism is commonly voiced, the evidence for its contribution to the clinical progression of disease is minimal.

Animal tumors consist of an admixture of cells with varying capabilities for achieving successful metastases (44). These conclusions were derived primarily from the heterogeneity of selected cell populations which can form successful metastases in animal models (45). Interestingly, the clonal diversity of metastases is greater in metastases that develop spontaneously from subcutaneous tumors than in lung colonies formed by intravenous injection of tumor cells (45). These studies in animal models are consistent with clinical observations that some metastatic foci are capable of extremely rapid growth, rapid development of a lethal tumor burden and death, whereas other metastases grow at a relatively slow rate. The observed variations in animal models correlate well with the behavior of various neoplasms in clinical situations.

Clinical data on the relative contribution of metastasis from metastases to the development of lethal body burdens are rare. The best observations are the distribution of metastases found at autopsy. The majority of these studies originate from Roswell Park Memorial Institute where they have found that there is commonly a pattern of key organ metastasis present when other metastases are present in anatomically related organs. The initial metastasis to the "key" organ is thought to be responsible for the development of the "secondary" metastases in the other anatomically related organs (46,47). Admittedly, this evidence is circumstantial but it does appear to support the hypothesis that a substantial source of the lethal tumor burden originates from established metastases in the "key" organs.

Animal models have clearly demonstrated that tumor cells continue to be shed from the metastases into the pulmonary venous (48) and cardiac (49) circulation following surgical removal of the primary tumor after development of spontaneous lung metastases. Experiments with parabiosed animals have also demonstrated metastasis from metastases (50). In these experiments, tumor cells were injected into the footpad of the donor animals. The resulting tumor was allowed to grow until spontaneous metastasis to the lung had occurred, and then the primary footpad tumor was removed surgically. Following surgery the donor animals were parabiosed to recipient animals and a common parabiotic circulation was allowed to develop. The animals were sacrificed in 2-3 wk and the presence of metastases in the lungs of the recipient animals demonstrated unequivocally metastasis from metastases.

We have developed two related murine model systems [intravenous (IV) and footpad (FP)] to study metastasis from metastases. These models employed implanted fetal organs as the "target sites" for secondary metastases. Implanted fetal organs have been used previously to evaluate the organ preference of various sublines of the B16 melanoma (51-53).

In the IV model, dispersed and elutriated (54) B16 amelanotic melanoma (B16a) tumor cells (> 95% viable and ≤ 3% host cell contamination) were injected i.v. into the lateral tail vein of C57Bl/6J mice. Five days later fetal organs from near term C57Bl/6J fetuses were implanted into the hind flank of mice previously injected with B16a cells. A time interval of five days was chosen as sufficient to allow the arrest and either destruction or successful extravasation of the tail vein injected B16a cells. [We and others (see Chapter 9; 55) have demonstrated that ^{125}IUdr labeled tumor cells are essentially cleared from circulation 48 hr after tail vein injection.] The animals were sacrificed 5 wk post fetal organ implant. The implants were dissected "en bloc" and processed for routine histology. Five

410

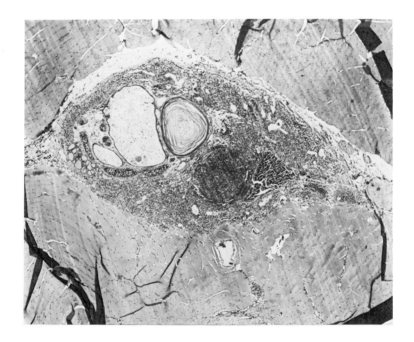

FIGURE 5. Fetal Lung Implant Surrounded by Thigh Skeletal Muscle. Note the bronchial structures with cartilage and squamous metaplasia. The lung parenchyma is atelectatic as it has never been expanded. In the center is a single secondary metastasis of B16 amelanotic melanoma. (Hematoxylin and eosin, magnification x 22).

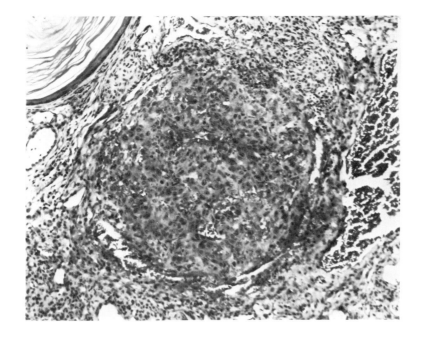

FIGURE 6.   Higher Magnification of the Secondary Metastases
Demonstrated in Figure 5. The adjacent unexpanded fetal lung surrounds
the neoplasm and in the upper corner is a bronchial structure which has
undergone   squamous   metaplasia.   (Hematoxylin   and   eosin,
magnification x 203).

hematoxylin and eosin stained sections (10 μ) were reviewed for the presence of Bl6a tumors and the number of metastatic foci were quantitated (Table 1). The areas (mm^2) of the implanted fetal organ and of each Bl6a metastatic foci were measured by microscopic morphometrics. Metastatic foci developed in the majority ($\geq$ 76%) of implanted fetal lungs (Table 1). These metastatic foci could only have arisen from tumor cells released from thoracic lung colonies.

Table 1. Metastasis from Metastases.

	Intravenous (IV) Model	Footpad (FP) Model
Number of animals	17	9
Animals with secondary metastases	13 (76%)	7 (78%)
Number of secondary metastases per animal	4 (1-11)*	5 (2-18)*

*Range of number of metastases/animal.

This model demonstrates that these pulmonary tumor nodules are themselves capable of releasing tumor cells into the circulation with the subsequent establishment of secondary metastases. Secondary metastases failed to develop in implanted fetal stomach, thymus, kidney, thyroid and esophagus. Implanted fetal testes developed secondary tumor deposits in a limited number of animals. Morphometric analyses revealed that the total area of metastases varied considerably among implants of comparable size. In the majority of the implants, the area of the metastases was considerably greater than the residual fetal lung surrounding the tumors. Ratios of the metastases/lung areas ranged from 0.3 to 12.7 with an average value of 3.2. In this model the establishment of secondary metastases is a reproducible event in which the volume of metastases represents an appreciable portion of the implanted fetal lung.

The tail vein injection of tumor cells to form pulmonary metastases has been appropriately criticized as an artificial system. Obviously, the preparation of single cells from solid tumors prior to tail vein injection bypasses a number of critical steps in the invasion and penetration of vascular channels by primary tumors. To further evaluate metastasis from metastases we utilized a spontaneous metastasis model. Tumor cells (dispersed and elutriated; 54) were injected into the footpad. Footpad tumors were surgically removed when 100% of the animals had developed pulmonary metastases. Five days post-amputation, a period felt to be sufficient for the arrest and either destruction or successful implantation of circulating cells, fetal lung tissue was implanted. Animals were followed for approximately three weeks and then the implants were removed and quantitated in the same manner as in the IV model (Table 1). Metastases were found in 78% of the implanted fetal lungs which is similar to the 76% noted in the IV model. The average number of metastases was similar but the metastases were considerably smaller in area (3.6 mm^2 compared to 17.9 mm^2).

The most striking feature in the footpad model was the great variation in the number and size of the secondary metastases in the implanted fetal lung tissue. The majority of fetal implants had from two to eight metastases with total areas varying from 0.008 mm^2 to 0.11 mm^2. However, one animal developed massive metastases to the implanted lung with 18 identifiably different nodules and a total metastatic area of 32.4 mm^2. This observation could indicate the heterogenous nature of primary and metastatic tumors, particularly in respect to the variation in the metastatic capacity of the various subpopulations (56,57).

In the B16a models (IV,FP), metastasis from metastases is a common occurrence. The B16a melanoma is a lung-seeking neoplasm and metastases from metastases eventually obliterate the transplanted lungs. Therefore, this model system may be useful for the preclinical study of antimetastatic therapies. Using these models, we have recently demonstrated that the antimetastatic drug nafazatrom (58) significantly inhibited metastasis to fetal lung implants (unpublished observation).

Although it is impossible to unequivocally demonstrate metastasis from metastases in humans, the Roswell Park studies (46,47) provide suggestive evidence that secondary metastases do occur in humans. Thus there may be potential for application of therapies which interfere with the metastatic cascade in some, if not all, human tumors with known or probable systemic metastases. Non-toxic therapies which lengthen the time span to development of lethal body burdens are at least palliative. Their use as adjuvants to conventional radiation therapy and cytotoxic chemotherapies may increase the number of "cures" by inhibiting the development of a lethal body burden of tumor cells.

ACKNOWLEDGMENTS

We would like to thank Gloria Greco for her typing of this manuscript, Ben True for his photographic work, and Jerry Meade and Deborah Moilanen for their technical expertise. Supported in part by NIH grants CA29405-5 and CA29997-4.

REFERENCES

1. Sugarbaker EV: Cancer metastasis: A product of tumor-host interactions. Curr. Prob. Cancer 3:3-59, 1979.
2. Fisher B, Slack NH, Bross IDJ: Cancer of the breast: Size of neoplasm and prognosis. Cancer 24:1071-1080, 1969.
3. Bedwani R, Vana J, Rosner D, Schmitz D, Murphy GP: Management and survival of female patients with "minimal" breast cancer: As observed in the long-term and short-term surveys of the American College of Surgeons. Cancer 47:2769-2778, 1981.
4. Grinnell RS: The chance of cancer and lymphatic metastasis in small colon tumors discovered on x-ray examination. Ann. Surg. 139:132-138, 1964.
5. Slack NH, Chamberlain A, Bross IDJ: Predicting survival following surgery for bronchogenic carcinoma. Chest 62:433-438, 1972.
6. Lindberg R: Distribution of cervical lymph node metastases from squamous cell carcinoma of the upper respiratory and digestive tracts. Cancer 29:1446-1449, 1972.
7. Keller R: Induction of macroscopic metastases via surgery. The site of primary tumor inoculum is critical. Invasion Metastasis 1:136-148, 1981.
8. Meyer JS, Friedman E, McCrate MM, Bauer WC: Prediction of early course of breast carcinoma by thymidine labeling. Cancer 51:1839-1886, 1983.
9. Barlogie B, Ruber MN, Schumann J, Johnson TS, Drewinko B, Swartzendruber DE, Gohde W, Andreeff M, Freireich EJ: Flow cytometry in clinical cancer research. Cancer Res. 43:2982-2997, 1983.
10. van Nagel JR, Donaldson ES, Wood EG, Parker JC: The significance of vascular invasion and lymphocytic infiltration in invasive cervical carcinoma. Cancer 41:228-234, 1978.
11. Crissman JD, Makuch R, Budhraja M: Histopathologic grading of squamous cell carcinoma of the uterine cervix. Cancer (In press).
12. Baak JPA, Kruver PHJ, DeSnoo-Niewlaat AJE, DeGraef S, Makkink B, Boon ME: Prognostic indicators in breast cancer - morphometric methods. Histopathology 6:327-339, 1982.
13. Spratt JS, Spjut HJ: Prevalence and prognosis of individual clinical and pathologic variables associated with colorectal carcinoma. Cancer 20:1976-1985, 1967.
14. Urban CH, McNeer G: The relation of the morphology of gastric carcinoma to long and short term survival. Cancer 12:1158-1162, 1959.
15. Steiner PE, Maimon SN, Palmer WL, Kirsner JB: Gastric cancer: Morphologic factors in five-year survival after gastrectomy. Am. J. Pathol. 24:947-969, 1948.
16. Beecham JB, Halvorsen T, Kolbenstvedt A: Histologic classification, lymph node metastases, and patient survival in stage Ib cervical carcinoma. Gynecol. Oncol. 6:95-105, 1978.
17. McGarvan MH, Bauer WC, Ogura JH: The incidence of cervical lymph node metastases from epidermoid carcinoma of the larynx and their relationship to certain characteristics of the primary tumor. Cancer 14:55-66, 1961.

18. Crissman JD, Liu WY, Gluckman JL, Cummings G: Prognostic value of histopathologic parameters in squamous cell carcinoma of the oropharynx. Cancer (In press).

19. Nakadate T, Suzuki M, Sato H: Quantitative study on the liberation of tumor cells into the circulating blood. Gann 70:435-446, 1979.

20. Weiss L, Mayhew E, Glaves Rapp D, Holmes JC: Metastatic inefficiency in mice bearing B16 melanomas. Br. J. Cancer 45:44-53, 1982.

21. Nealon TF, Nkongho A, Grossi C, Gillooley J: Pathologic identification of poor prognosis stage I ($T_1N_0M_0$) cancer of the breast. Ann. Surg. 190:129-132, 1979.

22. Weigand RA, Isenberg WM, Russo J, Brennan MJ, Rich MA: Blood vessel invasion and axillary node involvement as prognostic indicators for human breast cancer. Cancer 50:962-969, 1982.

23. Kodama Y, Inokuchi K, Soejima K, Matsusaka T, Okamura T: Growth patterns and prognosis in early gastric carcinoma. Cancer 51:320-326, 1983.

24. Baltzer J, Lohe J, Kopcke W, Zauder J: Histologic criteria for the prognosis in patients with operated squamous cell carcinoma of the cervix. Gynecol. Oncol. 13:184-194, 1982.

25. Stendahl V, Eklund G, Willen R: Prognosis of invasive squamous cell carcinoma of the uterine cervix: A comparative study of the predictive values of clinical staging Ib-III and a histopathologic malignancy grading system. Int. J. Gynecol. Pathol. 2:42-54, 1983.

26. Bell JT, Burney SW, Friedell GH: Blood vessel invasion in human bladder cancer. J. Urol. 105:675-678, 1971.

27. Copeland EM, Miller LD, Jones RS: Prognostic factors in carcinoma of the colon and rectum. Am. J. Surg. 116:875-881, 1968.

28. Talbot IC, Ritchie S, Leighton M, Hughes AO, Bussey HJR, Morson BC: Invasion of veins by carcinoma of the rectum: Method of detection, histologic features and significance. Histopathology 5:141-163, 1981.

29. Khankhanian N, Mauligit GM, Russell WO, Schimek M: Prognostic significance of vascular invasion in colorectal cancer of Dukes' B class. Cancer 39:1195-1200, 1977.

30. deMascarel A, Coindre JM, deMascarel I, Trojani M, Maree D, Hoerni B: The prognostic significance of specific histologic features of carcinoma of the colon and rectum. Surg. Gynecol. Obstet. 153:511-514, 1981.

31. Tannock IF: The relation between cell proliferation and the vascular system in a transplanted mouse mammary tumor. Br. J. Cancer 22:258-273, 1968.

32. Butler TP, Gullino PM: Quantitation of cell shedding into efferent blood of mammary adenocarcinoma. Cancer Res. 35:512-516, 1975.

33. Roberts S, Jonasson O, Long L, McGrew EA, McGrath R, Cole WH: Relationship of cancer cells in the circulating blood to operation. Cancer 15:232-240, 1962.

34. Liotta LA, Kleinerman J, Saidel GM: Quantitative relationships of intravascular tumor cells, tumor vessels, and pulmonary metastases following tumor implantation. Cancer Res. 34:997-1004, 1974.

35. Engell HC: Cancer cells in the circulating blood. Acta Chir. Scand. (Suppl.) 210:10–70, 1955.

36. Engell HC: Cancer cells in the blood. A five to nine year follow-up study. Ann. Surg. 149:457–461, 1959.

37. Liotta LA, Kleinerman J, Saidel GM: The significance of hematogenous tumor cell clumps in the metastatic process. Cancer Res. 36:889–894, 1976.

38. March MC: Tumor massage and metastases in mice. Cancer Res. 11:101–107, 1927.

39. Riggins RS, Ketcham AS: Effect of incision biopsy on the development of experimental tumor metastases. J. Surg. Res. 5:200–206, 1965.

40. Keller R: Induction of macroscopic metastases via surgery. Invasion Metastasis 1:136–148, 1981.

41. Turnbull RB, Kyle K, Watson FR, Spratt J: Cancer of the colon: The influence of the no-touch isolation technic on survival rates. Ann. Surg. 166:420–427, 1967.

42. Hart IR, Fidler IJ: Cancer invasion and metastasis. Quart Rev. Biol. 55:121–142, 1980.

43. Wheelock EF, Robinson MK: Biology of disease. Endogenous control of the neoplastic process. Lab. Invest. 48:120–139, 1983.

44. Fidler IJ: Tumor heterogeneity and the biology of cancer invasion and metastasis. Cancer Res. 38:2651–2660, 1978.

45. Poste G, Doll J, Brown AE, Tzeng J, Zeidman I: Comparison of the metastatic properties of B16 melanoma clones isolated from cultured cell lines, subcutaneous tumors, and individual lung metastasis. Cancer Res. 42:2770–2778, 1982.

46. Viadama E, Bross IDJ, Pickren JW: An autopsy study of some routes of dissemination of cancer of the breast. Br. J. Cancer 27:336–340, 1973.

47. Viadama E, Bross IDJ, Pickren JW: The metastatic spread of cancers of the digestive system in man. Oncology 35:114–126, 1978.

48. Ketcham AS, Ryan JJ, Wexler H: The shedding of viable circulating tumor cells by pulmonary metastases in mice. Ann. Surg. 169:297–299, 1969.

49. Ketcham AS, Wexler H, Chretien PB: The metastatic potential of experimental pulmonary metastases. J. Surg. Red. 15:45–52, 1973.

50. Hoover HC, Ketcham AS: Metastasis of metastases. Am. J. Surg. 130:405–411, 1975.

51. Kinsey DL: An experimental study of preferential metastasis. Cancer 13:674–676, 1960.

52. Sugarbaker EV, Cohen AM, Ketcham AS: Do metastases metastasize? Ann. Surg. 174:161–166, 1971.

53. Hart IR, Fidler IJ: Role of organ selectivity in the determination of metastatic patterns of B16 melanoma. Cancer Res. 40:2281–2287, 1980.

54. Sloane BF, Dunn JR, Honn KV: Lysosomal cathepsin B: Correlation with metastatic potential. Science 212:1151–1153, 1981.

55. Fidler IJ: Biological behavior of malignant melanoma cells correlated to their survival in vivo. Cancer Res. 35:218–224, 1975.

56. Mantovani A, Giavazzi R, Alessandri G, Spreafico F, Garrattini S: Characterization of tumor lines derived from spontaneous metastases of a transplanted murine sarcoma. Eur. J. Cancer 17:71-76, 1981.
57. Poste G, Doll J, Brown AE, Tzeng J, Zeidman I: Comparison of the metastatic properties of B16 melanoma clones isolated from cultured cell lines, subcutaneous tumors and individual lung metastases. Cancer Res. 42:2770-2778, 1982.
58. Honn KV, Meyer J, Neagos G, Henderson T, Westley C, Ratanatharathorn V: Control of tumor growth and metastasis with prostacyclin and thromboxane synthetase inhibitors: Evidence for a new antitumor and antimetastatic agent (Bay g 6575). IN: Jamieson GA, (ed.) Interaction of Platelets and Tumor Cells. Alan R. Liss, New York, pp. 295-328, 1982.

INDEX

422